In Search of the Medicine Buddha

DAVID CROW

JEREMY P. TARCHER/PUTNAM

a member of

Penguin Putnam Inc.

New York

2000

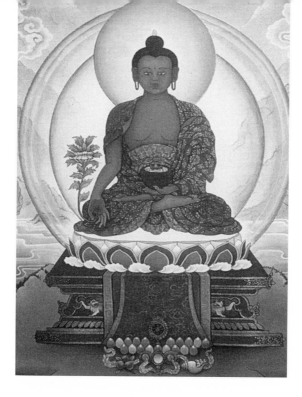

In Search

of the

Medicine Buddha

A Himalayan Journey

This book is dedicated to the Medicine Buddha, who resides within every heart and mind as the potential for freedom from all sickness and suffering; to the healers of every tradition who embody the deity's compassionate wisdom; and to the multitude of sentient beings within the plant kingdom who provide foods and medicines for humanity.

Photo of Dr. Sarita Shrestha by H. James Crow.
Photo of Fasting Buddha by David Howard.

Most Tarcher/Putnam books are available at special quantity discounts for bulk purchases for sales promotions, premiums, fund-raising, and educational needs. Special books or book excerpts also can be created to fit specific needs. For details, write Putnam Special Markets, 375 Hudson Street, New York, NY 10014.

Jeremy P. Tarcher/Putnam
a member of
Penguin Putnam Inc.
375 Hudson Street
New York, NY 10014
www.penguinputnam.com

Copyright © 2000 by David Crow

Library of Congress Cataloging-in-Publication Data

Crow, David, date.
In search of the Medicine Buddha : a Himalayan journey / David Crow.
p. cm.
ISBN 1-58542-030-1
1. Medicine, Tibetan.   2. Medicine, Ayurvedic.   I. Title.
R603.T5 C76   2000   99-086049
610'.951'5—dc21

Printed in the United States of America
1   3   5   7   9   10   8   6   4   2

This book is printed on acid-free paper. ∞

Book design by Jennifer Ann Daddio

CONTENTS

ACKNOWLEDGMENTS

This book is the result of many fortunate circumstances, the hard work of several dedicated individuals, and the generosity and kindness of numerous friends and family members.

Without the resources generously provided by my late mother, Arlene Watson, I would not have been able to fully devote my attention to this long endeavor.

If it were not for the tireless efforts and extraordinary editorial skills of my father, Dr. James Crow, I would undoubtedly still be wondering if this project would ever come to completion. His involvement in every phase of this work, from our Himalayan treks to the final revisions, has been one of the greatest joys of my life, worthy of a book itself.

It was the genuine and meaningful friendship of Jack Forem (and his wife, Roberta) that brought this book out of its darkest hours; it has been shaped and influenced in no small way by his commitment, patience, diplomacy, and writing skills.

My deepest appreciation goes to those Tibetan, Ayurvedic, and Chinese physicians and scholars mentioned in this book, as well as others who contributed but were not included: Dr. Ngawang Chopel; Dr. Lobsang Dhonyo; Dr. Ngawang Gyaltsen; Dr. Ngawang Soepa; Dr. Bishnuprasad Aryal; Dr. Kamadev Jha; Dr. Lokedra Singh; Dr. Narendra Tiwari; Dr. Sarita Shrestha; Dr. R. D. Mahatyagi; Dr. Uprenda Thakur; Dr. Ram Brikhya Sahu; Dr. Siddhi Gopal; Dr. Rishi Ram; Dr. Ishwor

Upadhaya; Dr. Man Sang Yu; Kiran Sankar; Kabiraj Kedarnath; Gopal Premi; and Raman Bandari.

Many people provided invaluable assistance during my sojourns in Nepal, including Gopal Upreti and the staff of Om Ayurvedic Research Center; Kedar Upreti and the staff of Himalayan Herbs, Pvt. Lmt.; Sonam Topgyal; Jamtso; Jigme, Yves Michaud; Indira Thapa; and the monks of Shelkar Ling, Boudhanath.

To my agent, Lynn Franklin, and her staff, I owe many thanks, as well as to those who carried this book from inception to fruition: Peter Weinberg (the "godfather" of this manuscript); Philip Goldberg (for early guidance and encouragement); Jeremy Tarcher (for seeing the potential of this story); Wendy Hubbert (for skillful development and astute editorial insights); and all those at Tarcher/Putnam who have helped at every stage.

Several special people deserve mention for providing me with a home during the long journey: Diane Ware of Hale Kalani, Volcano, Hawaii; Mark, Kathleen, and Ian Chambers for the use of their sacred desert caves; David Howard and Kay Brownfield for the many blessings of the Growing Edge, Big Sur, and the sailboat at the Channel Islands Marina; Lissa McConnell and John Campbell for the garden cottage in Cambria; Arun Deva the yogi for his Hollywood hideaway; and Bill and Ellen Walter for the comfortable couch and sympathy.

Ray Regan painted the Medicine Buddha used in this text; my father provided the photograph of Dr. Sarita Shrestha; and David Howard provided the photograph of the fasting Buddha. Nickki Hill supplied creative inspiration; Dianne Rini and Dr. Sarasvati Buhrman offered editorial assistance and facilitated Dr. Shrestha's coming to the West.

My wife, Gentry Gorg, nurtured the flowering of this book with passionate prayers and unconditional love.

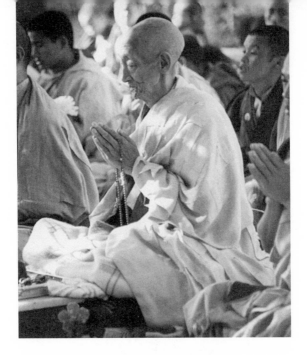

Introduction

The first time I flew out of Kathmandu was on the new moon of February 1988. I had just completed a year of study with Dr. Ngawang Chopel, a Tibetan monk-physician. Over the next ten years, I would depart from this Himalayan valley five more times, each time uncertain if I would ever return.

On that afternoon, amid the colorful festivities of Losar, the Tibetan New Year, I exchanged gifts with my old teacher, expressed my heartfelt gratitude for the wonderful instructions and kindness he had given me, then sadly said farewell. I left his monastery with white blessing scarves draped around my neck and bags of fragrant herbal medicines in my pack, and made my way one last time to the forested hilltops of nearby Pashupatinath.

Baby monkeys hanging from their mothers' bellies shrieked as I approached the upper terraces overlooking the Shiva temples and ghats along the banks of the Bagmati River. Between two burning pyres and surrounded by a lamenting family, a corpse was being prepared for cremation. Rain began to fall, the drops illumined by bright sunlight streaming through the jungle foliage. I looked back across the valley toward Boudhanath, the village that had been my home, and the white dome of its sacred Stupa. Strains of hypnotic music accompanied the rhythmic work of peasant women in the fields below as the Stupa sparkled in the distance. From its golden spire rose a perfect rainbow, arching across the yellow-green paddies like a ray from the eye of a Buddha, a bridge of memories, and a beacon of hope to guide me through the uncertainty ahead.

Here, in this vision before me, was the essence of Nepal: a magical land steeped in spiritual history, a medieval serfdom of toil and hardship, a world of timeless cultural treasures, and a place of disease and impermanence. This moment was the fruition of the prayer that had brought me to Kathmandu in search of classical Himalayan medicines and the teachings of Dharma, universal truth. I picked up my pack, heavy with woodblock-printed texts of ancient herbal formulas, manuscripts of alchemical secrets, silk pouches bulging with botanical remedies, and notebooks filled with my teacher's wisdom, and turned my mind toward America.

I had had modest but unusual professional ambitions when I applied to the American College of Traditional Chinese Medicine in San Francisco in 1980, where the door to Asian healing arts was beginning to open in the West. My interest was to follow in the footsteps of the "barefoot doctors" of China, the auxiliary health workers who provide medical care to the rural poor, using primarily acupuncture needles, moxibustion, and locally available herbs. My desire was to be able to make a living by sharing knowledge and giving comfort, using simple yet effective methods handed down through the ages. Without know-

ing it at the time, I was about to follow many of the same stages of training as physicians in the past, who studied the arts and sciences of massage, acupuncture, herbal formulation, dietary therapies, purification
practices, and meditational healing.

Walking through the door of traditional Chinese medicine, I encountered the world of Taoist thought, where mysteriously flowing chi
moves in tides and cyclic currents through the body's meridians and
acupuncture points. I watched as silver and gold needles, skillfully en-
livened by the master's hand, vibrated vitality back into the weary. I
breathed the wispy smoke of pungent artemisia glowing on the needle's
handle as the soothing warmth of fire and metal in conjunction spread
through invisible channels blocked by cold. I saw the play of the seasons across the landscape of the body, the influences of the stars in the
blood, the pull of the moon in the core of the womb. I heard tales of forest hermits practicing inner alchemy by guiding their breath in contemplative absorption, sustained by elixirs of longevity as they purified their
consciousness. I found clay pots simmering with families' secret brews,
flashing neon streets lined with windows displaying ginseng and deer
horn, old men reading pulses in humble quarters, and apprentices dispensing herbs from distant mountains out of old wooden cabinets.

It was during this period of study in San Francisco that I met Kalu
Rinpoche, an extraordinary mystic from the Tibetan Buddhist tradition.
Before taking birth, he had appeared to his future parents in dreams, asking to visit their home, and when he was born, it was said, the sky filled
with rainbows. An unusually wise and intelligent child, Kalu was regarded by the lamas of Kham as an incarnation of a highly developed
being. He entered monastic life at a young age, and—with a photo-
graphic memory, impeccable understanding, and exemplary discipline—excelled in his scholarly studies. His guru named him Karma
Rangjung Kunchab, Self-Arisen and All-Pervading.

Completing monastic training in his mid-twenties, Kalu departed
into the wilderness of eastern Tibet. Following the lineage of Milarepa,

the great "cotton-clad" yogi, Kalu lived a most austere and ascetic life. Travelers would find him dwelling under rock ledges open to the winter winds, or in cave hermitages, wearing only a thin cloth. Deep in the snow mountains he practiced the highest yogas and gained mastery over the currents of mind and body. He meditated continuously for fifteen years, nourished by the inner warmth of bliss, absorbed in wakeful dreaming, radiant with immense compassion for all sentient beings. When Kalu was about the age of forty, the monks implored him to return to the monastery for their benefit. He became renowned throughout the world as a master of contemplative practice who knew the true nature of reality.

I wept when I met Kalu Rinpoche, so powerfully did his presence arouse hope for myself and humanity. Already old, he calmly presided over an evening of Tibetan ritual, gracefully draped with golden saffron robes, voice resonant with a lifetime of prayers. He exuded warmth, and at the end of the ceremony I saw his extraordinary head glowing with light. Was it a coincidence that unseasonable showers fell that night, and rainbows filled the San Francisco sky the next day?

Then he was gone, back to his monastery in the misty mountains of Darjeeling. During his absence I graduated from acupuncture college and started my medical practice. He returned four years later to conduct ceremonies, give teachings, and initiate his advanced students into the traditional three-year meditation retreat. One day I sat with Rinpoche (Precious One) and told him about my interest in studying Tibetan medicine. He listened patiently, then pointed out that although it would be good to go to Asia to learn these things, it was more important to understand the Dharma, the compassionate truth that transforms any kind of medicine into spiritual practice.

Synchronistic events happen around those whose minds are wish-fulfilling gems. In response to Kalu's omniscient aura, I found myself transported from the mandalas invoked during ceremonies, to the mandalic neighborhood around the Stupa of Boudhanath. There, in a circular village under skies resonating with mantras, I found the first of my teachers, Ngawang Chopel. Over the coming years I would meet nine more distinguished physicians of Kathmandu, whose training and experience encompassed a vast range of Ayurvedic and Tibetan medical knowledge.

Many others would share their teachings with me as well, including monks, nuns, Rinpoches, alchemists, herbal technicians, temple-dwelling swamis, the King's astrologer, and silent chillum-smoking saddhus. Kathmandu itself was the greatest of teachers. Endless monsoon rains cultivate patience; hungry beggars and homeless children stir the heart in ways that eloquent discourses on the Dharma cannot; the horrific pollution of the streets demands the deepest equanimity; and nothing awakens a doctor's compassionate empathy for the suffering of patients more than being afflicted with illness himself.

Soon after my mentorship commenced, Dr. Chopel generously blessed me with his knowledge of Sange Menla, the Medicine Buddha. The emanation of Buddha as a celestial physician and mythical source of Tibetan medical lineages, Sange Menla resides in a pure realm, surrounded by wondrous geometric gardens of botanical wealth, curative animals, and wish-fulfilling gems. Of all the Dharmic gifts I was to receive and contemplate in my studies and travels, none has influenced me more than this vision of Sange Menla, representing an ecologically renewed world purified by love and governed by enlightened wisdom. Through my teacher's kindness and my own contemplative efforts, I came to see that, although shrouded with the veil of spiritual darkness, our world is in essence the mandala of Sudarshan, Beautiful to Behold, the kingdom of the lapis-bodied universal healer.

When one contemplates deities, patterns ripple through consciousness, weaving chronological time and linear space into a dance of archetypes. As one trains the mind to see the purity of the world, the deities' realms merge into waking perceptions, creating a subtle spell. This is especially true in the Himalayas, where sacred places are steeped in the accumulated psychic power of holy people performing such practices through the ages. As if in response to visualizing the Medicine Buddha's botanical paradise described by my teacher, plants began to appear. Soon herbs were everywhere in my rooftop apartment. They hung in bundles from the rafters, grew in pots on the floor, and filled indoor planters in the alcoves beneath the windows. They were stored in jars, stacked on shelves, and spread around whatever medicine-making project was in progress. High racks held hundreds of aromatic herbal distillations, glass-windowed cabinets displayed handmade pills and powders, and lab equipment sat on top of any available counter space. Layers of fragrances swirled through the rooms, food for the Buddhas and devas adorning the walls.

My growing pharmacy did not have to wait long for customers. When alchemized with thanks for their precious medicinal gifts, plants become delighted; then, seeking to fulfill their highest aspiration—to partake of human bodily consciousness—they attract those who need them. There is no shortage of illness in Kathmandu, nor of opportunity to study and practice medicine, for almost everyone is sick to varying degrees. Before long, people were arriving, their karma having drawn them to Boudhanath from all walks of life and corners of the earth, and they tasted the beneficial flavors of the jungles, alpine meadows, riverbanks, and farms. I went to them as well, walking along trails through misty forests above the clouds to villages and neighborhoods with names from antiquity, carrying bags of medicines from my teachers' pharmacies and my own apothecary. Later, I would export crates of these herbal treasures for my patients in San Francisco and Los Angeles, and eventually bring people from the West to share in these experiences.

I had come to Nepal seeking the renowned and potent Ayurvedic and Tibetan herbs from pristine habitats. As I traveled through the villages and countryside, I looked down from mountain peaks and up from dust-choked streets and alleys and saw environmental degradation spreading across the Himalayas, destroying the forests and threatening the existence of precious botanical species. I carefully recorded the words of my teachers as they described formulas that could cure much of humanity's suffering, but I knew these medicinal treasures were disappearing. Many of these plants and animals were from a vanishing world, their habitats encroached upon by civilization, their priceless gifts hunted more aggressively as their value increased. Where will medicines come from when the flowers, trees, vines, grasses, bushes, and wild creatures are gone? I wondered. In the course of our short human lifetimes, the botanical richness represented by the Medicine Buddha's iconographic kingdom is evaporating, and we are losing the companionship of nature's life-sustaining diversity.

Early in my travels and studies I learned how little one can do to alleviate illness and discomfort when food is poor, poverty deep, and streets awash with fetid sewage. As I journeyed between Kathmandu and my clinics in California, I could not escape a growing sense of futility in the superficiality of medicine, for even in the relative affluence of the West, many people cannot find the time and resources necessary for resolving their health problems. Holistic healing methods produce wonderful, reliable, and verifiable therapeutic results, but of what benefit are they if people cannot afford health-promoting treatments, remedies, or diets; work and home environments create diseases; and rest and recovery are impossible? What is the purpose of administering Ayurveda's profound detoxification procedures if the water, soil, and air are poisoned? If we continue contaminating the earth's nourishing elements, transforming them into disease-producing toxins, the finest of both modern and traditional medicines will ultimately be rendered impotent.

Over time, as I witnessed the clinical successes of plant-based medicines and struggled with the dilemmas of health problems affecting rich and poor, young and old, I found the mandala of the Medicine Buddha growing brighter in my mind. I began to realize that by harmoniously reintegrating human, plant, and animal societies, we can provide meaningful health care for everyone and avert the threat of global poverty, hunger, epidemics, and biological extinction that looms over our children's future. By compassionately caring for all life, we will have cures for our diseases, foods that cleanse and strengthen us, happiness for our minds, and peace for the earth. Now, the vision of Beautiful to Behold, like an exquisite drop of attar patiently distilled by a master alchemist, gently transforms my disenchantment into inspiration and hope for the renewal of this garden, once the paradisiacal home of our ancestors.

My generous teachers graciously shared their knowledge of classical medicine, and I was fulfilled beyond my greatest expectations. But Nepal is a hard teacher who gives insight into life and human nature in unexpected ways. I found myself faced with many ironies, contradictions, and perplexing mysteries. Why are the traditions of these gifted mentors neglected and suppressed by their own culture, even as they are beginning to be embraced by the modern world? If these medical systems are effective, why is there still so much sickness? If spiritual practices are beneficial for health, why do meditation masters suffer from entirely preventable ailments? Why are goddesses worshipped in every temple, but women treated as inferior incarnations, with serious health consequences for all of society? If prayer and religious devotion are the fabric of society, why are many men's hearts tragically hardened? Why are indigenous cultures abandoning the bounty of sustainable lifestyles and embracing the futureless consumerism of the West? Like a long and complex alchemical process, my real education began, and within the vessel of Kathmandu's worldly and spiritual paradoxes I found revealed the underlying universal principles of healing.

One cannot go far into Ayurveda without encountering alchemy; soon after, one comes face to face with mercury. I wished to learn about mercury's powers, and the shimmering silver water from the serpent realms granted my wish. What I found was as strange a paradox as the element itself, which is at once gaseous, metallic, and liquid. It is the semen of God, say the Himalayan alchemists, a universal essence with peculiar properties analogous to the human mind: when impure, it is deadly, but when purified, it becomes the greatest longevity- and enlightenment-bestowing sacrament. We must treat mercury with care and reverence, for its secrets, dangers, and benefits are more sublime, insidious, and subtle than we suspect. "It will increase the power of your thoughts," the King's alchemist cautioned, handing me a small bead of mysteriously solidified hydrargium.

Alchemy awakens the imagination, stirs the curiosity, arouses mystical longings, and inflames the hunger for gold. But there is nothing romantic about mercury. It is a virulent transgenerational poison that is rapidly accumulating in our brains and reproductive organs. In our medical ignorance we have made mercury the most widely implanted foreign substance in the body and have poisoned our water, soil, and food chain with its complex toxins. Ayurveda offers promising purification therapies for cleansing mercury from the tissues and reversing the physiological damage it has caused. Ayurvedic and Tibetan physicians also claim, based on a thousand years of accumulated empirical evidence, that when properly purified, compounded, and administered, mercurial drugs have curative powers relevant for diseases unresponsive to modern treatments.

I approach the subjects of mercury toxicity and mercurial medicines with ambivalence and trepidation. I have seen suffering caused by mercury, but rather than crusade against the industries responsible for its misuse, my purpose is to explore the possible remedies offered by Ayurveda. I have also seen the benefits of mercurial preparations used by my teachers, but I cannot advocate their use until their safety is confirmed by modern research. Mercury has taught me to be careful about what I ask for.

Although I have not witnessed the transmutation of mercury into gold, I have come to appreciate the symbolic relevance of alchemy. When guided by the heart, the human mind has the extraordinary capacity to refine nature's perfection; when separated from the organ of sentient wisdom, the mind is obscured by spiritual darkness, and the world suffers. In our confusion, we are using our divine powers to transform the earth's life-giving elements into alchemical horrors and creating a legacy of disease and biological destruction. Like alchemists playing with mercury in the hope of finding wealth, we have poisoned ourselves with the toxins of deluded ignorance and greed. The mercurial mind is a wish-fulfilling gem, within which we can instantly create either disease or healing. Where but in the three jewels of awakened consciousness, compassionate truth, and spiritual community can we find the heart-wisdom to practice the higher alchemy?

Somewhere along the way, as the echoes of my dreams unfolded into a journey through the elements of life, this book began to take form. The seed first stirred during candlelit monsoon nights, my imagination ignited by the exotic ingredients, complex preparations, and reputed curative powers of my teachers' formulas. The leaves of this manuscript opened in the warm sun of herb-gathering expeditions, grew with the friendship and dialogue of each new teacher, flowered in the application of their knowledge to my clinical work, and came to fruition in my meditative moments. As rain fell on the dark cobblestones and lush rice paddies of Boudhanath, I reviewed the teachings I had received during the day, gradually filling notebooks; now, as I sit in the tranquil quiet of this California coastal forest, it is done, and only a few words are left to be said.

I have written this book out of love for my teachers, gratitude for their knowledge and generosity, and a desire to help fulfill their compassionate aspirations. The world needs the healing benefits of Ayurveda and Tibetan medicine, and these traditions, in turn, need widespread support to survive and flourish. Classical healing systems, with their millennia of experience in diagnosing and treating diseases, are repositories of valuable insight into urgent medical problems. They have much to offer in treatment of chronic and degenerative diseases, immune enhancement, preventive therapies, alternatives to antibiotics, detoxification, and rejuvenation. More important, these holistic philosophies teach the interrelatedness of body and earth, inseparability of consciousness and matter, mutual dependency of male and female, and humanity's long evolutionary relationship with plants. We are sick, estranged, and longing for the sacredness of life, and the Ayurvedic and Tibetan medical traditions, with their deep respect for all living things, are a rich source of nourishing wisdom.

Classical medical systems can show us the path to collective well-being and global ecological health, for plants are the key to preserving and restoring what remains of the earth's once-abundant living wealth. As awareness and demand for natural food and remedies increase, opportunities for organic farming, sustainable forest management, and cultivation of herbal medicines are also increasing. All countries have unique botanical heritages that can be developed and marketed to raise standards of living, improve health, cultivate social harmony, and revitalize the spirit. Nepal and India, with their rich and diverse geographies, climates, cultures, and traditional medicines, offer unique plants whose therapeutic blessings are needed throughout the world. Nepal especially, with its historical role as provider of numerous species to Ayurvedic and Tibetan physicians, has the potential to become a model of sustainable ecology governed by spiritual culture. This is a vision shared by my teachers, who in their own ways understand how their medical traditions can alleviate much of the suffering that surrounds them.

The old men and women who carry the ancient knowledge of healing with plants are passing on. During the course of their lives, they have seen the ending of ways that have existed for centuries, and the relationships with nature that cultures have maintained for millennia. As these teachers and their heirs speak to us from these pages, let us share in their hopes and dreams and, remembering that we are the caretakers of this precious garden, envision our world as a sacred mandala of healing. The seeds of their teachings lie in our hands. What shall we do with this gift of life?

Big Sur, California
January 12, 2000

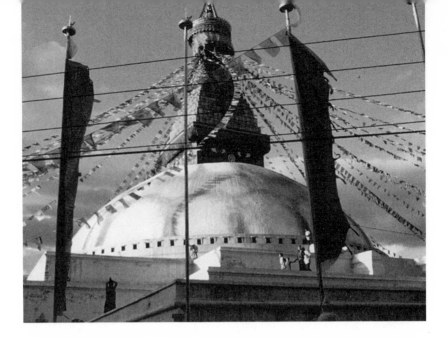

I.

THE MEDICINE BUDDHA

Wisdom without words

Born of inner silence

Carried within the heart

Dispensed with loving-kindness;

This is true medicine.

The Great Stupa of Boudhanath rises like a wish-fulfilling jewel in the eastern Kathmandu Valley. Its gold pinnacle is draped in bright fluttering silks and whispering prayer flags that call faithful pilgrims from distant lands. Around the upper tier, stone deities anointed with vermilion dance in cubicles blackened by years of candle offerings. Beneath its crown, gracefully painted eyes gaze in each of the four directions: north, toward the lost Tibetan homeland across the Himalayas; south, toward the jungles where Buddha walked; to the west, where Swayambhu Hill rises with its own Stupa and secret underground labyrinths; and east, toward the rising sun.

The geometric harmonies of the Boudhanath Stupa's dome are whitewashed by monks before religious festivals, then decorated with lotus petals painted in giant arcs of saffron water. On ceremonial nights the sounds of gongs and bells fill the air as ten thousand shimmering butter lamps transform its terraces into enchanted pathways of light. Prayers uttered in the presence of this monument to transcendence are answered, aspirations and wishes come to fruition.

Around the Stupa revolve the lives of the Tibetan community in exile. Their shops, homes, and monasteries overlook a cobblestone street filled with constant activity. People of all ages circumambulate the shrine from early dawn until late night, spinning prayer wheels, stepping over playing children, murmuring mantras. It takes about ten minutes at a leisurely pace to complete one round—longer if you are old and stiff, less if you are young and vital. The whole world is here: madmen and enlightened teachers, destitute beggars and wealthy patrons, maidens, mothers, and crones, seekers from all corners of the earth, the worldly and the world weary, all the faces of humanity moving together in prayer, appearing and disappearing like rosary beads with each step, each breath.

The Stupa had been calling me for a long time. It cast its net, woven from rays of monsoon sunrises and Himalayan moonlight, and spoke in voices of conch-shell trumpets and resonant chanting. Its eyes looked at me through painted deities and the faces of lamas who suddenly started appearing in my life in the West. The repute of the Tibetan doctors reached my ears; I tasted their medicines made from herbs and purified gems, small pills wrapped in silk and sealed with stamped wax. Like a sand mandala opening doors into realms of initiation, the Stupa spun its designs of destiny, and I was drawn into its embrace.

A light spring rain was falling as I stepped out of the Kathmandu airport, with no plans or prior arrangements. "You can't make anything happen in Nepal," I had been told before my departure, "but everything you want will manifest in its own way." Behind me was a busy clinical practice, a comfortable home, and all my possessions; in front of me was the chaos of dusty streets that unfolded as the taxi made its way toward the Stupa. I arrived in Boudhanath weary and excited, a Buddhist pilgrim, an herbalist seeking remedies from the Himalayan forests. I came in search of doctors who would instruct me in Tibetan and Ayurvedic medicines, who would share their knowledge and methods, their secrets. I had come to bring my aspirations to fruition.

I made my home near the shrine, in a colorful and exotic new world of spiritual and earthly paradoxes. Rows of monks in full ceremonial attire, wearing orange robes and crested yellow hats, circled the big white monastery outside my window, blowing long horns and beating huge drums. In the courtyard below, wrinkled old Nepali women sat in the hot sun, sifting sand and breaking rocks into gravel. Young children struggled up steep flights of stairs under sacks of cement. Outside the gilded shrines, beggars lifted their leprosied hands, eloquently revealing the Buddha's noble truth of suffering. The Stupa's eyes watched impassively as I walked along the cobblestones, devotion smiling through the dust.

The pungent aroma of herbs from the mountains greeted me as I entered the clinic of the local Tibetan doctor. The fragrant plants were stored in burlap bags stacked along the walls and in large metal bowls, waiting to be ground into powder. Several bookcases held a variety of glass jars filled with pills of different sizes and colors. On the balcony outside, young monks talked and laughed as they worked at preparing more formulas. Under a large portrait of the Dalai Lama sat an old monk dressed in maroon robes. He was listening quietly to a patient's pulse, eyes hidden behind darkly tinted glasses. His concentration was undistracted by my entrance or the presence of several other Tibetans waiting to see him. Here, in this room, was what I had traveled so far to find.

The morning before, I had awakened feeling feverish and weak and spent the day lying in the humid heat of my concrete room, looking out at Kathmandu's polluted brown sky. Outside, raw sewage lay in the medieval streets, mangy dogs and wandering cows foraged through piles of rotting garbage, the soot of cooking fires hung heavy in the air. That night, lightning flickered over the village and its dry rice paddies, then ancient sounds of monastic ritual drifted through dawn's thick fog into my restless sleep. Dizzy and nauseous, I made my way through the unbearable stench of the narrow alleys to the monk-doctor's residence.

The consultation with each patient took less than ten minutes. After asking a question or two to confirm his pulse diagnosis, Dr. Ngawang Chopel and his assistant filled a prescription from the modest pharmacy. I sat on a wooden bench, my head throbbing. When my turn came, the doctor gently took my wrist and pressed his attentive fingers to the radial artery. Its feverish pulsations were obvious and uncomplicated. "Bile," the old physician said in Tibetan, and began counting out the pills for my prescription. As I stood to leave, I expressed my interest in learning about his medicines and asked if he would consider taking a student. The doctor's assistant translated my question, which was met with a warm smile and an affirmative nod. "Come back when you are feeling better," he said.

I spoke no Tibetan, Dr. Chopel spoke no English, and neither of us spoke Nepali. Sonam Topgyal was the most qualified interpreter in Kathmandu. He was a professional translator, a teacher of Tibetan language at Tribuvan University, and had spent six years studying with a Tibetan doctor. After some friendly haggling over his fees and schedule, the intelligent young man agreed to become part of my educational journey. Sonam knew Amchi-la (Honorable Doctor), as he affectionately called him, and would enjoy hearing his teachings.

The next day we met outside the apartment building that served as the temporary home of Dr. Chopel's monastery, Shelkar Ling. The afternoon sun was baking the dusty streets; I still felt weak from my fever, but the doctor's pills had definitely been helpful. Several monks stood on the balconies making medicines. A couple of the younger boys came racing down the stairs to greet us, then cheerfully showed us the way to the doctor's room. We found him sitting in his small clinic, examining a patient's pulse. After the patient had left, Dr. Chopel shuffled out into the hall, opened his bedroom door, and invited us in.

The doctor's personal quarters were typically Tibetan. Small wooden couches covered with dragon-decorated rugs sat along three of the cement walls. A cabinet with glass windows held statues of Buddhas wrapped in white cloths. Thangkas of deities lined the upper walls, and rows of silver offering cups sat on the windowsills. All of Dr. Chopel's books and religious objects were clustered around the end of his couch, where he would sit and study or meditate when there were no patients.

The old man gathered his robes around him and climbed onto his seat, motioning for us to sit on the couch to his left. He sent a young monk running to the kitchen for tea as he made himself comfortable, sitting cross-legged on the orange and purple carpets spread over his simple bed. The monk returned with a tray of porcelain tea bowls and two thermoses of steaming tea. We had our choice of either sweet tea (made of powdered milk, sugar, and tea) or butter tea, the traditional drink of Tibet. I ordered butter tea, sipping it as Dr. Chopel, the monk, and some other faces peering through the door watched to see my reaction. It looked like chicken broth and tasted like tea cooked with salt and butter. Amchi-la grinned and asked if I liked it; the monks laughed and went running down the hall. The moment, and the tea, were delicious.

Dr. Chopel removed a long narrow manuscript from his cabinet and carefully unwrapped its yellow silk cover. This was the *Gyu Shi*, the *Four Tantras*, or "expanded treatises," which contained the core teachings of Tibetan medicine. The physician adjusted his tinted glasses and started his instructions.

"The origin of Tibetan medicine is Sange Menla, the Medicine Buddha," the old monk said. He spoke softly and deliberately, in a dry, high-pitched voice; the succinct and pithy instructions that followed contained a wealth of knowledge.

During the years when the early monastic order was being established by Sakyamuni Buddha, the practice of medicine by monks and nuns was restricted mostly to the religious community. Many of the Buddha's rules of monastic conduct, such as avoiding intoxication and eating only one meal per day, had health-promoting benefits, but relatively little importance was placed on health for its own sake. The emphasis of the teachings was on the practice of meditation and morality for achieving enlightenment, the ultimate state of freedom from suffering.

After the Buddha's passing, medicine gradually became an increasingly important aspect of Buddhism. This change was promoted especially by the later philosophical developments of the Mahayana tradition, which taught that, through service to others, one's own spiritual practice was enhanced. As a result, monks and nuns were responsible for much of the dissemination of classical medical teachings and practices throughout Asia. Along with this integration of healing arts into the Buddha's doctrine of compassion came the appearance of several physician-bodhisattvas, universal Buddhas who could be worshipped as deified forms of enlightenment. The first to appear were King of Remedies and Supreme Physician. These were later overshadowed by Bhaisajyaguru, Master of Remedies, who resided in one of the paradise realms; this was Sange Menla, the Medicine Buddha of whom Dr. Chopel now spoke. This new addition to the Buddhist pantheon gained immense popularity across Asia, and was later officially adopted by Tibetan medical schools as the source of the *Four Tantras*, the root texts that now lay on the table in front of my new teacher.

"Because people lack the spiritual fortune to see his pure form directly," Dr. Chopel explained, "Buddha entered into meditation and sent emanations from himself into the world. In this way he took incarnation in perceivable form for the purpose of benefiting beings."

In the magical world of classical medicine, the distinctions among historical, mythical, and archetypal events are blurred, and the lineages of human doctors, medical sages, and hermit healers intermingle with those of celestial divinities. As a result of this interdimensional aspect of Tibetan medical history, there are many explanations about who and what a deity such as Sange Menla is, and these have been the subject of research and debate through the centuries.

According to one of the unique doctrines of Tibetan philosophy, when a Buddha "turns the wheel of Dharma"—that is, gives teachings that elevate others to higher states of existence—he appears in the form of a deity; at the same time the world is transformed into a corresponding sacred realm, the abode of that deity. There are many versions describing the details of when and where the historical Sakyamuni Buddha, as Bhaisajyaguru, gave the teachings on medicine: one says that it occurred in northwest India; others describe it as one of several different heavens.

"While in meditation," Dr. Chopel continued, "rays of light emerged from the Medicine Buddha's heart. Under the influence of these rays, all beings throughout existence were cleansed of their deep ignorance and evil thoughts. Their diseases were cured, and the three poisons of delusion, hatred, and desire were pacified."

What my new teacher was describing was the series of cosmic events that precede every teaching of the Buddha as the powers of his enlightened mind begin to manifest themselves. These phenomena are recreated during Tibetan meditation as visualizations of different-colored lights shining from the energy centers of both the meditator and the invoked deity. The rays emanating from the meditator are used to purify the body, speech, and mind, while those imagined coming from the deity into one's body confer various levels of initiation.

"From that light," Dr. Chopel continued, "an emanation of Sange Menla's mind appeared as the sage Rigpe Yeshe [Wisdom of Science]. At this time many other Trang Sung [Those Who Speak Only Truth] appeared, as well as countless gods and goddesses, humans, and other beings, both Buddhist and non-Buddhist. Rigpe Yeshe remained in the sky and gave these teachings to the audience of listeners:

"O friends, know the meaning of what I tell you. If you want to live without being afflicted by sickness, or want to know how to cure sickness, you need to know the following medical system. If you want to prolong life, to do things in this life in accordance with religion, or to be rich and make worldly progress, you must study this system. If you want to be enlightened by removing the root of ignorance, or if you want to relieve the suffering of sentient beings throughout the six realms, you must study this system. If one aspires to be a person who is respected by the community and become a leader of the people, studying this text will also help with this kind of success."

At this point the Medicine Buddha emitted from his tongue multicolored rays of light throughout the ten directions, purifying the negativity of harmful speech, curing diseases caused by imbalances of the body's biological humors, and pacifying demons.

"As there were none among the followers who could ask questions," Dr. Chopel continued, "Sange Menla emitted from his tongue the form of Yi Le Ge [Born of Mind]. Yi Le Ge circumambulated the Medicine Buddha, prostrated himself, and requested teachings."

Dr. Chopel paused to clarify the meaning of the scripture. "This text is in the form of questions and answers between these two emanations of the Medicine Buddha's mind and speech," he said. I found this description of the origin of Tibetan medicine's most sacred books fascinating; I sipped my salty tea, took careful notes, and contemplated my good fortune to be able to hear this dialogue between two sages projected from the tongue and heart of a deity, who in turn was a celestial mirage born of a Buddha's meditation.

"Yi Le Ge asked, 'If this is really true, how does one study these things?' Rigpe Yeshe replied, 'These are known by studying the *Gyu Shi*, the *Four Tantras*, which teach the science of medicine.'

"The complete title of the *Gyu Shi* is *Dutsi Nyingpo Yenlag Gyepa Sangwa Men Ngak Gi Gyu*," Dr. Chopel explained. "This means *The Am-*

brosia Heart Tantra: The Secret Oral Teaching on the Eight Branches of the Science of Healing." An alternative translation of this long title is *Tantra of Secret Instructions on the Eight Branches of the Essence of the Elixir of Immortality*.

"Dutsi is nectar," Dr. Chopel went on, "which is water used by the gods. It has three qualities: if one drinks from it, it will cure disease without medicine; it is an elixir for prolonging life; and it frees one from attachments and therefore from suffering. This text exemplifies these three qualities. Nyingpo means 'the heart or essence' of dutsi. Yenlag gyepa means 'the eight branches of healing.' These are the branches of physiology and internal medicine; pediatrics; gynecology; diseases caused by evil spirits and ghosts; treatment of wounds caused by weapons and injuries; poisons; rejuvenation therapy for old age; and treatment of infertility and impotence.

"Sangwa means 'secret.' This text is shown to those who are eligible for hearing and seeing it; it is not shown to those who are ineligible. Those who are ineligible are people who wish to learn only for the sake of tasting or experimenting, people who wish to use the knowledge to inflict harm, and those who are motivated by desire for name, fame, and wealth. Men ngak has many meanings, one of which is 'the word which benefits.' It is instruction in the right way of doing things, showing what is to be done and what is not to be done. Men ngak also means 'that which is the essence of advice or instruction.' In general, when we give instruction or advice to someone, it is biased with personal likes and dislikes. This text is free from any defects of this type of duality."

Dr. Chopel paused to read the text. He then gave a brief synopsis of the opening statements that typically precede scriptural writings. "The first stanzas are a dedication to the Medicine Buddha, in the form of commending and praising his activities. Sange Menla is referred to as 'the one who elaborates or explains the pure meaning of the text without the slightest trace of fault.' Following this, the author offers prostrations."

The doctor then began elaborating on the main body of the text. The first section was devoted to invoking a vision of the pure realm that appeared around the Medicine Buddha as he taught the Dharma of healing to the exalted assembly.

"The place where the Medicine Buddha gave these teachings is free from defects, pleasant to look at and experience, and full of Truth. In this place is a palace made of precious medicinal gems that can cure all diseases; they are cooling to hot diseases and warming to cold diseases, fulfill all wishes, and ward off evil spirits. Around the four sides of the palace grow medicinal plants of every variety. All types of medicines are present, such as flowers, trees, grasses, mineral waters, precious gems, and animals. In the center of the palace is a throne, on which the Medicine Buddha is seated. He is surrounded by disciples of gods, sages, Buddhists, and non-Buddhists. Sange Menla sits in deep meditation, for the purpose of curing the innumerable types of sufferings."

Bhaisajyaguru's meditation embraces all beings throughout the expanse of space. From his forehead comes white light, which cleanses the nerves and detoxifies the channels of mind and breath. These rays remove afflictions of desire and bestow inner peace, contentment, and harmonious relationships. From the center of his throat shine red lights with the power to purify the blood so that afflictions of anger are pacified, fortunes are increased, and aspirations are attained. From the center of his heart radiate blue lights that absolve wrongdoings of the body and mind, increase spiritual awareness, and enhance the power of positive attraction.

This complex healing mandala, filled with elaborately detailed images, contains both important medical information in codified form for the student and doctor, and beautiful symbology with the power to elevate the mind and enhance the vitality of those troubled by illness.

In my mind's eye I could see the land described by my teacher. From the cold Snowclad Mountain of the north, where the power of the moon is strong, come sandalwood and camphor, gentian, and licorice, cooling medicines that pacify feverish diseases. To the south, where Thunderbolt Mountain rises and the solar energies prevail, grow hot medicines like peppers, cinnamon, and ginger, which rid the body of cold diseases. In the east, on Fragrant Mountain, grow different species of myrobalan trees, which have the power to cure all diseases of the body. In the west rises Cool Mountain, the source of such excellent drugs as nutmeg, cloves, and saffron, minerals and crystals, and medicinal waters from hot springs. Creatures of all kinds live in the forests, jungles, and meadows—peacocks, elephants, tigers, parrots, and bears—providing valuable remedies from their bodies. All around the palace of the Medicine Buddha, physicians are carrying on their noble practices, cultivating medicinal plants, preparing healing nectars, diagnosing patients, and administering therapies.

In the center of this kingdom resides Sange Menla, his omniscient mind coursing through the deep ocean of compassion. He sits on a throne of talking jewels that possess the power to remove all obstacles to health and happiness, in a palace made of gold, silver, and multi-colored pearls. Translucent and insubstantial, his deep-blue body is like a luminous rainbow, revealing his space-like wisdom and impartial love toward all beings. Graced with perfection, he sits in the lotus posture of self-mastery, wearing the saffron robes of a monk, the symbol of virtue's inner warmth. Fountains of blessings stream from his lapis fingertips, and cascades of sparkling lights fall from his mouth as he teaches. His left hand rests open in his lap, expressing mental equanimity; it holds a simple medicine bowl filled with the nectar of immortal life. His right hand extends in the gesture of supreme generosity, offering nature's gift of healing and renewal, a branch and fruit from the tree of the universal medicine.

Bhaisajyaguru is the patron deity of Tibetan medicine, the archetypal mentor of its physicians and students, and a source of healing for the sick. When preparing formulas, doctors recite mantras of the Master of Remedies: prescribing medicines and giving treatments is regarded as making offerings to the deity. Sange Menla is invoked with liturgical chanting and ceremonial music every day in Tibetan medical colleges.

The students are taught that medicines are gifts bestowed by the deity, mentors are his living embodiment, and books and teachings are his words. Across Asia and through the long span of centuries, the temples of Bhaisajyaguru have drawn those in search of health.

The Medicine Buddha is the mythological source of the Tibetan medical tradition. The sadhana, or spiritual discipline, of invoking the deity re-enacts his trans-historical origins. Accompanied by drums, horns, bells, and conch shells, the liturgy describes how he emerges from a sacred syllable representing Buddha's mind. His body, the palace of gems, the guardians of the ten directions, the retinue of sages and gods who appeared at the time of his giving teachings, and the mandala of nature's medicines are chanted into existence, to assist the visualization in the mind of the practitioner. The rays of light the Buddha emitted in past eons are generated once again for the benefit of all beings. After completing the visualization, participants of the sadhana make literal and symbolic offerings to the deity. They then meditate, maintaining a stream of concentration that is focused either sequentially or simultaneously on the healing lights, the syllables of the mantra, the deity imagined before them, and themselves as the deity. At the end of the practice, more prayers are made for universal healing, the visualized deity is dissolved into the body, and a state of meditative absorption is practiced for as long as possible.

This type of ritualistic, ceremonial, and multifaceted meditation is one of the unique characteristics of Tibetan Buddhism. It is a profoundly enriching contribution to the world's spiritual practices, and a source of divine blessings and deep healing.

Suffering and illness are directly related to the unstable nature of the mind. Chaotic and stressful thought patterns disturb the flow of life force in the channels and nerves, resulting in physiological disequilibrium. Balance can be restored by guiding the distracted mind back into an effortless state of flow using proper posture, smooth cycles of breathing, and gradually prolonged periods of steady visualization. Stabilizing wandering attention gives rise to many positive effects that are helpful for healing the body, increasing happiness, perceiving deeper reality, and resolving suffering. These effects are especially powerful when the mind is focused on a symbol of higher consciousness that inspires faith (such as a deity) and is soothed with the vibratory tones of a mantra. A state of relaxed concentration, such as that practiced in a deity sadhana, can induce positive physiological changes in the body, including decreased tension, sensations of lightness and expansion, heightened circulation, and warmth.

A more subtle but perhaps more profound benefit is the change of self-perception that occurs during the process of imagining one's physical form dissolving and being replaced with a rainbow-like ethereal body. In the first phase of the practice, the meditator envisions and feels the solid body becoming insubstantial like empty space; this is followed by mentally recreating oneself in the form of the deity, who performs the main part of the sadhana. In the final stages of the sadhana this process is repeated, first dissolving the visualization of the deity into oneself, then resting in the space-like emptiness of open awareness without giving rise to a concept of a self, and finally re-emerging into one's own body. This method of disassociating from ordinary perceptions, entering into emptiness, appearing as a deity, then returning through emptiness to the physical body teaches the grasping mind to liberate itself from habitual clinging to perishable outward appearances. Ultimately, the purpose of this type of meditation is to achieve spiritual freedom: by repeatedly projecting and withdrawing consciousness in and out of gross and subtle forms, the meditator recognizes that "reality" has an illusory, mind-created nature.

Deity meditation is the art of self-generating blessings by identifying with a divinity, and the inner alchemy of mentally creating a new form that symbolically embodies spiritual attributes. In a sadhana such as Sange Menla's, mythology is brought to life by outer ceremony and internal concentration, which awaken the vitality of the psyche and its magically transformative influences. Visualizing a deity who is adorned with auspicious attributes and surrounded by images of nature's beneficence, and is blessing one with rays of purifying light, affects the mental atmosphere in a positive way; this in turn brings numerous health benefits for patients, and intuitive wisdom for doctors. By focusing the contemplative imagination on sacred imagery with devotional attention, meditators learn to perceive the outer world as the pure realm of medicine, the body as the celestial palace, and one's own thoughts as the mind of the deity. This is the "Divine Pride" of knowing oneself as the deity and the outer world as the self-emanated pure realm.

"One of the first things that a student of Tibetan medicine learns," Dr. Chopel said, "is that everything in this world is potentially a medicine. We are taught to view the world as the mandala of the Medicine Buddha. There is nothing that cannot be prepared or purified into a substance that has medicinal value." The doctor then told a story about Jivaka, one of ancient India's greatest physicians, who attended the Buddha and his Sangha.

"When Jivaka was a young student he was much admired by his teacher and the other students. It seemed there was nothing he could not memorize or comprehend. His studies and learning seemed unsurpassed. One day his teacher decided to test his chief students. Bringing them together, he said, 'I am sending the four of you on a search. Please go out into the world and bring me back something that is not a medicine.'

"After a few days the first student came back, bringing an unknown plant. 'I have found this plant, which I believe has no medicinal value,' said the student. Taking the plant, the teacher examined its tastes and smells, then demonstrated how to prepare it into a medicine.

"After a week the second student came back, carrying a rotting animal part. 'I have brought this useless part of an animal carcass,' the student said. The teacher showed the student how it could be cooked and cleaned to produce a healing substance.

"After another week the third student came back, bringing a rock. 'I have found this rock, which I believe has no value,' he said. The teacher instructed him in the alchemical procedures that rendered stones and minerals into medicinal nectars.

"After a long time, Jivaka finally returned, empty-handed. 'I have searched everywhere,' he said, 'but could not find anything that was not a medicine.' With this test, he again demonstrated his superior understanding."

About four hours after we had arrived at Dr. Chopel's office, he announced that the day's lesson was over. Sonam and I unfolded our cramped legs, put our shoes on at the door, and thanked the doctor. He casually waved us away as he gently wrapped the scriptures back into their colorful cover, telling me to return at the same time tomorrow.

Outside, children were playing in the street, people stood talking in doorways and walkways, and an occasional cow wandered past. Down the alley I could see the early evening crowd gathering around the Stupa while lightning pierced the sky around the edges of the valley. Saying good-bye to Sonam, I decided to join the revolving circle of prayer.

The descending darkness found me walking with the faithful as we made our devotional rounds of the shrine, my mind full of the rich imagery of Tibetan myth and medicine. I thought of my new teacher's final comments as I walked along the black slate path past the alcoves of prayer wheels. There are stories that have come down through the ages, he had said, about people who have come face to face with the Medicine Buddha. The deity appeared directly before those fortunate ones, giving magical elixirs that instantaneously cured their diseases.

I looked at the people around me. Some were praying at the altar of the wrathful Protector, Mahakala; others made supplications to the giant golden Maitreya Buddha or gave offerings of incense in the shrine rooms of monasteries along the cobblestone street. Old nuns did full-length prostrations on the flagstones, mothers helped their children light butter lamps, monks chanted from scriptures. It was not difficult to imagine the encounters with the Medicine Buddha that Amchi-la had described. In this land where deities live among people, anything was possible.

When the Buddha taught, our world became a celestial abode. The power of his articulated wisdom made it possible for those present to see beyond mundane reality, into the inherent purity and cosmic presence that eternally surround us. The mandala that appeared around him is a vision of humanity's potential: enlightened mind in harmony with nature, working for the benefit of all. It is the archetypal pristine world inhabited by beings living in a golden age of spiritual achievement: heaven on earth. It is our world, after the gloom of ignorance and confusion of mental defilements have been removed by the lights of purifying awareness, and the glorious prosperity of nature renewed by treating the earth as a sacred garden of medicine.

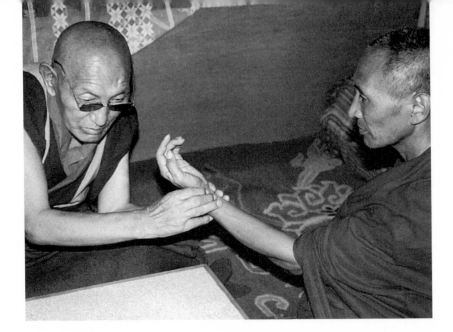

II.

THE TREE OF KNOWLEDGE

For a bodhisattva attempting to achieve enlightenment there is no greater obstacle than illness! When living beings are burdened with an ailing body, the spirit cannot be at peace. How can perfection be achieved under such circumstances? The bodhisattva who strives for enlightenment must therefore first heal the afflictions of the body.

GANDAVYUHA SUTRA

Dr. Chopel's office was similar to the clinics of many village healers: a simple desk, a concrete floor, and bookcases lined with jars full of pills. It was humble to the point of being bare, except for the intricate aromas emanating from the repository of handmade medicines. The routines of the doctor's medical practice were simple, consisting primarily of an in-depth pulse diagnosis that determined a prescription of herbs. Amchi-la would sit cross-legged on a bench behind the desk, his back to the windows overlooking the rice paddies. His presence was serious yet gentle, and his patients responded with quiet humility. The doctor would offer words of practical and spiritual advice as he counted out his prescription from the bottles on the shelves.

These pills were the classical medicines of Tibetan antiquity. They were medicines from the earth, made with hands guided by generations of knowledge, and blessed with prayer. The formulas dated back through the years; some had been passed down many centuries. The pharmacopoeias preserving this medical knowledge were scrolls of woodblock-printed texts, stacked alongside the bags of raw herbs. They called for common ingredients like easily accessible spices and herbs, as well as rare gems or hard-to-find botanical species. Some formulas were simple, comprising only a few substances; others were complex, with a hundred or more ingredients.

Other medicines contained alchemical preparations made from purified mercury, sulfur, iron, copper, coral, and pearls; the doctors of old utilized every imaginable crystal, salt, gem, and mineral for its therapeutic properties. These ingredients had to be purified using tools and complex techniques handed down through the generations; some substances required months of daily labor before their poisons were fully removed. The days and nights of the alchemist-doctors and their students were filled with meditative work, in laboratories equipped with mortars and pestles, grinders, stills, iron pots, clay urns, kilns, and fireplaces.

With stone pestles, they would gently rub the precious substances brought from the veins of the earth and bottom of the sea, steadily and carefully mixing them with other minerals and plant substances. As each process worked its effects, the medicine in progress released another of its poisons, to be washed or distilled out of the mixture. In some procedures, more months would pass as the triturated powders were repeatedly distilled and re-mixed until ready for human consumption. The purified essence of the original ingredient was then combined with others to create the final formula. Centuries of experimentation, clinical practice and observation, inspired insights, accidents, and divine revelation were contained in the tiny herbal pills that filled the shelves of Dr. Chopel's pharmacy. His remedies were the multiflavored fruits of the ancient lineages of iatro-chemists, the physicians who alchemized their own medicines.

In his younger days Dr. Chopel went into the wilderness to gather his own herbs, bringing back the best plants in their prime stages of potency. Now he relied on what he could purchase from the herb markets at Asan Tol in Kathmandu. As in the old days, the laborious process of preparing the botanical ingredients for medicine was done by the monks and apprentices of the monastery. When a formula needed to be refilled, the doctor weighed out the herbs on a large balance scale, then poured them into metal bowls; the plants' fragrant bodies were then pulverized in mortars and sifted through screens. Most modern pharmacies producing Tibetan and Ayurvedic medicines have grinding equipment to speed up this work, but traditional herbalists know that the heat generated by machines damages the volatile substances of the plants and weakens their potency.

Once the herbs were finely powdered, they were mixed with water or decoctions of other ingredients to make a thick paste. A special measuring spoon was used to determine the right amount of paste for each pill. The monks assisting Dr. Chopel would sit together and roll pills by hand, talking and laughing as they worked. As each pill was completed, it was added to the others on wicker trays and set out to dry. Several days later, when the pills were hard, two monks poured them into a sheet and rolled them back and forth, holding the cloth closed at both ends to form a tube; this polished the pills for longer storage. Finally, they were counted and poured into jars next to the doctor's desk.

Amchi-la would inform me whenever special ingredients arrived, as when a small bag came from Tibet: purified gold, which went into his formulation of the "Great Purified Moon Crystal Pill." This extraordinary remedy was originally compounded from thirty-four ingredients, including herbs like saffron and nutmeg, minerals and metals processed for human consumption, and such animal substances as the gallstone from an elephant. It was used to counteract poisons, kill parasites, and pacify chronic fevers. "It is hard to make these medicines completely in the traditional way," Dr. Chopel explained. "Many of these ingredients are no longer available, especially the ones unique to Tibet." Like other herbalists facing shortages of important ingredients, Dr. Chopel sometimes had to use substitutions or make formulas without key ingredients.

Amchi-la's fascinating pharmacy was filled with the medicines I had been seeking. Inside an old Ovaltine jar were tiny black pills of gentian and other bitter roots, to destroy bilious conditions and rejuvenate the liver from hepatitis. In another were large brown pills of aquillaria wood and warming spices, calming to the mind and nervous system. Other pills were made of pomegranate seed and limestone, whose flavors cleanse mucus from the stomach, or sweet sandalwood and cooling flowers for pacifying fevers. Dozens of bottles lined the doctor's shelves, while still more medicines lay stacked in bags around the edge of the room or hidden away in cupboards.

Waiting close to the doctor's elbow were the rinchen rilbu, precious pills, sent from the Tibetan Medical Institute in India or carried over the Himalayas from hospitals in Lhasa. Each pill came wrapped in brightly colored silk, tied with a thread, and stamped with a wax seal. There was the "Wish-Fulfilling Gem Pill," reputed to cure seizures and paralysis; the "Great Accumulation Pill," which destroys poisons in the digestive system; the "Great Iron Pill," which treats eye problems; the "Old Turquoise Pill" for cooling liver inflammation; and "Coral 25" for fevers in the brain and bones. The rarest of these was the "Great Black Cold Pill," formulated with over a hundred ingredients.

This simple clinic, with its medicines from Himalayan jungles and mountains, Indian tropics, and Nepali hillsides, was a familiar atmosphere, permeated with the presence of the plants and their hidden powers. It was reminiscent of my own clinics, which had been well stocked with botanicals from both East and West, stored in a large wooden cabinet built in the old apothecary style. This cabinet was like the ones I had used as an apprentice in Chinatown, during my first formal education in Chinese medicine.

The bricks of chrysanthemum flowers lay stacked behind the glass counter, wrapped in brown paper and tied with twine. They made a sweet tea that was popular with the old women who came into the herb shop, who used the flowers in their home remedies. The resident doctor added them to his calligraphed prescriptions to cool fevers and soothe inflamed eyes. Every few weeks the bin in front where the loose flowers were kept would run low. Each brick then had to be untied and broken apart so the pressed flowers could be fluffed up. Like soft sunbursts, they spread their yellow pollen across the brown paper as they came apart, releasing fragrance brought from across the sea. Whenever it was time to refill the bin, the perfume of Chinese gardens filled the store.

The simple chore of preparing the chrysanthemums was a pleasant task that took about an hour. Since it was usually given to the novice apprentice, it was natural that the newcomer would be asked to do it. I picked up the first brick, cut the twine, and opened the package of sweet flowers. My herbal education had started.

The proprietor of the herb store, Dr. Man Sang Yu, was a respected herbalist in the Chinese community. He was not interested in taking me as a student, his wife informed me, but I persisted in my visits and spent regular sums of money on the exotic medicinals that filled the big jars and rows of drawers at the Yang Sang Company. Eventually, the doctor gave in and allowed me to join the staff behind the counter, who spent their days weighing out the prescriptions he wrote for his patients.

Dr. Yu had other chores for the white boy. Sometimes he would just hold up a broom and point to the floor, since he spoke no English and I knew no Chinese. Other times, when the store was quiet, he and his assistants would open drawers in the huge pharmacy and pull out herbs so I could become familiar with their names. One of the older men who worked there spoke English and would comment on their functions, saying something like "Cleans the system," "Good for the woman," or "Stops pain." I took meticulous notes, amusing and irritating everyone with my curiosity.

After a week I was promoted to the job of cutting ginseng and dong quai roots. They were heated slowly in a toaster oven, just enough to soften but not enough to scorch. Each root was then laid precisely at the cutting edge of a giant hinged blade and quickly cut into thin slices. The roots were succulent and gave off an aura of wholesomeness. The ginseng was the red Korean type that came packaged in colorful tins. The slices glowed translucent amber, smelled earthy and warm, and sold for good money. The dong quai was fibrous and stretchy, smelling pungent as it came away from the knife. These were the two greatest tonic herbs of Chinese medicine, known throughout the world for their restorative powers.

When not filling prescriptions, unpacking shipments of herbs, grinding fossilized "dragon" teeth in a mortar, or washing dishes, I explored the drawers and bins of the shop's hidden interior. Medicinal wasp nests, cicada skins, dried snakes, toad venom, fragrant spices, dried seahorses, glittering crystals, and other strange marvels lay beyond the more obvious commercial herbs. One of the pharmacists told me that the doctor had a safe in his office containing even more precious medicines, like powdered gems and pearls. It was a pharmaceutical wonderland.

As the months went by, I brought my friends and classmates for consultations and herbal treatments. After asking only a few questions and touching their pulses, Yi Sang (Mr. Doctor) would write out his formulas and send them out to the counter to be filled. While I apprenticed there, filling hundreds of packages, I recorded almost everything the doctor prescribed. The results were typical of Chinese herbal formulas: mostly beneficial, sometimes miraculous, occasionally nauseating. Although communication with the doctor was limited, I was able to gradually learn the most important attributes of the herbs: their tastes, their heating or cooling influences, and some of their important uses. Years later, when starting to formulate my own medicines, I came to fully appreciate the degree of sophistication this quiet doctor's prescriptions revealed.

"I am taking the monks on a trip to the mountains tomorrow for the purpose of visiting some holy places and doing puja. Why don't you come with us?" Dr. Chopel closed his text and peered up from his tinted glasses. "We are leaving by taxi early in the morning. Meet us at the Stupa gate."

We gathered in the yellow light of sunrise at the brightly painted entrance to the Stupa's cobblestone circle. The fruit vendors were opening their stalls, and people on their way to work whistled for taxis into town. Soon the buses and trucks would begin their noisy rounds, covering everything with dust. The young monks assembled together, carrying thermoses of salty tea and cloth bags filled with food, religious texts, and musical instruments; the older monks ran around hiring a fleet of taxis, haggling with the Nepali drivers. Our destination was Par Ping, a mountain south of the Kathmandu Valley, where Buddhist saints once meditated in caves and the black goddess Kali lives in her south-facing shrine at the confluence of three rivers.

Our little caravan wound through the city. The narrow streets were filling with people: farmers carrying baskets of vegetables, shopkeepers opening their doors, old men and haggard women with worn-out bodies, young girls in the brief flowering of their youth, dark-skinned children playing in the dirt. Men on motorcycles weaved through the traffic, their sari-wrapped wives perched sideways behind them, foreheads decorated with crimson tikas. Idle men in sunglasses smoked cigarettes in the choking smog, bent laborers carried giant loads, schoolboys walked arm in arm, pale tourists wandered through the maze of hawkers and things to buy. Dogs scavenged in gutters, pigeons flew from their homes behind ornately carved shutters and temple rooftops, coming to rest on the morning laundry hung out to dry. The air was full of sounds and scents: bicycle bells and rickshaw horns, honking cars wedged between vendors' stands, aromas of incense, sewage, and tobacco, hacking coughs, Nepali music. Cows stood in the road, oblivious to the commotion.

We entered the countryside, traveling into a deep gorge toward the steamy southern plains of the Terai region. In the primordial dawn of Kathmandu's history a lake filled the valley until Manjushri, the region's guardian deity, cut this cleft in the mountains with his flaming sword. Now a river cascaded through the chasm, past red earth houses clinging to rocky terraces parched with pre-monsoon thirst.

After about two hours we arrived at Par Ping. Our destination was the mountain's peak, which was accessible by a steep stairway overlooking the gilded roofs of Tibetan monasteries. The monks clattered up the steps with their supplies, emerging in a pine and rhododendron forest on the upper slopes. Every tree was draped with prayer flags, new and old, colorful and faded, which filled the air with mantras and images of Buddhas. We unpacked our bags and unraveled huge rolls of fresh flags to hang; soon the breeze was lifting our prayers into the sky.

I wandered away to a shady place and sat looking at the scattered dwellings far below. Sounds of farm animals and the smoke from cooking fires rose from the valleys that rolled away in the hazy distance. Images of village life drifted through my mind: men hauling bags up steep stone steps, girls washing clothes at fountains, women in fields, everyone carrying the heavy weight of medieval agriculture. Somewhere in the distance to the north were the snowy Himalayas, looking down on this place of fertility and life, disease and death. Soon the monsoons would arrive with dramatic lightning, thunder, and torrential downpours to bring the crops back to life. Everything would be transformed into mud, and waterborne diseases would flourish. After the final rain and before the onset of winter, the land would be fresh, green, and ready to harvest. Gradually winter would descend, finding people wrapped in thin shawls against the cold fog.

In the shadows below, the goddess of the old religion stood at the rivers' confluence, holding her sword of merciful ego-destroying wrath; it was rumored that she still spoke occasionally. At the base of the mountain, springs of blue water dripped through red rock cliffs, then flowed quietly through a series of small pools. Fish were gliding in their shady turquoise world among floating leaves and reflections of over-hanging trees. Giant roots extended from the cliffs above, entwined around protruding boulders; over the centuries the rain had covered them with colored calcifications, transforming them into giant coiling snakes. Cool stone courtyards led to ancient meditation caves where hermits were absorbed in contemplative practice. In one cave a Tibetan monk was reciting liturgy by the light of a smoky butter lamp; in an-other an old Hindu baba with flowing white hair and beard was sitting motionless, absorbed in trance, thin from fasting, and naked except for a loincloth. On the walls of the caves were imprints made by adepts to demonstrate their mastery over phenomena—teachings in the form of handprints and footprints in solid stone, transmissions across time to re-mind us that the solidity of the world is merely an illusion.

I lay in the comfort of the forest floor, absorbed in this dance of eter-nity and impermanence. On the slopes below, the monks were perform-ing puja, invoking Buddha's blessings with chanting, blaring horns, and crashing cymbals. I thought of the past several weeks, and the insights my teacher had shared with me. In his early talks, Dr. Chopel had de-scribed how physicians of the past had intimate knowledge of the plant kingdom. Once, and even now in some places, doctors wandered through mountains and jungles gathering potent drugs.

Physicians of old were also botanists who knew the identification of numerous plants, their habitats, and details of their uses. Taking herb and mineral supplies back to their workshops and laboratories, they be-came chemists, extracting, purifying, and blending the medicinal substances into their final form. As alchemists, they researched and developed elixirs for extending life and enhancing consciousness, performing complex procedures with the metals, minerals, gems, and poisons collected during their travels. Many physicians have been priests, priestesses, shamans, and philosophers who understood the deepest workings of nature unseen by most, and who achieved spiritual realization as a result of their contemplations. Much of their healing work was linked to ceremony and worship.

From tropical rain forests, with their profusion of vegetation, to open prairies, from coastal mountains to deserts, on every continent and in every age, every culture throughout history has relied on the plant kingdom as its primary source of medicine. Physicians once got their clothes and hands covered with healthy dirt digging for roots. In Amchi-la's part of the world they walked through the dripping rhododendron forests of Annapurna, bags loaded with freshly harvested plants. Following the changing seasons, they wandered in the quiet valleys of Solokumbhu, searching for rare herbs with miraculous effects, and ordinary herbs with common and reliable results.

Through the ages, the vast woodlands of Tibet, the dense jungles of Burma and India, and the misty foothills of the Himalayas have been the outdoor classroom for groups of students who followed their teachers on gathering expeditions. Their sojourns in the wilderness were filled with meditation, prayer, and hard work. Back home in pharmacies and laboratories, they tended slow-cooking fires, watching the transformation of crude drugs into purified forms. Their wisdom came from centuries of intimate contact with the environment and from extensive written and oral lineages.

According to Amchi-la, every physician should be well acquainted with the wilderness his drugs come from. "The strength and power of a medicine depends on where the plant grows," he said. "A species growing in one valley may have very different qualities from the same species in another valley or on a mountainside. This is because of differences in soils, other plants in the environment, and influences of the sun and moon. Those that are exposed to more direct sun have a greater degree of fire element, while those in shady moist areas have more water element."

The doctor then described how these elemental influences change the medicinal properties of the herbs: "In Tibetan medicine, it is said that all tastes originate from the five elements, each element contributing its own properties to that taste. Because of the different elemental combinations, plants acquire different tastes, which determine their functions. If the earth and water elements predominate, the taste is sweet. If fire and earth dominate, the taste is sour. If water and fire predominate, the taste is salty. If space and air predominate, the taste is bitter. If fire and air predominate, the taste is spicy. If earth and air predominate, the taste is astringent. The properties and uses of medicines in curing disease are dependent on the ingredient's individual taste, strength, and nature."

Amchi-la's teachings were derived from the Sankhya system of India. Sankhya, meaning "enumeration," is one of the philosophical foundations of Ayurvedic and Tibetan medicines; it is the study of the universe's proto-elements, the archetypal forces that form our world and direct its movements. This ancient contemplative science holds many keys to understanding life, which have awakened insight into Creation's processes within the minds of physicians, philosophers, and mystics for millennia. It is an art that requires no technology other than awareness and sensitivity, for the macrocosmic patterns underlying nature's activities are woven into the microcosm of one's body and senses, waiting to be discovered.

For doctors, the mahabhutas, great universal elements, are the language of homeostasis and health, or disequilibrium and disease. For herbalists, they are the play of seasonal energies unfolding within the cycles of plants' lives, giving roots and leaves their unique flavors, smells, and biochemical actions. To alchemists, the unceasing transmutations of the elements reveal the secrets of spirit within matter. To astrologers, the mahabhutas are the dance of celestial influences streaming from the sky into our lives. To the mystic, contemplation of the elements can lead to realization of the Absolute, the interconnected unity that circulates throughout everything; knowing the true nature and origin of the mahabhutas can carry one into omniscience and eternity. This deep philosophy of fire and water, earth, space, and air can never be fully fathomed; it can only point the way to ever-widening realization.

"In the past, when a student went out with his teacher," Dr. Chopel told me, "he would learn many things that helped him to identify the best possible medicines. All the different parts of the plants were known, and what conditions they were good for. Different parts of plants should be harvested at different times of year: the flowers and leaves in spring and summer, the roots and seeds in fall. Students would spend a lot of time with the plants and would learn from direct experience of tasting and harvesting which were the best to use. The greatest doctors were those who understood the ways of the wilderness and knew about the individual plants in their environment."

The ways of the physician-naturalist are receding into the past. More and more, the gathering of plants is done by local villagers, who sell their harvest in the markets and through brokers to herb companies, while doctors increasingly rely on manufactured products for their patients. Clinics such as Amchi-la's, where all the medicines are handmade by the doctor and staff, are decreasing in number; those where the medicines are made from ingredients collected by the doctor in the traditional ways are even more rare. This trend is leading to the loss of both valuable botanical species and priceless medical knowledge.

And what had been Dr. Chopel's experiences gathering herbs? I wondered. "We used to take horses into the forest and stay for several days. Before gathering the plants we would have a fire puja, to make offerings and chant prayers. As we gathered the plants we would clean them and pack them, then take them back to the monastery for drying and preparation. Local farmers would bring herbs and different crops to the monastery for our use. We also got many important herbs from traders, who brought them from India and China."

Gathering herbs and preparing them by hand was once the foundation of medical practice. It was a livelihood that involved physical exercise, prayer, and solitude in the beauty and grandeur of the wilderness; these were as healthy for the doctor's body and soul as the herbs were for the patient's. Doctors learned the curative effects of the plants by smelling their aromas and tasting their flavors as they harvested and prepared the ingredients for their formulas, benefiting from their healing powers in the process. These activities shaped the physician's worldview and guided him in his relationship with nature and society. By getting on his knees and grasping the stem of the plant he seeks on behalf of others, a physician realizes that it is the earth itself, and the body of a living being, which are selflessly given for the benefit of the patient. Reflecting on his humble role, the wise physician understands that there is frequently little he can do to remove the deeper levels of sickness from another person, but that within the medicinal constituents of the marvelous being he holds lies the essence of nature's vitality, giving itself to those in need. Without a doubt, plants are the expression of Creation's highest love.

Amchi-la's living memories opened my eyes to traditional herbalism and the ways of the old physicians as a spiritual livelihood based on profound knowledge of the earth's resources. I saw that supreme medicines are the consummation of nature's generosity, hard work, intelligence, and compassion. Those who prepare their own medications know that this undertaking is a noble art and science.

The afternoon sun sent dusty beams through the rhododendrons as I left my contemplations and turned my attention to the activity of the monks on the mountain slope below. Their puja was finished and they were packing away their long trumpets, cymbals, drums, and texts of liturgy. We climbed down to the road and waited in the evening shadows for a bus to take us home. The young monks laughed and yelled as we raced through the countryside, hanging out the windows to see if those of us on the roof would get brushed off by low branches or left behind as we sped around the hairpin turns over the gorge. It was dark when we arrived in Boudhanath, and the sky was heavy with clouds. As I stood on my balcony looking across the village, moist winds began to blow. Soon a warm rain was falling.

My studies with Dr. Chopel continued into the monsoon season. The dramatic lightning of late afternoons changed into evening downpours, then daytime showers, until Boudhanath and its Stupa were continuously veiled in drifting curtains of rain. Families gathered to plant rice in the paddies below my windows. The men struggled with heavy wooden plows pulled by reluctant water buffalo as women stooped to plant the young sprouts in the prepared fields, singing as they worked knee-deep in mud. The crops grew brilliant green under the gray sky, an occasional bright umbrella passing on the slippery paths through the fields.

Every afternoon I would leave my apartment, descend three flights of stairs to the cobblestone courtyard where children played, push open the tall iron gate, and depart for another session of teachings. Sloshing through mud, I hiked past the madman living under piles of plastic and newspaper, busy talking to his invisible companions. Below Dhilgo Khentse Rinpoche's gilded monastery, water poured from flooded terraces across the trail. I would stop at Sonam's house to inquire of his whereabouts, then continue along a narrow street lined with greenery, trash, and brick walls. At Trangu Rinpoche's I entered a busy corridor leading to the Shelkar monks' concrete house, usually finding some of the younger ones hanging mischievously over the balcony railings.

"The *Tsa Gyu* is the *Root Tantra*," Dr. Chopel said, continuing his teachings on the *Gyu Shi*, the *Four Tantras*. "In the classical version it has six chapters. The *She Gyu* is the *Explanatory Tantra*, with thirty-one chapters. The *Men Ngag Gyu* is the *Teaching Tantra*, with ninety-two chapters. The *Chi Me Gyu* is the *Later Tantra*, with twenty-five chapters. In addition there is a summary chapter, followed by a final chapter advising future students to study the texts; this brings the total number of chapters in the *Gyu Shi* to one hundred fifty-six. These texts are the basis of Tibetan medicine; in order to become a doctor, one must understand them.

"When studying Tibetan medicine, the student first learns the *Tsa Gyu*. The *Root Tantra* is also known as the *Mind Tantra*. It is the 'seed,' without which nothing develops; without this Tantra there are no other medical teachings. It is explained very concisely, but it contains much knowledge."

Dr. Chopel paused and reached into his cabinet, bringing out a rolled-up cloth. He gently unrolled it to reveal an ornately painted diagram. "The Medicine Buddha is a supremely skillful teacher," he said. "To make his teachings easily understood he used the analogy of trees with roots, trunks, branches, and leaves. The *Tsa Gyu Dong Trem*, the *Tree Showing the Root Tantra*, is a diagram that is a summary of all the information in the *Root Tantra*. In order to teach Tibetan medicine, the iconography of this tree is used as a mnemonic device. This chart is like a field of land that becomes the source of all medical resources when cultivated. It is said that when one knows this chart well, he or she understands the basic principles of medicine."

The doctor laid the painting over his desk and pointed out the trees of knowledge, with their trunks, branches, and leaves. They were painted in a flowing antique style and labeled with a delicate script. "This is an old thangka brought out of Tibet," he said. "I also have another here, done more recently." The newer scroll looked like a simplistic diagram of harsh colors compared to the faded and intricate work of the original.

"The trees showing the *Root Tantra* grow in three different types of soils," Amchi-la went on. "From these soils grow nine different trunks from three main roots. Altogether there are three roots, nine trunks, forty-seven branches, two hundred twenty-four leaves, two flowers, and three fruits. These are all illustrated in the medical thangkas, scroll paintings showing the Tibetan system of healing."

What Dr. Chopel was describing was a series of extraordinary paintings commissioned by Sangye Gyamtso, the Regent of the Fifth Dalai Lama. These 79 scrolls were used to illustrate the *Blue Sapphire*, a commentary written by Sangye Gyamtso in 1688, which systematically explains the medical information presented in the *Gyu Shi*. For centuries, the *Gyu Shi* has been the Tibetan equivalent of other great encyclopedic works created by ancient Chinese, Greek, Persian, and Indian physicians, and the scrolls accompanying the *Blue Sapphire*, with their exquisite imagery, have been the basis of Tibetan medical philosophy and education. The painting in front of me was a condensed version illustrating all nine trunks together; in the original version the nine trunks are divided into a series of three separate paintings.

Dr. Chopel began describing the tree of knowledge and how its various trunks and branches relate to medical practice. "The first root is called the 'root of the body's natural condition and the basis of disease,'" he said. This referred to teachings on the physiology of the healthy body and the disturbances caused by imbalances in the biological humors.

"This root has two trunks, those of sickness and health. The left trunk is that of the healthy body, which has three branches. The first is the branch describing the activities of the three bodily humors. Its leaves are blue, representing the Air or Wind humor, yellow for Bile, and white for Phlegm. The formation of the body is dependent on these humors, as is the development of diseases. In the beginning these three elements are the cause of the body, in the middle they are the cause of sickness, and in the end they are the cause of the course of illnesses and of death."

I looked carefully at the tiny calligraphed inscriptions and iconographic imagery painted on each leaf as my teacher pointed to the graceful curve of the first trunk. The leaves showed figures standing or sitting, with diagrams traced on the bodies to explain how the three humors functioned. There were five leaves of each of the three colors, corresponding to the five different divisions of each humor's physiological action.

The next group of leaves showed a variety of body parts, including muscles and bones, and fluids such as blood and sperm. Above them was another branch, with figures urinating, defecating, and perspiring. "The second branch is the branch of constituents that form the body, such as blood, muscle, fat, bone, and marrow," Amchi-la explained. "The third is the branch of body wastes. The human body is constructed from these elements, and is dependent on them. Because the body is created and formed from these elements, it is impermanent. How the human body is born and dies depends on these elements. These three branches are also interdependent."

At the top of the tree, two brilliantly painted majestic flowers opened, with rainbow-colored fruits in the midst of their petals. "The two flowers represent long life and good health, with freedom from disease," Dr. Chopel said. "The fruits are the realization of Buddha's teachings that give us spiritual and material wellbeing and the unsurpassed enlightenment that liberates us into the blissful body of light. By being without disease, we can use our bodies and lives to enjoy the Dharma, wealth, and happiness, and to prepare to enjoy these things in future lives."

What a beautiful way to illustrate the highest goal of healing: spiritual liberation and the joyful path to union with the Ultimate. What does it feel like to be "liberated into the blissful body of light"? I wondered, looking at the flowers painted in bright mineral and vegetable hues. They spun open like swirling novas of illumination, emitting kaleidoscopic waves of grace. It is said to be like walking through a veil of indescribable jewel raindrops, and awakening from the world of the dead.

My teacher leaned forward to point to the next trunk as he continued his explanation. "The right trunk is the trunk of pathology, and its leaves show the various kinds of diseases." One group of leaves depicted the specific channels affected by the aggravated humors: a dancing skeleton showed that bones were affected by Wind; a woman squatting to defecate showed how Phlegm humor affects the feces. Another branch showed the various phases of life when the humors become predominant. One of its leaves showed an elderly man leaning on a stick, revealing that old age is the time when Wind is predominant in the body; another showed people harvesting grains, to illustrate how the Bile humor arises during the autumn months. On another branch, scenes of death by weapons, bodies consumed by fevers, and demonic possession were drawn on the leaves; this was the "branch of results that bring fatality." On the bottom branch of this trunk were two leaves, one showing a woman enveloped by swirling flames, and the other a man surrounded by icy blue water; these were the two ultimate states of all diseases, which are either hot or cold.

There were sixty-two leaves on this trunk, each one representing a complete topic of oral instruction and commentary. My mind drank in the symbols ornamenting this arboreal metaphor, wondering how long I would have to wait to know the meaning of the two men fighting with swords, the wild-haired demon dancing in front of the meditating yogi, the man and woman in a sexual embrace, the mountain peaks covered with snow clouds, and the other intriguing images hanging from this Tree of Knowledge.

The *Tsa Gyu* contains the core of Tibetan medical philosophy. From the *Root Tantra* come the branches of learning that include medicine and mysticism, meditation and psychology. It has been passed down since ancient times, studied, venerated, and commented on by generations of physicians. Amchi-la's teachings on this classical treatise, using the beautifully illustrated scroll he had brought from Tibet, brought together his clinical practice, scholarly training, meditative realizations, and life experience. Hour after hour, page after page, for many months

I would receive profound, insightful, and provocative commentaries dealing with the essence of life, death, suffering, healing, and spiritual liberation. More than any other traditional medical knowledge I had previously received, the instruction that flowed from my teacher during these afternoons would satisfy my mind, influence my medical work and worldview, and leave me intrigued by its possible applications and thirsty for more.

From Dr. Chopel's astute and pithy instructions on the "branch of root causes of disease," I would learn how all suffering and physiological disturbances are ultimately caused by ignorance and emotional confusion. Weeks would pass as my teacher informed me of how the secondary factors of climate, diet, conduct, and psychological factors influenced the state of health by causing the biological humors to increase or decrease. As the monsoon clouds drifted across the sky, Amchi-la patiently explained the "branch of doorways to disease," increasing my knowledge of how illness enters the body, followed by the "branch of residing places" of the three humors, and then the fifteen leaves of the "branch of channels through which disease travels." When we discussed the complex "branch of reversing of diseases," Dr. Chopel's knowledge provided fascinating and important insights into how mistreatment of illnesses causes diseases to mutate, and I recognized many common conditions that are the result of suppressing symptoms, such as fevers or pain, with synthetic drugs. All of these teachings, along with many others, were based on only one of the nine trunks.

The "root of identifying disease through examination and diagnosis" opened a new direction of study, and Dr. Chopel began instructing me in the methodology of Tibetan diagnosis. In his discussions of the "trunk of diagnosis by sight," my teacher provided detailed descriptions of how to examine the signs on the patient's tongue to determine the condition of the biological humors and internal organs. This skill is also an important part of traditional Chinese medicine and, until very recently, a standard diagnostic technique of Western doctors as well. Pulse diagnosis, done by palpating the radial artery at the wrist, is also universally used by doctors in all cultures; my instructions in the Tibetan version were based on the "trunk of diagnosis by touch." These teachings were accompanied by marvelous stories describing the skills of past Amchis, such as their ability to diagnose a patient's condition by reading the pulse of a relative, to prognosticate the exact time of death, or determine the sex of an unborn child. Listening to my teacher's accounts, I was both inspired and intimidated; how could I hope to learn such things if I could not even be sure that the pulse I was feeling was that of Wind, Bile, or Phlegm, the most basic diagnostic requirement?

After many lengthy discourses, we arrived at the third root, the "root of methods of curing." This root has four trunks, which describe the various methods used to cure diseases. They include the "trunk of diet," which prescribes specific types of foods to be used or avoided to regain health; the "trunk of activity," which explains the conduct and environment recommended for cure; the "trunk of medicines," which elaborates on the different kinds of herbal preparations; and the "trunk of auxiliary treatments," such as moxibustion, bloodletting, massage, and herbal baths.

Dr. Chopel's generous teachings skillfully introduced me not only to the fundamental concepts of Tibetan medicine contained in the *Tsa Gyu* and the Tree of Knowledge but to important principles of Ayurvedic medicine from India as well. Much of the information contained in the *Root Tantra* concerns the three biological humors, which are also the basis of Ayurvedic diagnosis and treatment.

The Tridosha theory of Ayurveda is one of the most important contributions traditional Asian medicine has made to the world. Originating from early Vedic philosophy, it is a method of viewing the body that is at once holistic, specific, practical, and based on a realistic understanding of anatomy. Poorly translated as "three humors," the doshas are biological entities that encompass interrelated yet diverse physiological functions, providing a system that unifies symptoms and signs into clear patterns for diagnosis and treatment. The language of the three humors helps classify the effects of herbs, foods, and treatments so they may be properly applied as the antidote to states of disequilibrium. One aspect of Tridosha theory that is becoming popular in the West is its application in categorizing individuals into physical and psychological constitutional types. This important aspect of Ayurveda recognizes the individuality of every patient and provides an essential understanding of how diagnosis, treatment, and prevention vary from person to person; this is a fundamental element of medical practice that is frequently neglected by modern doctors.

The concepts of humoral medicine, along with other aspects of Ayurveda, were transmitted into Tibet by scholars and physicians over a period of many centuries, starting around 700 C.E. These ideas, along with the Buddhist worldview that was being introduced by mystics from India and China, became integrated into the preexisting indigenous system of herbology and shamanic healing and have remained the basis of diagnosis and treatment within the Tibetan medical system. Tibetan doctors attribute the *Gyu Shi* directly to the Medicine Buddha; scholars postulate that it is probably the work of an ancient Tibetan physician who based its humoral philosophy on the Indian principles. The Tridosha theory and other doctrines from Ayurveda permeate all classical medicines of Asia and can be found in different forms in Greek, Persian, and Chinese medicine. Although widely dispersed and influenced by many cultural developments throughout the Old World, their origin was probably ancient India.

The Tridosha theory is both simple and extraordinarily complex and subtle. According to this medical model, bodily functions are said to be governed by three major processes. The first is the Air humor, which is composed of the gases of respiration and digestion; it also includes aspects of the nervous system that control movement, circulation, and pressure. The second is the Bile humor, the digestive juices centered in the liver and small intestine; this also includes aspects of thermogenic, enzymatic, and catabolic activities. The third is the Phlegm humor, the mucous secretions centered in the stomach and mucous membranes; this also includes structural, anabolic, and fluid-regulating functions. Each of these humors can become excessive, deficient, or corrupted, can travel through improper channels, or can become blocked and stagnant. The study of how to recognize the internal behavior of these bodily liquids, gases, and enzymatic transformations through observation of symptoms and external signs, and then successfully bring them back into a state of equilibrium, is the work of a lifetime and as sophisticated in its own way as any modern scientific method.

My studies of the biological humors started with vata, a term that has been translated as "Air," "Wind," and "Current." Its origin is in the early Vedic belief that all movement in the universe is the effect of the unseen power of wind. The patterns of its behavior, as Dr. Chopel explained them to me, corresponded in many ways with the Chinese medical teachings I had received concerning chi, life force. I began seeing and analyzing parallels, similarities, and differences among Ayurvedic, Chinese, and Western medicine.

"In order to understand diseases of Wind, we must examine their manifestations," Dr. Chopel explained. "The general symptoms of Wind affect both the mind and the body. Those that affect the mind and emotions include unhappiness without reason, especially after dark; unhappiness that causes insomnia, especially early in the morning; frequent sighing, depression, irritability, anger, and inability to concentrate.

"Wind causes various types of pain symptoms. These occur mostly in the chest and upper back, in the joints (especially of the knees and elbows), and pain that moves around the waist. It can also produce muscular stiffness or contraction of the extremities, pain around the liver, or pain in the bones. Pain that moves from place to place is characteristic of Wind. Other symptoms include yawning, stretching of the limbs, poor sleep, giddiness, sudden tinnitis, feeling chilled and shivering without having a fever, a shallow dry cough with bubbly mucus, dizziness, lethargy, dullness, and cloudy vision."

"'Blood Wind' is an accumulation of blood and Air in the upper back and shoulder region, which causes pain and high blood pressure," Amchi-la said one afternoon. He was giving teachings from a text of Tibetan diagnosis and herbal formulas, and we were discussing the relationship among respiration, circulation, and blood pressure. "It appears with general Wind symptoms as well as ache in the upper back and breathing problems. It is caused by any kind of work that disturbs the body and mind, or by being excessively hot from the sun and then drinking a lot of alcohol, or by doing excessive physical labor. All of these factors cause an increase of impure blood. The disease occurs when the impure blood becomes diffused and spread out into the upper part of the body by the 'All-Pervading Air' (circulatory pressure). The resulting conflict between impure blood and Air causes constriction of breathing and obstruction of the blood vessels of the back and chest." My teacher then described the preparations of herbal formulas that were used to reduce hypertension.

At times the symptoms Dr. Chopel described were unfamiliar and made me wonder if they were diseases known only in Tibet. As the weeks passed, however, I began realizing that many of these humoral syndromes offered a clear diagnosis and treatment approach for chronic degenerative and iatrogenic diseases I had seen in the West. As I saw the potential goodness and urgent relevance this ancient system of medicine held for modern people, I frequently thought of my patients back home and how Tibetan medicines could benefit them. With every new teaching came more insights and revelations into the medical understanding and accomplishments of the Tibetan healers, a deeper appreciation and increased respect for my old teacher's wisdom, and a great inspiration to share it with those seeking alternatives to unhealthy modern medications.

Dr. Chopel's lessons on the *Tsa Gyu* provided an extensive overview of the entire Tibetan medical system, as well as in-depth instructions in the details of clinical applications. The material was in many ways similar to the education I had received in my studies of Chinese medicine and would later encounter again in the philosophy of Ayurveda. Although it contained universal principles of healing, the teachings of the *Tsa Gyu* were also uniquely Tibetan: the diseases and their cures were described in the language, symbols, and metaphors found only in the extraordinary confluence of Indian Tantra and alchemy, Buddhist psychology, indigenous shamanic demonology, and Taoist physiology that developed in the "land of snows." The process of extracting the essential medical information in a way that was relevant to the concerns of my patients in the West would be an ongoing yet deeply fulfilling challenge for years to come.

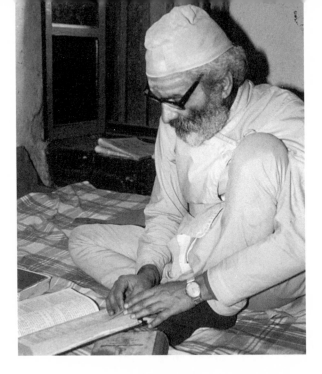

III.

THE BRAHMIN'S
INSTRUCTIONS

The Sages went to Dhanvantari, the physician of the gods and celestial beings in the

heavens, and prayed, "O Lord! Diverse sorts of pains arise from the body and mind.

We are very sorry to see humanity, though full of resources, act as if quite helpless

when afflicted with sickness and calamities. They remain apathetic, and shout words

of despair. We wish to learn Ayurveda from you, to cure the diseases of these pleasure-

seeking people, to protect our own bodies, and for the good of Creation."

Dhanvantari replied, "It is wonderful to meet you, dear students. You are well versed in many sciences, so you are excellent disciples for receiving this knowledge. Ayurveda is necessary to cure the diseased and protect the healthy."

DR. KAMADEV JHA

What is Ayurveda? The more one learns about this healing philosophy, the more unfathomable it becomes.

Derived from the root ayus, meaning "life," and veda, meaning "knowledge," Ayurveda is commonly translated as "the science of life." This ancient study, derived from the religious scriptures of the Brahmin caste of Aryan people who conquered India, can be simply defined as "the classical medicine of India" or "the traditional healing system of the Hindus."

Ayurveda is a comprehensive and highly effective approach to healing the physical body of illness. Yet the vision of its creators, the physicians and seers of old India, goes far beyond the treatment of diseases. It emphasizes prevention of sickness, which implies wholesome conduct, balanced society and family life, clean environment, and mental well-being. Ayurveda also recognizes that disease is sometimes an inescapable part of life, and provides spiritual guidance leading to inner freedom and transcendence of the discomfort inherent in the human body. The Science of Life is ultimately not only for the benefit of humans, because its knowledge extends to the care of plants, soils, and animals, and covers topics included in botany, agriculture, forestry, pest management, and livestock raising. "Ayurveda is for all of life," I would hear many times during my studies.

Even this description cannot convey the breadth and depth of what this Science of Life encompasses, nor can it reveal its long history through cycles of golden eras and subsequent degeneration. One may experience the wonderful effectiveness of Ayurveda's medicines and treatments, listen to the wisdom expounded by its practitioners, study its secrets in depth, and still not know exactly what Ayurveda is. While at first appearing simplistic, even naive, to a modern medical mind, it is actually highly sophisticated and profound.

Although Ayurveda contains an extensive corpus of writings that preserves its central concepts and methods, this life science takes as many forms as there are practitioners interpreting and applying its wisdom. These individuals comprise a wide spectrum of viewpoints about what Ayurveda means, from the conservative Brahmin elder who rejects all aspects of modernization and believes the alchemical transmutation of gold is a literal fact, to the recently graduated younger physician who rejects the mystical aspects of his tradition, and is more interested in using allopathic medicines and analyzing herbal formulas with modern laboratory equipment.

In recent times Ayurveda has been simultaneously suppressed in the land of its origin and exposed to the modern world. Both of these developments have brought about unprecedented mutations in the way its knowledge has been preserved, transmitted, and interpreted. The Western interest that is stimulating a resurgence of Ayurvedic medicine has its own scientific worldview and economic motives, which are also redefining what the Science of Life means. It is possible that orthodox Indian and Nepali physicians, who take pride in preserving its traditional methods, would find the Ayurveda of a few generations ago fundamentally different in many ways from what they now practice; they would certainly find their beloved medical system even further removed from what trend-conscious commercialism is promoting as Ayurveda in the West.

One of the difficulties in defining Ayurveda is that its boundaries merge into and incorporate many other related sciences. Yoga is one of Ayurveda's therapeutic modalities; yoga is also a complete and systematic science of its own, which in turn borrows from Ayurvedic principles. The Science of Life is inextricably entwined with the mythology, history, and worldview of the Indian subcontinent and Himalayan regions, so its branches intermingle with those of astrology, the ritual magic and deity worship of Tantra, and alchemy. As such, it is difficult to separate the different threads that weave together Ayurveda's vast tapestry, for each makes its unique contribution, yet is so closely bound together with the others as to sometimes be indistinguishable.

Yoga, the path of becoming united with God, is one of the great influences on Ayurvedic medicine. Both disciplines share the Sankhya system of enumeration as a common philosophical basis. This brilliant wisdom, which is the foundation of Ayurvedic physiology and diagnosis, describes how all phenomena unfold from the unmanifest Absolute down to the pancha mahabhutas, the five universal elements perceived by our gross outer senses. Yoga has also contributed important healing therapies to Ayurvedic medicine. Many of the purification practices utilized in Ayurvedic clinics were originally developed by yogis, who understood that removing toxins from the physical body not only cured and prevented diseases but also accelerated spiritual development.

Yogis perform exercises that are both simple and cost-effective, yet reach into the core of the organs to remove impurities and activate physiological functions. Using only dilute salt water and a series of abdominal stretches, the exercises wash out the convoluted "conch shell" of the gastrointestinal tract by sequentially opening the valves and flexures where disease-causing waste matter can become blocked. Yogis practice therapeutic vomiting or swallow rolls of cotton to pull out excess phlegm from the stomach, the root of many digestive and respiratory conditions. Using nasal insufflations to energize the brain and increase cerebral circulation, yogic healers can treat various ailments of the eyes, ears, nose, and throat, as well as increase mental capacity. They pour warm salt water into one nostril and out the other, activating the sinus cavities and their connections to the brain, desensitizing the body to external pathogens, and eliminating allergic reactions. The respiratory calisthenics that yogis practice to bring about physiological alterations to enhance meditation have been adopted by Ayurvedic doctors and modified for such purposes as controlling asthma attacks.

Many of these therapeutic regimens are routinely used in Ayurvedic clinics, and the postures of hatha yoga and their health benefits are now world-famous. Other disciplines remain obscure, mysterious, and legendary, such as kaya kalpa, body regeneration, which is reputed to allow one to live hundreds of years; this intensive and prolonged yogic undertaking is said to cause the old tissues, including hair, teeth, and skin, to be completely sloughed off and replaced with new growth, rendering the body youthful again.

Tantra is another of the great rivers that water the fertile soil of Ayurveda. In its more sophisticated forms, Tantra is a yogic path that can purify the obscurations within consciousness which breed ignorance and suffering, so that the intelligence of enlightened wisdom may manifest. To accomplish this noble aspiration, ordinary appearances are replaced with divine visualizations, ordinary sound is transformed into mantra, and ordinary mind is purified by identification with deity-consciousness.

These transmutational aspects of Tantra are highly alchemical in nature. Like the alchemist's alembic, the physical body is considered a vessel containing a microcosm of the universe, within which the currents of prana, life force, circulate according to ingrained ego habits. Many of the visualizations used to control these pranic flows and release their trapped potential are purely alchemical procedures, such as igniting mystic flames within the solar plexus to distill and melt drops of "bliss nectar" from the brain, thereby purifying the gross and subtle defilements of awareness. Alchemically prepared mercury is also a component of Tantra; it is consumed as a longevity drug and to enhance psychic concentration, and is used as a ritual sacrament. Conversely, Indian alchemy is strongly influenced by Hindu Tantra. The stages of mercurial preparations are preceded by invocations and prayers to Shiva, the King of the Yogis, accompanied with mantras of various deities, and guided by astrological calculations. Both paths are based on devotional relationships among God, guru, and disciple, and shrouded in secrecy. The goals of both are identical: good health, longevity, wisdom, power, spiritual and material wealth, and enlightenment.

Alchemy has nourished many fields of study. The labors and experiments of alchemists through the ages have contributed not only to the development of Ayurveda but to many areas of modern medicine, science, and industry. Essential oils, used for perfumes, preservatives, flavoring agents, and medicines, are a multimillion-dollar global business, which traces its roots back to the distillations of alchemists. The history of alcoholic beverages also begins with fermentations bubbling in alchemists' vats. Chemistry and metallurgy owe many of their advances to the research of alchemists, who produced acids, salts, metallic compounds, and other substances in their beakers and ovens. The modern era of synthetic pharmaceutical drugs began with the isolation of chemically active compounds from plants, an evolutionary step that rested upon the alchemical methods of herbal preparations. In their search for gold, alchemists through the centuries have bestowed upon humanity wealth in countless forms.

Alchemy has played a major role in the development of the Ayurvedic pharmacopoeia, and many of the formulas used in routine clinical practice are the result of alchemical experimentation. Ayurvedic medicines are divided into two major categories, herbal and mineral, both of which have been shaped by alchemical research. Poisonous plants are subjected to purification processes that began among tribal people and were then further developed in the alchemists' laboratories. The use of minerals, metals, gems, and crystals as medicines is a direct consequence of alchemical studies. Rasa Shastra, medicinal alchemy, was introduced to Ayurveda in the second century by Nagarjuna, who discovered ways of purifying mercury that render it a medicinal substance.

Ayurveda can be simplistically equated with herbal medicine, but again the boundary between what constitutes the Science of Life and other medical and spiritual disciplines is undefined. Ayurveda utilizes India's and Nepal's unique botanical resources according to its own philosophical system, but there is no clear delineation between the ethnobotanical knowledge of indigenous tribal people, the family recipes handed down through generations of village doctors, and the formulas used by academically trained physicians. The role of herbs extends beyond purely Ayurvedic use, since many plants are utilized in Tantric ceremonies, as part of yogic purification practices, and in different stages of alchemical work.

As complex and undefinable as it may be, Ayurveda is above all else the art of utilizing the blessings of nature and spirit to restore balance of body and mind. As such, it is filled with aesthetic beauty that is pleasing to the senses. It is the unctuous warmth of smooth oils, fragrant with jungle woods and tropical flowers, spread on dry skin and massaged into tired muscles; it is luxurious billowing steam drawing disease-causing toxins from the organs and tissues. Exotic smells of herbs harvested in rain-forest valleys permeate its clinics; its workshops are filled with the sounds of pestles pounding fresh roots in stone mortars and of physicians chanting prayers to protecting deities for guidance and inspiration. Ayurveda's knowledge is preserved in ancient manuscripts containing precious formulas, beautifully inscribed on palm leaves in languages disappearing into antiquity. Old physicians, educated during another era in different ways of perceiving life, listen quietly to the undulations of their patients' pulses, reading the secrets of the body in the currents of the blood. Alchemists watch fires burning in earthen hearths, metals and minerals in blackened pots slowly transforming into ashen oxides that subdue serious diseases, as the Himalayan stars turn overhead. For those who follow Ayurveda's long and well-traveled road, its sights, sounds, smells, and flavors gradually seep into the heart and soul to become a collage of sensual knowledge.

The Science of Life is a vast repository of medical experience, spiritual wisdom, and cultural history. It is a system of highly effective healing methods, profound physiological concepts, and humane clinical principles. Ultimately, Ayurveda is a source of wonder and inspiration about the miracle of life, a utopian vision of what natural medicine could mean to the world, and a path to understanding and resolving the difficult challenges confronting humanity.

Dr. Kamadev Jha is a well-known Ayurvedic physician of Kathmandu. He practices medicine in an office at the end of Asan Tol, across the street from the Old Palace. His name means "God of Love." To find him, one passes behind the displays of carved masks and scroll paintings sold by street vendors, through a courtyard and up stone steps, into a room with a ceiling so low that all but the shortest must stoop down. The doctor sits on cushions on the floor of his clinic, surrounded by patients as he practices his art.

If you are seeking diagnosis and treatment, Dr. Jha will read your pulses and examine your tongue, eyes, and hands. If you have spent time in Nepal, the doctor will probably say your liver is weak and you have parasites, and then instruct one of his sons to dispense medications wrapped in small pouches of paper. You may get bitter powdered herbs, pills of purified minerals, or a bottle of liquid, which will usually be beneficial. Those in need of Tantric magical healing will be escorted into his ashram, filled with religious icons, candles, and incense. Should you find yourself strolling down the shining cobblestones during an evening rain, check to see if the doctor's light is still on; he will be happy to read the fortune inscribed on the palm of your hand.

I found the doctor in his customary repose, discussing philosophy with a handful of visitors. He greeted me enthusiastically and inquired about my interests, stroking his full beard and smiling broadly.

"What would you like to know?" Dr. Jha asked. I told him I was seeking teachings about Ayurveda.

"I am an expert in all the branches of Ayurveda," he replied.

"I am very interested in pancha karma and the yogic purification techniques."

"Ah, good," the doctor said. "I am an expert in pancha karma. I know all the different stages of this kind of work."

"I am specifically interested in herbal recipes for these therapies."

The doctor smiled. "I have many recipes. We can examine the texts together."

"I would also like to know about vajikarana," I said.

Dr. Jha laughed and adjusted his blanket around his knees. "Ah, yes, vajikarana. This means 'to make like a horse.' It is the process of making healthy semen. I can also teach you this."

"I am curious about alchemy and the use of minerals," I went on. Dr. Jha jumped up and went into his little ashram, reemerging with a large bag, which he proceeded to unpack in front of his audience. All the major minerals and metals were there: beautiful specimens of bright yellow sulfur crystals, shining purple cinnabar, deep blue copper sulfate crystals, and others.

"I know everything about their preparation," the doctor exclaimed. "I will show you every step, and how to test for toxicity and quality when finished."

"Have you ever seen the alchemical transmutation of gold?" I asked.

"Yes, yes! That too! That is a very long and dangerous process, but I know how it is done, and have seen it myself. You come every day and I will teach you everything. You can even start right now if you like."

I was elated. "How shall we begin?" I asked.

"You can help my son clean up the pharmacy room," he replied.

"Ayurveda is a branch of the Atharva Veda," Dr. Jha said. "This Veda also includes the science of mantra and astrology." The guru was sitting on his cushion, preparing a wad of chewing tobacco during a rare break in the flow of patients. As a professor at the Ayurvedic university, he had no need to refer to the texts for this introductory material.

"There are three types of medical knowledge: knowledge of the causes of diseases; knowledge of symptoms and signs of diseases; and knowledge of medicines. Their source is the Self-Begotten Lord Brahma, who remembered these three sciences without study. In the Vedic texts, these are categorized into two groups: supporting the healthy, and curing sickness. Therefore, these three sciences are used not just for patients but also for those who are healthy."

The doctor packed the tobacco into his lower lip and continued his discourse.

"Ayurveda has eight branches: the study of the ear, nose, and throat; surgery; diseases that afflict the whole body; diseases caused by demons; toxicology; pediatrics and gynecology; rasayan [life promotion]; and vajikarana [aphrodisiac therapy]."

Outside, people wandered up and down the lanes of Asan Tol, the sound of their conversations punctuated by bicycle bells. The guru brushed tobacco crumbs from his palms and went on.

"Ayurveda categorizes diseases into two groups, mental and physical. Physical diseases are cured primarily through purification practices and sedative medicines. Mental diseases are cured with gyan, the knowing of God, and vigyan, research into God through concentration practices. Physicians who are not concentrating on God cannot cure diseases in general, especially mental diseases. Only those involved in religious practice can cure mental diseases."

I wrote down my teacher's words, looking up periodically to watch his lively expressions. Dr. Jha was wearing the style of cotton pants and shirt typical of Nepali babas, which give a man an appearance of part nobility and part boy in baggy pajamas. He sat cross-legged on the maroon mats, showing no signs of discomfort in the legs, knees, or back, even after a long day. Other than the common sallow-gray shading from Kathmandu's toxicity, the doctor's complexion was remarkably robust. It is curious, I mused, how a man in his sixties can live in this damp, tropical environment, among epidemics of parasitic and infectious diseases, chew tobacco despite having a gastric ulcer, and yet be able to tolerate this crowded and dirty place better than most foreign travelers.

The doctor considered his next topic, then resumed. "The definition of health, according to Ayurveda, is when the three biological humors of Air (vata), Bile (pitta), and Phlegm (kapha); digestive fire and enzymatic functions (agni); waste products (malas); tissues (dhatus); soul (atma); and mind (manas) are in balance."

The tobacco took effect and Dr. Jha began chanting in Sanskrit, lovely melodic verses containing pithy instructions. In response, a light breeze wafted through the room, carrying spicy-sweet odors of incense and candle smoke from the shrine room. Every few lines, the guru stopped and translated the words of Charaka, one of the greatest physicians and scholars of ancient India.

"The good physician has four qualities. There are also four qualities of the patient, four of the attendant, and four of medicines. There are thus sixteen qualities that affect the treatment.

"The physician should have a thorough understanding of medicine, practical experience, sound logic and justification of the diagnosis and treatment, and a good relationship with the patient that inspires faith.

"The patient should be mentally stable, have faith in the doctor, be willing to follow the doctor's advice, and have the willpower to be cured.

"The attendant should be soft in nature, punctual in times of administering medicines and treatments, have good behavior and conduct toward the patient, and know the proper method of medication.

"The medicine should be easily available, affordable, presentable in various forms, and have no side effects or toxicity."

How clear, simple, and wonderfully true are the words of the ancients, I reflected, as the guru's voice rose and fell in the sacred language of the old gods. How difficult it is for doctors and patients to encounter the conjunction of all these conditions conducive to recovery, and how fortunate when it occurs.

My Ayurvedic education with Dr. Jha had commenced after our first meeting. I came from Boudhanath several times a week, stayed until afternoon, then returned to the monastery for class with Dr. Chopel.

I quickly learned that Dr. Jha was an interesting character. Widely knowledgeable in the field of Ayurveda, scholarly and erudite in his expositions, he could lecture spontaneously for long periods, reciting quotes from the scriptures by heart. His confidence in his treatments was immense, and he claimed to have cured numerous cases of cancer and AIDS. He was steeped in Brahminic attitudes and charged with a strong aura of psychic energy, a result of devotion to the deities living in his ashram.

My first lesson at the doctor's office was reminiscent of my studies with Dr. Man Sang Yu at the Yang Sang company: how to properly fold the paper packages the herbs were dispensed in. It was a classical approach to education, a form of apprenticeship that serves both the student and teacher; the student receives valuable experiential knowledge, while the doctor benefits from the free labor. In traditional clinics where medicines are prepared by hand, there are many chores to be done. In Dr. Chopel's monastery it was the monks who performed this work, and in families of Brahmin doctors, the sons. As testament to the effectiveness of my new teacher's specialty, he had eight of them.

Punshavan karma is a specialized branch of Ayurvedic gynecology, which can be described as a Tantric-botanical prototype of genetic engineering. Using a combination of herbs and mantric prayers, the practitioner attempts to influence the sexual development of the embryo. The result is a child of the sex desired by the parents.

Dr. Jha is a famous purveyor of punshavan karma. A sign hangs outside his office declaring SEX CHANGE OPERATION in Nepali and English. Although somewhat misleading, what the doctor's shingle refers to is an herbal formula, kept a family secret, that many Nepali women want.

To prepare this medicine, Dr. Jha starts with cow's milk, adds freshly harvested secret herbs, and pulverizes them in a mortar until they attain a thick, creamy consistency. The mixture is then strained through cheesecloth, and only the liquid is used. To administer the medicine, the pregnant woman lies on her back, and the doctor injects thirty to forty drops into her right nostril. She is sent home with a more dilute form of the preparation to drink. Following this protocol during the early stages of pregnancy will allegedly influence the hormones in a way that will bring a baby boy.

"Why would women only want a baby boy?" I naively asked the doctor.

"Giving birth to a girl is considered inauspicious as well as expensive," he answered. "She will need to have a husband bought for her when she grows up, and there will be less help around the house when she goes to her future husband's home. Having a boy, however, brings not only the future bride's dowry but another set of helping hands into the family when he marries."

I saw Dr. Jha in many forms over the course of my studies, not unlike the multiple appearances of the deities he worshipped. Sometimes he had a full white and gray beard, sometimes he was clean shaven. Sometimes he looked robust and healthy, at other times emaciated and sickly. Sometimes his hair was long, and sometimes he had a shaved head. Two things never changed: he always wore sandalwood paste and tika markings across his forehead, and he always said he was happy.

Like his changing appearance, the doctor's moods toward me were also fickle. Sometimes he was a veritable fountain of teachings, at other times I would receive little attention. On the days when the guru was not inclined to teach, I spent my time with his eldest son, Muna, who worked as his father's pharmacist. While rain fell on the mossy roof of the Old Palace outside, we sat on cushions, filling prescriptions and discussing the functions of the formulas.

Ayurvedic physicians through the ages have developed a large number of medicinal preparations of all types, including pills, powders, syrups, confections, wines, salves, oils, and decoctions. The pharmacopoeia ranges from the simplest compound, consisting of only one or two ingredients, to medicines containing dozens. They may be easy to make, needing only some grinding of dry herbs, or exceedingly difficult, such as the complex procedures and months of labor required to purify minerals, metals, and gems. When used properly, these medicines both cure and prevent diseases.

One does not have to search far through Ayurveda's vast repertoire of medicinal preparations to find living remnants of ancient alchemical lore. Many of the procedures and tools used to make formulas have been virtually unchanged for centuries and are derived from a view of life that dates back to another era. The methods and techniques of Indian alchemists and physicians were similar to those of their counterparts in other countries of the Old World, from Europe to the Far East. Much of the philosophy that guides medicine-making in Ayurveda is universally found in other alchemical lineages as well.

For example, the influence of natural elements is a foremost consideration in the minds of those who alchemically prepare remedies. Some medicines are based entirely on gathering subtle vibrations from the earth's environment, like the dew—formed under auspicious celestial events—collected by the old European alchemists to be used in special ways. Ayurveda also utilizes the powers of the elements by exposing medicinal preparations to sunlight or moonlight, using special types of metal or earthen crucibles, and cooking with particular kinds of fuels.

One simple technique utilizes the healing power of water, sunlight, and colors. Glass jars of different colors—dark blue, sky blue, red, green, and yellow—are filled with pure water and placed on a wooden platform exposed to sunlight. At the end of the day, the jars are stored inside a cabinet, with each one in a separate compartment. This type of water is described as having subtle yet powerful effects, and can be used for a number of health problems. The yellow water is used for digestive problems; for diarrhea, a combination of three parts yellow water and one part red are used. For headaches the yellow water is mixed with the green. Blue water is used for treating fevers, and if the patient is strong, the dark blue can be used. If vata is deranged in the body, a combination of three parts yellow and one part red is prescribed, and if the vata is causing pain in the joints, the red water is used with massage.

Another alchemical medicine made with celestial influences is called pisti. Pistis are made from coral and pearls from the sea, gems such as ruby and emeralds, quartz crystals, and limestone. The ingredients are cleaned, pulverized, and triturated with herbs to remove their poisons. Once purified, they are again put in a mortar and triturated with rose water. After being completely reduced to a fine powder, the mixture is then exposed to the rays of the full moon. It is thought that the medicinal ingredients, in combination with rose essence and lunar energy, attain a particularly potent cooling power. Pistis are especially useful in treating various types of fevers, inflammatory conditions, and hemorrhagic diseases.

According to the European tradition, an alchemist who prepares extracts of herbs is practicing the "spagyric art," which is considered a lesser form of transmutation than the higher alchemy of working with metals, or the highest spiritual alchemies. These alchemists seek to remove from the body of plants, purify, and then recombine the three primordial elements, described metaphorically as mercury, sulfur, and salt. These are not literal metals and minerals, but rather represent the three phases of extraction of active ingredients within the herb. Mercury represents the volatile, vaporous, nebulous, insubstantial quality of a plant, which is found in the essential oils extracted by steam distillation. Sulfur represents the hot, fiery, active principle, which is the alcohol produced by fermentation of the plant following the distillation. Salt represents the earthy, solid substance in the herb, the mineral salts found after calcining the dregs that remain after the fermentation process has been completed. Medicines prepared in this way contain all the various active ingredients that can be extracted from a plant, as well as a subtle and profound synergy that has been added by the labor of the alchemist; by removing these three universal principles in their pure form and then recombining them, the alchemist is doing the "great work" of improving upon nature's perfection.

Ayurvedic herbal alchemy utilizes two of these spagyric procedures to prepare a form of medicine known as arka. Arkas are created by placing fresh herbs in water and allowing them to lightly ferment. This fermentation liberates the essential oils and other ingredients from the body of the plant. When the fermentation has reached a specific stage, the whole mixture is placed in a copper still and steam-distilled through a cooling tube into a collecting jar. The result is an aromatic water, which can be taken internally, composed of the purified fermentation products: the watery constituent known as a hydrosol, and essential oils.

Arkas have several advantages. They are long-lasting, easy to dispense, and can be mixed with other arkas to create specific formulas according to the needs of the patient. With only a small number of arkas, a physician can prescribe combinations that successfully treat a wide range of problems. They are easy to take, pleasant-tasting, and rapidly assimilated. Their primary mode of action makes them excellent medicines for digestive disturbances.

The composition and use of Ayurvedic preparations reveal the underlying medical philosophy and theoretical understanding that formed them. When the compounds are analyzed, it becomes apparent that their creators had a brilliant comprehension of how the body works and how it should be treated to restore equilibrium. A complete and systematic knowledge of physiology, pharmacology, and pharmacognosy is contained in the logic of these formulas. Their applications reflect a sophisticated methodology of diagnosis and prescription, principles that are common to Tibetan and Chinese medicine as well.

In general, Ayurvedic medicines, like most holistic therapies, are "soft" by nature. This means that the effect of a medication is gentle and well-balanced, so as to not disrupt any bodily system. This assures the physician and patient that a prescription will not cause harm. Being "soft," however, does not imply that a formula is slow, weak, or ineffective. Medicines used for symptomatic relief can work almost instantaneously, while those treating deeper levels of imbalance correct problems gradually and thoroughly. In the treatment of acute illness, Ayurveda does utilize many powerful drugs; to avoid potential side effects, these must be prescribed only by highly skilled physicians.

Many medicines are formulated to simultaneously treat both the symptoms—the stem of the illness—and the underlying causes—the root. For example, many formulas with laxative effects also strengthen bowel functions. Compounds that treat phlegmatic conditions work both on the lungs and on the cause of excess mucus, the digestive system. Those that increase vitality and virility regenerate the entire body, unlike stimulants that create artificial energy that can lead to depletion. Medicines that treat infections attack the microbial pathogens, cleanse their toxins, and boost the immune system. Strong antibiotic or antiseptic herbs are balanced with digestives to minimize stress to the intestinal tract.

There are many benefits in using the holistic medicines created by the ancient physicians. They treat the entire body and rarely produce serious side effects. Well-balanced medicines do not aggravate the root condition while temporarily treating the stem. Being mostly nontoxic or minimally toxic, well-made classical Ayurvedic medicines will not create chemical poisoning, allergic reactions, immune suppression, or chronic degenerative conditions. Unlike synthetic compounds, many botanical medicines have the power to cleanse the liver and tissues of toxic accumulations. Other preparations are nutritive, strengthening, and immunity-enhancing—crucial functions that allopathic drugs cannot perform.

Besides being valuable to patients, these medicines benefit the doctor as well. By using medicines that cause no harm, a physician will enjoy good therapeutic results, a clear conscience, and positive relations with patients. This is the highest fulfillment of the art and science of medicine.

Gopal Upreti was a dreamer. I knew this the moment he started talking, one wet, gray afternoon in downtown Kathmandu. He had taken me aside at Dr. Jha's, where we were both apprenticing, and asked me to accompany him somewhere for tea and conversation. We ended up at the Cafe Cabin at Asan Tol, an old hangout left over from the days when Western hippies mingled with Nepali saddhus, smoking hashish on street corners. Parting a beaded curtain in the doorway, we entered an upstairs room and sat beneath clouds of tobacco smoke and incense. Wrapped in the warmth of steaming chai and sitar music, I listened as Gopal told me of his unusual aspirations.

There was something intriguing about the bearded young man who sat across the table from me, smoking Kukuri cigarettes and talking with a thick accent. He had a quiet voice that sounded suspiciously conspiratorial, but spoke with conviction about matters that were of serious interest to me. He was a student of Ayurveda, he said, and had studied with many doctors and yogis.

It did not take long for Gopal to get to the reason he had brought me here. He leaned forward and spoke so softly I could barely hear him. "I want to do research in alchemy," he said. "There are formulas that destroy diseases quickly, and I know how to make many of these. But there is something more important than this. The powers of mercury and other metals can bring us much success in this life. I don't believe in technology. If we have the right powers, we can use telepathy instead of telephones and can travel from place to place quickly without planes or cars. I know saddhus with many powers, and we can study with them if you want." Gopal also wanted to establish some connections with a Westerner for future business. "We can export herbs to the U.S.," he said. "I have family members who work in the customs and airport, and we can set up a company for this kind of work."

Gopal needed financial help to manifest his dreams, which included building an alchemical laboratory for transmuting mercury into gold. I listened attentively but made no commitments as my new acquaintance outlined the various scenarios, some reasonable and some utterly fantastic, that he imagined we could embark upon as partners. This unusual character, who appeared to be both an eccentric mystic and a worldly businessman, seemed to have much to offer me in my quest for traditional medical knowledge. Having a Nepali partner as a guide and translator would open the doors to many Ayurvedic adventures, I thought, as Gopal described how he wandered from place to place, learning about medicine, mythology, and philosophy from the saddhus and doctors he encountered. Our meeting left me curious about the role this person would play in my future, as we went our own ways into the dampness of the evening.

I began spending time with Gopal. We traveled to the villages around the Kathmandu Valley, visiting temples, shrines, and places of natural beauty. There were old alchemists to meet and observe, holy men to pose questions to concerning the nature of life, ceremonies and festivals to see, and books to translate and ponder. Wherever we went, the people knew "Gopi" and made us welcome.

Climbing through moist forests, we harvested well-known medicines, coming back to town loaded with plants like the purple chirata (*Swertia chirata*), which destroyed fevers, or the thorny kanta kare (*Solanum xanthocarpum*) and bushy vasak (*Adhatodha vasaka*), which stopped cough and cured respiratory conditions. Long nights were spent chopping, cooking, grinding, and stirring herbal preparations, later dispensing them to anyone in need. During our travels I carried a bag of Dr. Jha's and Dr. Chopel's medicines and my acupuncture needles. These journeys were the fruition of my earliest medical aspirations, to follow the footsteps of the Chinese "barefoot doctors," dispensing low-cost, uncomplicated natural remedies, for the simple satisfaction of helping others. There was no shortage of opportunities to give our modest treatments, and even when our meager resources could do little for our patients, the response was pure gratitude.

When not exploring the distant horizons of Nepal, Gopal lived at home in Kathmandu with his parents and brother. They all wanted him to make something of himself, to be a responsible man following in the footsteps of his businessman father. But Gopal had little interest in such things. "I am a Dharma man," he would explain. "All I want in this life is to practice my disciplines so I can get out of samsara [the whirlpool of existence]." A devout Hindu, he would often disappear for days at a time, reappearing with a freshly shaved head or bright tika blessings painted on his third eye, indicating he had been to a religious festival or on retreat in some shrine. In response to my questions about his absence, he would say something like "Don't worry, Master. This prayer and concentration work is very important to our success as healers."

One day Gopal returned after a long absence. He informed me that his mother had decided it was time for him to marry, had found him a wife, and had put a sudden end to his life as a single man. He seemed embarrassed about the whole affair, explaining that it was an arrangement of convenience, since his mother needed help around the house. Neither marriage nor the subsequent arrival of his two children over the next three years changed Gopal's convictions. If anything, family life intensified his yearning to be free of samsara, which I interpreted to be the irritations of mundane domesticity. Gita, his lovely young wife, spent her days at home, raising their children while her husband was off in jungle caves with mystics.

As Gopal and I explored the local villages it became evident that my neighborhood in Boudhanath was one of the dirtiest places in the Kathmandu Valley. Every day my senses were assaulted by fetid smells of rotting garbage, open sewage, vile dust churned from unpaved streets, dead animals, and thick exhaust from cars and trucks. I needed a retreat in a quiet place with fresh air, where I could study, meditate in solitude, and recover from the chronic sore throat, repeated fevers, and irritability that came with living in Kathmandu. We began traveling to more remote areas, along muddy rutted roads filled with rocks, across ridges with Himalayan views, through forests perfumed with green fragrances, seeking a hideaway from the oppressive pollution of the city.

Gunje is a small village on a steep mountainside rising from the northern Kathmandu Valley. Smoke seeps through the thatched roofs of a handful of red earth houses, their rough wooden doors and windows open to an expansive sky. Across the valley, far away yet majestically clear and close, rise the snow peaks of Lang Tang. Footpaths wind along rock walls and edges of serpentine terraces, past ochre-colored cottages, and across ravines with streams falling into the depths below. In all directions there are panoramic views of tiny farms, dense forests, and Himalayan glaciers floating in the clouds. Ancient stone stupas stand in clearings, the inscriptions of their sacred mantras overgrown with moss. High in the cliffs overhead are caves where yogis live in retreat, and on a distant ridge stands a small monastery with prayer flags flying. In the afternoon, clouds drift down, enveloping the trees with dripping mist and making the walkways treacherously slippery.

We found our cabin on a distant ledge. It sat away from the other houses of the village, surrounded by tall corn, with a small spring bubbling from the ground nearby. It was a typical mud house with a thatched roof, wooden shuttered windows, and a narrow ladder climbing to the sleeping loft. We rented the cottage from Asabir Tamang, the headman of Gunje. He smiled as he pocketed a roll of rupees, then warned us not to go walking at night, because leopards and boars came out of the forest.

Yellow firelight illuminated the homes scattered across the hills, where the villagers were preparing meals of rice and dal. I reclined on the rough mats of my humble dwelling, breathing the aromas of the fresh straw roofing and hand-smoothed earth walls. Gopal sat listening to his thoughts, savoring the silence of the evening. Our first day on the mountainside had not been what I expected. Instead of solitude and time for quiet reflection, it had been the big social event of the village. But now it was over, everyone had left, and the terraces were empty and dark.

"And so, friend," I said eventually, "how is it that you came to be interested in Ayurveda, the Science of Life, and began to know the things that you do?" Gopal took out his tobacco pouch as he considered my question, thoughtfully rubbing the resinous herb in his palm before rolling it.

"When I was nineteen, I was in school," he said quietly, amused by his memories. "I was feeling very bored. I didn't know what to do, didn't have any ideas, and was failing my exams. My father told me, 'You cannot read, you are a foolish man, and you are ruining my prestige. You should leave and just go where you want.'"

Gopal brought a candle flame to his cigarette, momentarily framing his features with orange light and swirling smoke.

"One day I met a man named Kaji. He is a disciple of the guru Ajambar, and a very truthful and special man. I went to Pashupati, where he was living, and all day we would talk about religion. Kaji was the first part of my spiritual journey." I waited, watching as my curious friend exhaled another stream of thick blue-gray vapor.

"Kaji was the man who taught me about Tantric medicine. One of the treatments is called kajakut. We write different mantras and the patient's name, using sandalwood paste and a jasmine stick, on a special plate. The patient and Tantric practitioner must both purify themselves on certain astrological days. Then they meet, and the practitioner writes and chants the mantras and gives offerings to the fire. This kind of tantra works for spiritual injuries, difficult diseases, menstrual problems, and other things. I have tried this many times for different patients and get good results."

Gopal went on. "I spent seven years this way, going to different jungles, spending time with different monks, meeting different yogis and pandits who described religion and mythology. After seven years I had learned many things, and no longer felt bored with my life. I was growing up all the time. I was thinking: How can I improve my heart, my soul, take care of my spiritual injuries?

"Kaji told me a story about a famous disciple of Ajambar," Gopal said. Our shadows flickered on the mud walls behind us, listening. "One day this poor man came home and discovered that his wife had left him for another man. He was very embarrassed and disturbed, and thought, 'Now there is nothing left for me in this life.' He became very detached

---

from this world. He went to Ajambar and said, 'I want to be a monk. I have nothing to do and no materials to support myself.' The guru said, 'If you want to be a disciple, that's okay. If you want to be a monk, I can make you one.' He instructed the man to bring him three skulls. From these he made a bone mala. He gave the new disciple the prayer beads, a mantra, a begging bowl, and a trisuli [the trident of Shiva]. Then he blessed him.

"Ajambar said, 'From now on you are a monk. Now your guru is Fire, who will take care of you. This pot is for your food, which God will give you. Go stay in the jungle, away from this illusion. Always live like this.' So the man went to the jungle. It was a very big jungle, and there was no one living around for many miles in all directions. He made himself a small hut and lived there."

Gopal squatted on his heels, leaning into his cupped hands and rocking slowly.

"Continue your story," I urged my friend, even as sleep descended around us.

"One night while the yogi was meditating, a tiger came. It walked up to the man and grabbed the back of his neck in its jaws. The yogi wasn't afraid or nervous. He looked at the tiger and said, 'You want to eat me? Go ahead.' The tiger let go and sat watching as the yogi chanted his mantra. When dawn came, the tiger left.

"That night the tiger came again. It stayed all night, and in the morning went hunting for its food. This happened every night for months, and the yogi and tiger became friends.

"The yogi spent three years living in the jungle. He never slept lying down, only sitting in meditation. His lower body became paralyzed, but his upper body was very straight, and powerful. Some channel was open and he could see everything, everywhere. He had achieved siddhis [supernatural powers]. The yogi didn't care about that, and just continued his work.

"Finally, his guru brought him back to his ashram and they began traveling from place to place. Wherever they went, many people came, and there was suddenly much food and money. Nothing was difficult, because the siddhi was there. Whatever money they received, they gave to poor people and ashrams. This kind of yogi can know our thoughts. This comes from being very close to the heart and seeing perfectly."

The evening chill crept in through the cracks of our rustic hermitage. A moth spiraled around the candle. I lay on the hard bed of fresh earth floor, wondering what it would be like to have unimpeded awareness. The village below lay untouched by time, the Himalayan sky untainted by city lights. From the spring came soothing music, the Milky Way rippling in its pools.

We drifted into reveries, thinking of tigers tamed by the power of meditation and mystics attaining perceptions of higher consciousness. Outside, the windows of the surrounding houses were black, our neighbors asleep after another arduous day of toiling in the fields. The terraces fell away into invisible valleys below. Our little cottage clung to the contoured shoulder of the mountain, a tiny speck of haloed candle-light riding a shadowy dragon through oceans of space.

Gopal laid out his blanket. The candle burned down. Something rustled in the grass ceiling. Solitude arrived unseen, like a sensitive spirit waiting for the noise of our inner dialogue to subside. I lay, empty, the elixir of rest sweetening each breath. Images moved across the diamond surface of my mind, of doctors with forgotten powers, sacred names of God traced in sandalwood with holy instruments, fires of worship. The mountain whispered mysterious thoughts through the terraced gardens of my dreams.

Dawn greeted us with silver light on the peaks of Lang Tang. I had never seen the mountains so close, or so dramatic. They were just over the next valley, rising into the heights. Here was the home of Shiva, a great blessing to behold. I sat wrapped in my blanket, drinking in the clarity of the air, thinking how inspiring it would be to live with these snowfields for a front yard, forever changing colors and shapes as the seasons pass. Leaning comfortably against the shuttered windows of the loft, I dozed intermittently while the rays of the sun turned the sky pink and lavender, then gold, and finally the bright yellow of a full sunrise.

When I rose, Gopal was downstairs talking to our neighbors. I looked out the window and saw more people arriving. "What's going on?" I called to Gopi. "These people are asking for medicines, Guruji," he replied. "Some of them have walked a long way to see us this morning." I smiled as my dream of solitude evaporated like the mists above, realizing that our little mountain house had become the local clinic.

Life in the mountain villages is filled with hardships that ruin people's bodies at an early age. The climate is either bitter cold, blazing hot, or wet to the bones. Everything is vertical, up or down, on foot, with a full load on the back. Men, women, and children work at back-breaking chores every day. The poverty is deep, resources are scarce, and nutrition is poor. There is one doctor for every ten thousand people, and a long trek is usually required to visit a clinic. The country has a 40-percent infant mortality rate, and the average life expectancy for men and women is forty-two years. The people of the hills, like those who now waited patiently outside our door, endure a rugged life.

There were old men, stiff and arthritic from a lifetime of working the terraces. Their skin was frail as dry paper, their sleep disturbed by pain. Women brought their malnourished babies with bloated bellies. They had their own complaints, of continuous menstrual bleeding, anemia, fatigue, and tumors in their abdomens. There were children covered with scabious rashes, and others who had fallen on the steps, their faces bruised and bleeding. There were young women with severe scoliosis, and old women hacking chestfuls of phlegm. Everyone had digestive complaints and incredible stories to tell after taking anthelmintics (worm-killing medicines).

Gopal and I went to Gunje periodically until the late monsoon rains closed the mountain roads. In the mornings we would sit on the front step of our rustic abode, talking with the village people, listening to their pulses, and learning about their health. I bought medicines from Dr. Chopel and Dr. Jha, telling them about the cases we were seeing and asking for their advice. We carried some basic allopathic drugs, but our pharmacy consisted mostly of traditional Ayurvedic and Tibetan formulas. I also brought my acupuncture needles, which nobody had seen before. I would rummage through my bags of medicines and find something to send the patients home with, or take them upstairs and give them massage, acupuncture, or a treatment with liniments or medicated oils. When our medicine bag was empty we would walk back down the mountain into Kathmandu, tired but satisfied with our sojourn.

The people who visited our little clinic needed food, rest, warm clothing, and sanitation. Simple herbal preparations and acupuncture were not going to improve the overall quality of their lives much. Nonetheless, good things happened and people felt better. Maybe it was just the expression of caring, or maybe the treatments provided relief, but a number of families continued to come into Kathmandu even after Gopal and I stopped trekking to Gunje. After walking for hours in the rain, they would arrive at my door asking for medicines and treatments. Sometimes they brought me bundles of herbs to exchange, and once a gallon of mountain honey.

"Today I will teach you about makaradwaj," Dr. Jha said. He stood up and walked into his ashram, stroking his beard as he went. He emerged a moment later with a stack of books and informed me that these were the texts of Rasa Shastra, medicinal alchemy.

"What does makaradwaj mean?" I asked.

Dr. Jha laughed robustly and answered, "Crocodile sex!" I knew that the name referred to one of the ingredients listed in the classical aphrodisiac formulas of antiquity: crocodile testes. I laughed with his guests and asked if he took this famous preparation. The doctor smiled and said, "This is for men with no sexual energy. I don't have that kind of problem." He chuckled as he sat back down and pulled his blankets around him, then made some comments in Nepali to his guests that caused more laughter. "I give many men this medicine," he continued, "and I know it gives very good results." He opened one of the larger books that he had brought out and began teaching about makaradwaj.

"This medicine requires one month to prepare," he said. "Most of this time is taken up by doing the preliminary purifications of gold and mercury. The actual firing itself takes seventy-two hours. It requires a special kind of heat and cooking apparatus to make the evaporated mercury and gold blend with each other. This is done inside a bottle called a kajkupi.

"First, we take one tola [ten grams] of gold and beat it slowly into fine leaf. This is then cut with scissors into small pieces and purified. The way this is done is to take the pieces of gold and heat them in the fire until red hot, then submerge them in a series of different substances. There are different recipes for this, but they usually use sesame oil, cow urine, curd, vinegar, dal, and other things. Then we take eight tolas of totally purified mercury and rub it in the mortar with the purified gold. When these are completely blended, we cook the mercury and gold with 120 grams of purified sulfur. This is done in the usual way of making kajjali [black sulfide of mercury], by rubbing in a hot mortar with a hot pestle. In this recipe we rub this kajjali with the juice of the cotton flower, the root skin of ankot, and the juice of aloes for four hours. This is kept in the sun until dry and then put into the kajkupi."

Dr. Jha paused for a moment and referred to one of his other books.

"What is a kajkupi?" I asked.

"The kajkupi is a glass bottle that is wide at the bottom and has a narrow neck at the top. The minerals go inside the kajkupi, which goes into an earthen pot that is completely packed with sand. The pot is sealed with mud and cloth and then fired. Controlling the heat is very important for makaradwaj. This is why the kajkupi is buried in the sand: it heats up very slowly and evenly.

"We also have to use a special technique when firing. Cow dung is used, and for the first four hours the fire is mild. Then the fire is increased to medium heat for four more hours, and finally a hard fire is built. This burns for sixty-four hours. After this the fire is allowed to go out and the pot to cool completely. When we open it we find the makaradwaj crystallized around the inside of the neck of the kajkupi. To get it out, the neck is broken carefully."

Dr. Jha peered from behind his bifocals and paused. I stood up and walked to his medicine cabinet, returning with the doctor's jar of makaradwaj. It glistened inside the container, tiny crystals of effervescent ruby purple, shiny and metallic. It looked very similar to shards of cinnabar, but of the deepest hue.

"There are several varieties of this medicine, but they are all prepared in basically the same way," Dr. Jha continued. "If we use one quarter part of gold for every part of mercury this is called 'simple' makaradwaj. If we use equal amounts of gold and mercury it is called 'siddha makaradwaj,' and is more powerful."

Makaradwaj is a form of HgS, mercuric sulfide. It is chemically the same as cinnabar, but the two are claimed to have entirely different properties. The alchemical explanation for this phenomenon is that mercury has the property of absorbing the actions of other substances with which it is sublimed. During sublimation the mercury acquires a potent efficacy and is then regarded as a valuable tonic.

Makaradwaj is mixed with a number of different herbs and minerals to create various formulas. In one recipe makaradwaj is triturated in a mortar for three days. Powdered cloves, nutmeg, and saffron are then added, and the mixture stirred with the juice of betel leaves for another three days. Camphor and musk are added and the trituration repeated.

Pills are then made from the paste, dried in the shade, and stored in glass bottles. These pills are taken in the morning and afternoon, on an empty stomach, with boiled and cooled cow's milk and rock sugar. This particular preparation is considered excellent for promoting digestion, metabolism, positive health, and longevity. It creates a good complexion and is an effective sex tonic. Because of its aphrodisiac properties, one of the synonyms of makaradwaj is Kama Deva, the god of sex.

The guru continued his discourse, describing how makaradwaj is administered for several obstinate and otherwise incurable diseases. "In Ayurveda we say that life is the mixing together of the soul and the body. Makaradwaj is very good for supporting life. When people are dying, makaradwaj is given in one-grain doses to stimulate the heart. If the heart is failing, one rati is mixed with two ratis of purified coral and two ratis of purified pearl and given three to four times a day. It is also very good to mix this medicine with musk and take with honey, as a stimulant."

A young couple had wandered in during the doctor's teachings. He put down his book and took off his glasses, inviting the woman to come forward so that he could read her pulses. They spoke briefly, confirming that she was recovering from some unmentioned illness. Dr. Jha instructed his assistant to give her a refill of medicines and then returned to his lecture.

"Makaradwaj can be mixed with sitopaladi," the doctor went on. "In this form it will cure tuberculosis, acute bronchitis, diabetes, and impotence. It will increase virility and cure all kinds of diseases. It can be taken with green and brown cardamom and honey or cream two times a day for giddiness and loss of memory. For impotence and frigidity one rati is mixed with two ratis of musk or one rati of saffron and taken two times a day with honey or betel leaf.

"This medicine should be avoided in cases of hypertension and mental diseases, because it increases vata. It is used primarily for low ojas [nutritional essence] and prana. The 'life prana' resides in the heart and lungs; the 'activity prana' resides in the genitals. Therefore we use this medicine when the prana that supports life is collapsing or when weakness of the genital prana causes loss of activity."

Dr. Jha completed his comments on makaradwaj. "We must remember that the most important requirement of mineral and metallic medicine is that the practitioner follow instructions carefully. When mercury is impure, it causes toxicity in the organs and tissues. When prepared and used correctly, this type of preparation will cause no trouble."

We spent the rest of the evening discussing alchemy and the importance of purification procedures in the making of classical medicines. "The greatest mineral medicines are those that have been transformed into nectar by one thousand cookings in the fire," Dr. Jha said. "A physician who prepares his medicines in this way becomes a 'nectar-handed' physician. This kind of healer is one who has incorporated his philosophical understanding into his whole practice."

Dr. Jha smiled widely and held up his smooth brown palm. "When you become a 'nectar-handed' doctor, it makes no difference whether you give gold or ashes: your patient will feel that you have given them nectar." I smiled in response to his words, and Gopal thoughtfully agreed, "Yes, Guruji."

The guru continued. "Challenging cases always require philosophy in our medical practice. If we are greedy for knowledge, this is a good habit. Being greedy for money is a bad habit. Ayurveda says that we should have many types of knowledge, and then the mind will be matured. This means all the types of Ayurvedic knowledge, words, and sciences. Ayurveda teaches us that the veins, arteries, and vital organs are very complex, that the tastes, properties, and active principles of the herbs and minerals are so varied, and the final effects in the body are so refined, that the intelligence becomes puzzled. An Ayurvedic student should repeat every teaching one hundred times and then practice it one hundred times. Only then is it possible to master the different kinds of medical knowledge."

Dr. Jha stretched and smiled, concluding his evening discourse. "One day you will feel what I am feeling now, at sixty-eight years of age. More maturity, more pleasure in this philosophy of Ayurveda."

I thanked him sincerely, and departed with many smiles and Namastes.

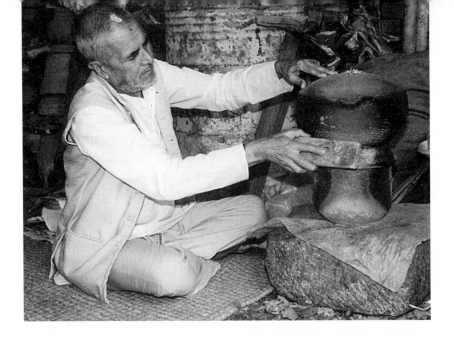

IV.

THE KING'S ALCHEMIST

I shall make the entire world free from poverty

by perfectly processing mercury.

NAGARJUNA

In the quest for health, healing, and happiness, the practice of medicine has always been inextricably entwined with magic and mysticism. Even modern allopathy seeks the elusive "magic bullet" and uses the mystique of science to evoke within the psyche an aura of medical power. Ayurvedic and Tibetan medicines, whose roots reach into the fertile soils of Tantra, alchemy, shamanism, and yoga, interweave science and the supernatural, showing us how to effectively activate the healing capacity of the mind and spirit. The diverse branches of these traditions utilize proven therapeutic techniques such as meditation, visualization, prayer, chanting of mantras, trance, and faith, all of which have been explained by modern science yet can produce effects beyond the confines of rationality.

Alchemy, known in Ayurveda as Rasa Shastra, the science of mercury, is a unique blend of medicine and mysticism. Medicinal alchemy is an academically recognized field of study that is taught in every Ayurvedic university in India. This well-known and publicly practiced branch of Rasa Shastra utilizes a variety of purified substances, including mercury, for preventing and curing diseases. The mystical branch of Rasa Shastra is based on this "iatro-chemistry" but uses primarily mercury; the goal of this tradition is complete rejuvenation of body and mind, leading to jiva mukti, spiritual liberation within this lifetime. It is within this lineage, shrouded in secrecy but filled with a history of miraculous events, that we find the ancient search for a means to transmute base metals into gold.

The two levels of Rasa Shastra, one commonly practiced and the other legendary, are closely related yet vastly different. The science of preparing mercury for medicinal use is derived from the experiments of mystical Tantric alchemy, and both involve purification of the mercury's toxicity. The two sciences can be described as inner and outer, higher and lower. Used together, the two disciplines can lead to complete fulfillment of life's purpose: the lower, outer practice of producing elixirs for good health and longevity gives one the necessary life span to complete the higher, inner alchemy of transmuting consciousness and achieving jiva mukti. What is commonly regarded as alchemy, the transmutation of base metals into gold, is only one of the extraordinary phenomena that can occur in the later stages of this art.

Rasa Shastra, with its blend of mystical and medical insights, is a source of valuable knowledge as well as the subject of skepticism and ridicule. Medical alchemy and mercurial medicines have been widely accepted and utilized for over a thousand years on the Indian subcontinent, but many modern Indians and Nepalis reject their own Ayurvedic tradition because of its magical aspects. For scientific-minded allopathic physicians of Kathmandu, who in many cases question even the medicinal value of herbs, discussion of paranormal exploits of Tantric alchemists is sufficient reason to view Ayurveda as a whole with scorn and contempt. For some Ayurvedic doctors, who have received instruction in Rasa Shastra as part of their medical training, subjects such as levitation and changing mercury into gold are explained as either a form of science we no longer understand, or a reality that transcends ordinary perceptions. For a classical alchemist—or for someone like Gopal, whose worldview seems to be left over from a seventh-century past life—assertions of alchemy's fantastic possibilities are taken not only as literally true, but as a higher form of truth.

Alchemical philosophy is far more widespread than Ayurveda, which was limited until recently to the Hindu culture; Rasa Shastra is only one of many tributaries feeding the great ocean of alchemical arts and sciences. Alchemy's ancient teachings have reached many lands, its cryptic language mutating under the influence of the religions it has encountered. For Europeans, alchemy was cloaked in the imagery of the Christian Church; for Persians, the geometries of Islamic cosmology; for Chinese, the poetry of the Tao; and for Hindus and Buddhists of the Indian subcontinent, the esoteric twilight language of Tantra. While simplistically regarded as the search for gold, alchemy soon reveals itself to be far more than the science of transmuting metals. The further one delves into alchemy's arcana, the more difficult it becomes to define. It is estimated that over 100,000 volumes have been written about this subject over the last 2,000 years, yet there is no agreement among scholars as to what these books are referring to.

Entering the labyrinths of alchemical knowledge, one finds oneself in the dreamlike archives of the subconscious, where mysterious living symbols dwell. It is a world where the phoenix rises from its own ashes, snakes endlessly consume their tails, and multicolored dragons hover in flames. Kabbalistic ladders climb through celestial spheres, culminating in the unutterable. Mandalas of the cosmos illustrate the divine geometry of the human form, and emerald tablets speak of the unity of higher and lower worlds.

A Tibetan yogi blows a thigh-bone trumpet, calling demons and hungry ghosts to feast on his own flesh and blood, which have been transformed by compassion into oceans of food and drink; this is alchemy. Medieval ceremonialists in secret circles of initiation rites consecrate talismans with planetary rays; this, too, is alchemy. A Christian priest consecrates bread and wine, changing them into the body and blood of Christ. An Indian yogini and her consort enjoy the bliss of sexual union, transmuting the currents of desire into flaming seeds of mind-energy that melt open the chakras of the etheric body. Rows of Buddhist monks sit for days reciting prayers, colored threads carrying the vibrations from their hearts to urns of medicines below huge altars. A Taoist hermit gently circulates his breath up and down the microcosmic orbits of the spine, nourishing the slowly blossoming golden flower of awareness. A Gnostic adept patiently tends the fire in his laboratory-shrine, seeking resurrection in the unfolding of colorful metallurgic transformations. The distiller watches drops of exquisite attar, gently coaxed from fresh rose petals, fall into the bottle. All of these are alchemy, the path of finding the light of spirit within the darkness of matter.

Although it is nearly impossible to define alchemy comprehensively, some things can be said with certainty about its history. There is no doubt that alchemical philosophy has attracted the attention of some of the most highly respected, creative, enlightened, and influential individuals throughout history, including saints and seers, scientists and physicians, artists, kings, emperors, and popes. It is also undeniable that centuries of laboratory research in the quest for gold have produced many valuable contributions to chemistry, metallurgy, medicine, the arts, and other fields. Alchemical history is also filled with intriguing accounts of great charitable works, such as construction of hospitals, support of religious communities, and promotion of political causes, financed with large fortunes of mysterious origin. One of the most famous examples from the Indian tradition is that of Nagarjuna, who allegedly supported a large Sangha of Buddhist practitioners with alchemically produced gold. Another curious aspect of alchemical history is the passage of laws banning the making of gold. An alchemist in ancient China could be publicly executed for manufacturing gold, and gold-making in sixteenth-century England was outlawed by Henry IV; similar laws exist in India even today. A cost-effective method of producing gold would lower the value of the metal; this in turn would render the riches of the wealthy worthless.

Countless individuals through the ages have sought alchemy's secrets for gold alone. But why would a shiny metal be the goal of the mystics who fill the history of this tradition? Such lofty spiritual minds undoubtedly understood the relative worthlessness of money. In the cultures where alchemy flourished, such as the Hindu Tantric setting that gave birth to Rasa Shastra, the pursuit of wealth was viewed by ascetic seekers as a form of bondage to this world and a cause of misery at every stage: in the beginning one suffered trying to acquire it, in the middle one suffered trying to maintain it, and in the end one suffered when it was inevitably lost. According to the sages of Rasa Shastra, the use of alchemically manufactured gold for personal profit was a great sin that brought heavy consequences. Stories are told around alchemists' cooking fires of the curses that God inflicts upon those who use gold for worldly gain.

One who is able to learn the ways of mercury, say the scriptures of Rasa Shastra, is patient, tolerant, and forbearing. His mind is stabilized, so nothing affects him. He prays continuously to God, has devotion and love for the goddesses, and uses mantra siddhis, invocation powers. He knows many different classical scriptures, is never lazy, and always follows the Dharma. This kind of man can be a responsible disciple of mercury, and the mercury can use him for Rasa Shastra's selfless, spiritual work. According to these standards, an alchemist who craves gold has failed even before beginning the work.

The highest purpose of Indian alchemy is not the transformation of base metals into gold but the achivement of jiva mukti, and emancipation from all suffering. Rasa Shastra philosophy believes that without a healthy and well-functioning body, one cannot perform the yogic practices that bring the mind under control, and without control of the mind, comprehension of ultimate reality is impossible. In order to achieve jiva mukti, it is necessary for the body to be free of diseases, to have a full lifespan, and not to be burdened with the hindrances of physical aging; these conditions provide the basis for stabilization of the mind. Even so, neither a healthy body nor a stable mind alone can bring about jiva mukti: only when sustained together and used for prolonged spiritual practice can they produce enlightenment.

In both Tantric alchemy and Ayurvedic medicine, highly purified mercury is used as a rasayana, a rejuvenation and longevity drug, to give strength and vitality to the body and the wisdom of detachment to the mind. Rasayan therapy using purified mercury is believed to nourish all the layers and sheaths of the body, including the sheaths of food nutrients, prana, psychic functions, intellect, and spirit. This deep rejuvenation and nourishment of the entire being leads to the achievement of health, according to Ayurvedic philosophy: equilibrium among the biological humors, digestive fires, waste products, and tissues, and happiness of spirit and mind. A person living in this state enjoys a full life span, without decay of the sensory or mental powers, and has a painless and joyful death.

Shodhana, the alchemical purification of mercury, accomplishes three primary purposes. The first is rendering the metal nontoxic to the body. This is achieved by removing the mercury's opportunistic impurities and toxic properties, then preparing it into a form that can be assimilated and metabolized by the cells. The second purpose is to increase the potency of the mahabhutas so the mercury becomes a vehicle of all the universal elements, not just the earth element that dominates metals. Finally, mercury's physical and chemical properties are modified so that its evaporation temperature is raised, making it capable of withstanding high heat, and its molecular structure altered so that it can digest and assimilate other metals.

When the stages of shodhana are complete, mercury possesses remarkable healing virtues. It is then further processed until it has become so energetically potent that it can be used as a seed of atomic transmutational force. This quintessence of mercury is the philosopher's stone, which, claim the alchemists, has the power to change base metals such as ordinary mercury into gold. If the atomic energy of the mercury has been prepared sufficiently to affect the molecular structure of other metals, it is deemed suitable for producing rejuvenation effects in the human body and mind that are profound enough to lead to jiva mukti.

Before the purified mercury can be used for purposes of rejuvenation, the channels of the body must be cleansed of their impurities. This is done using the methods of pancha karma, or the five purification processes, which include oil massage and herbal steam baths, therapeutic vomiting, laxatives, medicated enemas, and nasal insufflations. During these treatments the yogi is given a special diet, and herbs that stimulate digestion and metabolism. After the stages of pancha karma have been completed, more herbs are administered to sequentially remove excess salts, excess acids, excess alkalis, and parasites from the body.

Once the body has been properly prepared for rasayan therapy, the alchemically purified mercury is administered in increasing doses for periods of up to several months. During this time, and throughout the rest of one's life, strict dietary, social, and religious disciplines must be followed to ensure the success of the treatment, and to avoid the serious consequences of disturbing the new metabolic balance and enhanced awareness. Rasa Shastra claims that one who has performed this practice will live a full life span, without the usual signs of deterioration such as graying of hair and wrinkling of skin. If used in conjunction with other practices such as yoga and meditation, an individual who has been strengthened and rejuvenated with this rasayana therapy may then reach the ultimate goal of jiva mukti. It is for this reason that most of the Sanskrit names for mercury are synonyms of Lord Shiva, indicating that the liquid metal is regarded as God's essence. Mercury's most common name is parada, meaning "that which helps achieve salvation."

Dr. Bishnuprasad Aryal had been an alchemist in the court of King Mahendra. He had learned the arts of Rasa Shastra from his guru in Benares and knew how to prepare elixirs for longevity and sexual power. Judah Samser, the Prime Minister of Nepal, who had many wives and concubines, brought Dr. Aryal into the palace to provide him with aphrodisiacs for continuous erotic pleasure. For twenty years the alchemist compounded formulas from mercury, gold, gems, and herbs. When he left the service of the royal government he continued to practice medicine at his home in Sanepa, in a room filled with exotic substances and antique spagyric equipment. It was here that I met him, more than sixty years after he had begun his career.

Gopal had been studying with Dr. Aryal for a year and was eager to introduce me to his guru. "He is fully traditional, very conservative, and does things the same way his father did," Gopi said as we walked up to the doctor's gate one sunny morning. "He only eats fruits and drinks tea, and will not accept food from anyone. Before eating he changes his clothes and does puja. He doesn't trust anyone's medicines and never uses those from the market; he makes all his own in small quantities for his patients."

Dr. Aryal sat on the floor behind a low table, surrounded by alchemical treatises and bottles of medicines. He was thin and intense, with a serious manner that demanded respect. His high forehead was marked with a red tika, and beneath his short-cropped gray hair a streak of sandalwood paste was visible. We sat quietly while the old man read the pulse of a Nepali woman seated across the table. He listened attentively to the waves in the artery, his thoughtful, deliberate movements reminding me of the care required of those who prepare, from poisons, medicines for kings.

When finished, the doctor looked up and welcomed us, his concentration softening into a warm smile. "This is shring bhasma [calcined deer horn]," he explained as he began measuring out his patient's prescription. "It is for jaundice caused by parasites." He slowly laid out several neat rows of the pure white powder onto pieces of paper, meticulously folded each bundle, put them into a small bag, and handed them to his patient. They discussed the prescription and the woman's diet as she counted out a few rupees, then said farewell. Dr. Aryal cleaned off his table and sat quietly, giving his full attention to Gopal and me.

What unusual treasures fill this cavelike room, I marveled, looking around at the jumbled accumulation of jars and bottles. Bags of herbs and minerals hung from the low rafters of the ceiling; bookcases and cabinets held more secrets. Old laboratory equipment sat stacked in corners: measures and weights, crucibles and pots, mortars and pestles. Books were piled here and there, some obviously ancient; what wonders of medicine and alchemy lay between their ragged covers? Hindu deities looked down from the walls, dimly illuminated by thin rays of light from a small window. Tiny wisps of smoke escaped from a censer, traces of the fragrant offerings used during morning puja.

Gopal and I sat patiently, respectfully waiting for the teacher's words. The guru wore only a thin white cloth, open at the front, revealing the Brahmins' cord worn across the right shoulder and under the left arm. He showed no signs of being cold, even though a penetrating chill emanated from the concrete floor and surrounding shadows. There was a fireplace in the wall, but it was filled with more bottles of medicines.

Dr. Aryal decided to show us some of his treasures. He opened a drawer and brought out a small dry fruit.

"Lord Shiva was the first Ayurvedic physician," the alchemist said in an intriguingly melodic, desiccated voice. "In front of his garden is the original haritaki tree. You can't find this kind, because it is two joined together, and very rare. I have a sample."

The old man handed me the fruit from God's garden. It was about the size of a small plum, shaped like a cowry shell, with a dark green-brown skin, slightly grainy texture, and a groove where it had started to divide. I knew myrobalan (*Terminalia chebula*) from my studies of Chinese herbology, and something of its Ayurvedic use. It is rarely used in Chinese formulas, but widely consumed on the Indian subcontinent. It is so highly esteemed that it is said to come from heaven. There are seven types of haritaki, six of which grow on this earth. The seventh is the golden variety, which has the power to cure all diseases; this variety is available only to those who can travel to the devas' realms. Tibetan doctors consider myrobalan supreme among drugs, and call it Men Chog Gyal Po, the King of Medicines. It is the fruit of immortality that rests in the bowl of the Medicine Buddha.

Myrobalan is described as having all the tastes except salty, but when eaten it produces mostly a strong sour and astringent flavor that becomes a sweet aftertaste. The classical texts say this is one of the best herbs for producing an overall wholesome effect in the body, never causing any harm. The list of ailments haritaki treats is endless, because it can be used in all conditions. It is one of the most famous rasayan herbs, used to promote longevity and increase wisdom; it nourishes the brain and nerves, removes toxins, and regulates the digestive tract. I turned it slowly in my fingers, wondering where the alchemist had come across this specimen.

"This is silajit," Dr. Aryal said, producing a jar filled with a tarry black substance. "I purified this medicine fifty years ago, in the King's palace. If taken with milk, it benefits all diseases. Its main activity is to support the ojas."

I remembered the first time I had seen silajit, in Dr. Chopel's pharmacy. It was a piece of black material, resembling sticky asphalt, which I had found in the back of one of the cabinets. "It's mineral pitch," Amchi-la had explained. "It is the sweat of iron ore veins that come to the surface in rock mountains. When the sun heats the rock, it causes this tar to bubble out. It is a very good medicine."

Silajit is an extremely important medicine of Ayurveda. It is used for diabetes, hypertension, gastrointestinal disorders, stones in the gall-bladder and kidneys, hyperacidity, anemia, and liver disorders. It is a diuretic and a famous medicine for urinary tract infections. It is described as a superior tonic, a rejuvenator of vitality, a cleanser of the kidneys, and a regulator of blood sugar. If used regularly after middle age, silajit helps prevent diseases of the heart, liver, and kidneys, and can help shrink enlarged prostates. It is given in combination with guggul (*Commiphora mukul*) to patients recovering from heart attacks, to clear and strengthen the blood vessels. Silajit is a renowned panacea, one of the few drugs that simultaneously nourish and detoxify the liver. "There is no known curable disease that is not benefitted by the use of silajit," says the Ayurvedic materia medica. Besides being appreciated by countless doctors and patients, it is also favored as a snack by monkeys.

To prepare silajit, raw mineral pitch is mixed with water and kept in a clay pot in the sun. After three days the adulterants settle to the bottom, and the rich black cream on top is poured into another pot. The residue that has settled is again mixed with water, and the remaining silajit rises again. The liquid extract is dried in the heat of the sun, then mixed sequentially with decoction of triphala, decoction of bringraj (*Eclipta alba*), and cow's milk. It is again dried in the sun, which makes it ready for medicinal use.

It is difficult to find good silajit. I had seen various grades in other clinics, including Dr. Jha's, but nothing compared to this alchemical work of art that Dr. Aryal now presented. It was thick, smooth, and resinous, like molasses or barley malt, and had a flavor that was not only palatable but pleasing. Its bitter, acrid taste, reminiscent of cow urine, was present, but secondary to a sweetness and richness that made one desire more. This was true, high-quality medicinal silajit. Although he had a large jar of it, Dr. Aryal laughed when I asked to buy some; he would only part with about four ounces, and for a steep price. The doctor poured it slowly into an empty chewing tobacco tin, which I packed away in my bag, curious what the customs agent would say when I returned to the West. "This for your personal use?" she would ask incredulously, face contorted in repugnance as its fragrant bouquet met her nose.

"And what are these?" I asked, taking some small dry cakes out of a clay pot on the floor.

"That is black mica in the process of becoming pure," the doctor replied. Reaching into his cabinet, he brought out several pieces of the shiny smooth stone, showing us its original form. "When we purify mica, we first dissolve it into liquid. Then we remove its toxins with the help of herbal ingredients. After this the liquid is dried into cakes, which are then given multiple firings. Those have already been fired fifty times, and still require more." The alchemist took out a strong magnifying glass and peered intently at one of the cakes. Inviting us closer, he instructed us to look at its surface, where small grains of crystal could be seen. "These must be fired until all the crystalline material has disappeared," he said.

"How are the firings done?" I asked.

The guru rose from his seat and invited us to the outdoor laboratory. Several mud-lined holes of different depths and shapes had been dug into the ground. "There are many types of firings, which are given different names according to the size of the hole and the length of the fire." Dr. Aryal pointed to one of the larger underground ovens. "This is called goja poot, which means 'elephant-size firing.' We fill the hole with cow dung patties, put the mica inside sealed earth pots, put those inside the cow dung, and then cover everything with more patties and rice hulls. This fire burns for three days; this is one firing." Mica, he added, could require up to a thousand firings. When done, it would be a superb remedy for respiratory ailments and immunological deficiencies.

We returned to the clinic and continued our explorations. Dr. Aryal opened another drawer, removed an alien-looking object, and placed it on his desk for us to examine. I recognized its shape: it was the most famous of all Hindu symbols, a circular base holding a phallic column. Even though it represents the male and female organs in union, and all the procreative and regenerative powers of Creation this implies, it is referred to in the masculine as the Shiva lingam, God's penis.

What could it be made of? I wondered. It was solid but had a liquid appearance. The alchemist urged me to pick it up. It was smooth, cold, and heavy, with a peculiar slippery graininess in its texture, metallic and silvery yet soft.

"Guruji has made this from pure mercury," Gopal explained. "To solidify mercury is a very difficult job."

"What purpose does this have?" I asked.

"It is used in Dharma practice," our teacher replied. "It is the life force of Shiva. I do puja with it, and give it incense. Its major use is for praying. If you solidify mercury, you will become a successful man, and any siddhi you want will come quickly."

The object glistened in my palm, shimmering with metallic opalescence. What powers were locked inside this wish-fulfilling drop, this solidified liquid, this sacramental presence of the Creator, who opens the doors to every imaginable accomplishment?

"In order to properly study this alchemical art, you must work full-time for many years," the doctor explained, putting the mercury lingam back in the chest. I found the prospect of that type of research very appealing, and offered my services to the guru. He smiled his acknowledgment and invited us to help him prepare medicines in the future.

Rising from his seat, the old man escorted us into the warm sunlight of the courtyard. As we were leaving he handed me a gift, a packet of tiny seeds to grow back home in the West. "This is called tribij," he said.

"Three seeds a day will cure hypertension." Wishing us well, he lifted the latch on the high iron gate and sent us on our way.

The sunny warm days that follow the monsoon are a busy time for herbalists and alchemists of Kathmandu. The rains bring a profusion of greenery to the countryside, and the intense sunlight makes various preparations possible that could not be done in the stormy wet season. From September until the end of the year, optimum conditions exist for the harvesting and preparation of herbal formulas and for doing the labors of mercuric transformation. One radiant morning Gopal and I entered the courtyard laboratory of the royal alchemist, and were soon joined by Dr. Aryal and Raman Bandari, an Ayurvedic technician who would be helping us extract and distil mercury in the coming days.

The first step in every mercurial preparation, whether for ordinary medicines, high-level rasayanas, transmutation, or jiva mukti, is to produce chemically pure mercury. Because mercury easily forms amalgams with other metals and gathers opportunistic debris from the environment or marketplace, it must be thoroughly cleansed before being subjected to shodhana, alchemical refinement leading to nontoxicity. One of the preferred alchemical methods for accomplishing this is to extract the mercury from its ore, cinnabar. Dr. Aryal and Raman were ready to start this simple procedure.

We began by reducing hingula (cinnabar) to a fine powder. Raman sat on the brick floor of the laboratory, pulverizing the heavy vermilion-colored ore in a black stone mortar. I examined the shiny pieces that were waiting to be ground.

"Does hingula come out of the ground in this form?" I asked.

"It comes like this from the mine," Dr. Aryal replied. "Nowadays they make artificial hingula in the marketplace. They powder low-quality cinnabar, put it in a pot with water and sulfur, make it airtight, and it forms one piece. The cinnabar we are using is pure, so the quantity of mercury extracted is higher."

"Does this come from Nepal?"

"From the eastern mountains," the doctor said. "They only mine a small quantity, because there is not a large market here."

"Is it dangerous to handle hingula?"

"In the mineral form it is not poisonous externally," Dr. Aryal said. "Sulfur and other minerals are mixed in. Mercury has hundreds of different forms, ranging from nontoxic to toxic. It recombines and mixes in different ways, so it depends on what form it comes in."

When the cinnabar was powdered, we sliced fresh limes and squeezed their juice into the mortar. Raman skillfully pushed the pestle across the shiny mixture in the oval-shaped stone. His hands moved with a natural grace, born of decades of intimacy with the mineral kingdom.

"We rub the cinnabar with lime juice," Raman explained. "Then it has to dry in the sun. This is called bhavana, processing with sunlight. The juice evaporates, and we repeat the process three times. The hingula reacts with the citric acid, which causes the parad to leave quickly. It opens the hingula."

Raman was a tiny gnomelike man, wrinkled with age and alchemical experience. He had a dry, reedy voice, and rarely spoke. His eyes were lost in the deep grooves of his old Newari face, glassy black pupils that left one unsure if he could actually see. He was soft, gentle, and humble, almost childlike, and it was easy to be deceived into thinking he was just a simpleton laboring for a few rupees. But Raman had given decades of service to many Vaidyes, Ayurvedic physicians, both in private practice and government posts, and was exceptionally skilled. He was highly esteemed as an Ayurvedic technician and alchemical assistant, and known to have a refined intuitive sense of how to work with the plant and metal kingdoms.

We sat on the cobblestones under the awning of the laboratory, the day passing slowly as we took turns triturating the cinnabar. The bright sunlight dried the paste once by afternoon; by tomorrow this phase would be complete.

"How did you study Ayurveda?" I asked Raman.

"I have been involved more than forty years," the old technician replied. "In my childhood my father used to make Ayurvedic medicines. At that time some of the good Vaidyes here in Kathmandu taught me by having me help them do this and that. By laboring I got knowledge and experience. I still don't have much understanding, but I am doing my best."

The old man looked up from his work, squinting with a puckered smile.

"I will do my best for Ayurveda until my death," he said. "I want to produce good medicines for every home and village. If I had money, I would give them to all the people free, just to help. I'm helping by nature."

Raman continued rubbing the moist cinnabar, rhythmic strokes of the heavy pestle sliding across the vermilion paste. How many days has the old man spent doing this kind of simple, contemplative, tedious labor? I wondered.

"Did you ever do any other kind of work?" I asked sometime later.

"I am a musician for God," Raman answered. "I play flute and harmonium. I have knowledge about traditional music for religious ceremonies. I also sing classical songs."

Dr. Aryal spoke up. "Whenever I produce parad, Raman-ji is the helper. He knows about the heat, what the mercury needs, and there is no need to tell him anything. He has a kind of receptive power. Looking at him, nobody would know." Raman muttered some retort, and the old men chuckled to themselves.

The next day the preliminary work with citric acid was completed. The dried powder would now be put into clay cooking pots, called dhamaru yantras, for distillation. Raman meticulously scooped the cinnabar out of the mortar with a spoon and weighed out separate packages of two hundred grams each. When finished, we began mixing clay with well water in a bowl.

"Now we will put the hingula in the dhamaru yantras," Dr. Aryal explained. "Then we put the two halves together and wrap the lips with mud cloth. It must be sealed so no air can escape."

When the clay was mixed to the right consistency, Raman poured each of the packages of cinnabar into a separate pot, placed another pot upside down on top of the first, and held them together while we wrapped slimy mud-soaked cloth around the rims. When completed, we carefully lined up the yantras to dry in the sun before firing. The alchemist sent us away, telling us to return when the sun went down.

Gopal and I returned to Dr. Aryal's house around eight in the evening. The old man was resting in his quarters, so we waited in the courtyard. A waxing moon hung between ivory clouds, and crickets made music in the grass. A short time later our teacher joined us, and the next stage of the mercury preparation began.

We started a small fire in the hearth and carefully put the dhamaru yantra in place. It sat like a giant mushroom over the flames, an earthen urn containing the orange-red powder that would soon relinquish the silvery metal.

"We fire for eight hours," Dr. Aryal explained. "The heat has to be light, not too high, and we must keep wet cloths on top of the pot. Otherwise the yantra may burst."

Raman began soaking cloths in water, wringing them out, and putting them on top of the yantra.

"The parada turns to gas and accumulates in the top of the pot, in the form of a black powder that looks like sweat," Dr. Aryal continued. "Tomorrow we will take that powder out and put it into a bowl. When we rub it, the pure liquid mercury will come out."

We rolled straw mats over the brick floor and stoked the fire in the hearth. Gopal opened a vial of sacred ashes given to him by a yogi, and blessed us with an application to our foreheads. Dr. Aryal made himself comfortable on the rough mats. Our night passage had started.

The doctor spoke quietly in the hush of the evening. He talked about the fire and the need to keep its temperature even. He explained that the success of this work was dependent on the powers of concentration and sustained attention. Mercury's connection to the mind was also important to those who used mercurial drugs. "If patients do not practice meditation while using mercury medicines, they will not experience their full power," the alchemist explained.

The fire crackled softly as the neighborhood went to sleep.

"Mercury is connected to the Nagas, the serpent deities of the underworld," Dr. Aryal continued. "This is because mercury comes from the earth and is attracted to moist places. But mercury is all-pervasive. It is inherent in the five elements, our breath, the light and our eyes, the mind, and the prana, the origin of the mind. Everything in this world is a reflection of mercury, and connected through it."

The alchemist's words were profoundly accurate. This mobile, odorless, dense liquid-metal-gas is universally present. It is found in the oceans and seas, throughout the atmosphere, and spread through the galaxies. It evaporates into the sky from natural and man-made sources, returns to the ground in rainwater, and is revaporized again. It becomes concentrated in the flesh of creatures and plants, and chemically bonded to other substances throughout the mineral kingdom. The final resting place of mercury is believed to be the ocean floor, bound within sulfur's molecular embrace.

In my mind I could imagine the mercury's silvery face, its ripples making an endless journey through our world. Rising from the moist nether realms of miners' tunnels, it enters the light of this human domain. Evaporating like dew, the metal's gases rise on exhalations of the soil, drawn upward on spiraling currents of warmth that pull soaring birds toward the sun. Mercury falls from the clouds, tiny crystals cascading through curtains of raindrop beads hanging from the sky's airy palaces, seeking the hidden recesses where waters flow through genera- tions of darkness, bonding with other elements in its search for the sul- furic ovum of the earth. How remarkable that the alchemists describe mercury's source as the Naga world, the mythical subterranean realm at the bottom of the ocean, and see its subtle omnipresence connecting our consciousness to all life.

The silence of the evening deepened. Gopal rolled a smoke, shared it with Raman, then sat staring into the embers. Inside the blackened pots, the mercury was waking, coiling upward like a vaporous dragon.

"There are two kinds of work with parada," Gopal said. "Medicinal work is the ordinary level, making medicines like we are here, purifying mercury to make kajjali or makaradwaj. Mercury like this is very power- ful for curing disease, but it does not have any spiritual power. It is only background work. The real work of mercury is called dibir rasayan, which means 'cosmic alchemy.' This is a special kind of labor, and a very great way of giving devotion."

Dibir rasayan, as Gopal referred to it, was the path of the Tantric al- chemists, who approached mercury as the ultimate sacrament. Their laboratories were shrines and temples, and their work an immensely spiritual undertaking, for they saw in mercury's mysterious transmuta- tions nothing less than the keys to enlightenment. It was a dangerous path, which has led some to illumination and wisdom, and others to their death. The simple procedure that now unfolded in Dr. Aryal's rus- tic laboratory was merely a preliminary stage in the preparation of Ayurvedic drugs, a common process performed for centuries in every Ayurvedic family pharmacy and company in India and Nepal.

"To worship mercury and please the gods with dibir rasayan, we must have a pure sadhana," Gopal continued. "We do not behave like this, coming in here with shoes on, talking and telling stories. When cosmic alchemy is done it must be in a special place; many pujas are per- formed, many mantras are chanted, and special religious songs are sung. That is the highest level of medicine, and there is nothing beyond it. A man who does that work will quickly gain many siddhis and will be respected in all the worlds. He can do many things to the mercury."

That fantastic alchemy, so secret and legendary, was Gopal's passion in life. As much as he enjoyed the diverse subjects of classical medicine, they were only preliminaries. "All these studies of Ayurveda are very good," he said. "It is good to understand the three doshas and know many things about herbs. But we must remember that there is no end to this knowledge. Through the labor of Tantric alchemy we can come face to face with God; then we can simply touch a patient and cure them."

We sat in silence, absorbed in our own thoughts, as the contents of the yantra underwent their transformation. Dr. Aryal rose and bid good night, leaving us to tend the oven and contemplate our work. The hours passed slowly, carrying us toward dawn. Our work followed the rhythms of the hearth fire—mostly long stretches of meditation, punctuated with cups of hot chai. The evening smelled of damp earth and hearth smoke.

Gopal continued, quoting the words of God according to the scriptures of alchemy. "Shiva said to Parvati, 'O Devi, with this rasayana, the body will quickly develop internal strength. It will give self-control and wisdom. If you wish to leave the illusion of this world, then your mind should be connected to this science. It is a bridge. Whatever blessings of the Dharma that come from giving wealth freely and kindly to poor people, making pilgrimages, seeing statues of deities, and other such practices, we can also get from this art. If a man's heart meditates on parada, it will remove the negativity and accumulated bad karma that has affected him from lifetime to lifetime; he will be given life, money, health, good digestion, wisdom, strength, youth, and every kind of good luck. This Rasa Shastra is famous throughout every galaxy. It makes one holy, pure, and successful.'"

Raman moved softly through this timeless alchemical scene, gently replacing the cloth on top of the yantra. He stooped to feed the fire, the tiny flames revealing his elfin shadow. Soon we would let the embers die out, and the mercurial dew would form as Venus rose in the eastern sky.

"This rasayan theory of Rasa Shastra is brought from heaven," Gopal continued. "If you know how to use mercury properly with mantra and tantra, it can help us with everything; nothing is impossible with mercury. It is popular with the gods in heaven, the rishis, and divine beings. They always pray to parada to cross over this illusory world and ocean of disease."

Far away, some dogs were barking. Gopal fell asleep; Raman sat motionless, melting into the darkness as he listened to the mercury. I stretched out on the cool bricks and wondered what was happening inside the yantra. It began to rain gently, the drops making soft melodies on the tin roof of our simple laboratory. Deep in the womb of the night, the mercury was beginning its mysterious transformation inside the clay pot. I pulled my blanket around me, smelling its rough woolen fragrance. The earthen floor was luxurious against my weary flesh.

I rose at dawn after sleeping intermittently. The fire had died out and the parada had made its journey, leaving the cinnabar, vaporizing upward, and congealing into a sweaty powder in the top of the yantra. The sun warmed the courtyard as snowy Himalayan peaks rose from the morning clouds around us.

We began the final stages of the extraction by gently cutting away the layers of cloth and baked mud from the rims of the pots. When the pots were separated, Raman gently tipped the upper one over a bowl. A black-gray powder emerged. When all the material had been collected, the old technician changed it back into liquid. Simply by touching it with a spoon, he transformed the dry substance into mercury. Raman traced patterns in the mineral dust, leaving shiny trails. When it was all rubbed, the bowl contained flowing mercury. We washed the brilliant liquid metal with water, filtered it, and poured it into a jar, to await the next alchemical transformation.

The moon was stirring a cauldron of milky clouds. In the valley below, the alchemist talked with his apprentices as they prepared medicine.

"Once my guru and I were staying on a riverbank in the jungle," Dr. Aryal was saying. "One day a saddhu appeared, carrying only a small bag of possessions and a pot with a plant in it. He joined us in conversation, and there was much good feeling between us. After a while he said that he would like to make a feast for the poor people of the area. We thought this was a fine idea, but nobody had any money. The saddhu said, 'I trust you. I will show you something very secret.' I was sent to the village to procure a handful of copper.

"When I returned, the saddhu took out a small metal bowl and some natural sudhagi [borax] from his bag. He placed a thin layer of borax in the pot, then some copper, then some leaves from his plant. He repeated this layering several times, then placed the bowl in the fire. After some time a bright blue flame began to burn inside the crucible. After a few minutes the saddhu removed the bowl and let it cool. It was filled with pure gold. 'Take this to the village and sell it,' he instructed me. Not wishing to attract attention, I divided it into four smaller pieces and sold it. After this we offered a great feast to the poor people of the town.

"The three of us stayed together on the riverbank for several days. Finally, my guru decided to ask the saddhu about the plant that had changed the copper into gold. 'This plant is called jari,' the saddhu replied. He gave us directions to a particular valley where it grew, and how to find it. That night he disappeared.

"My guru and I decided to make our way to this valley. When we arrived we inquired about finding jari. The people laughed at us, telling us that jari simply meant 'plant' in their language. 'Jari is everywhere,' they replied."

Dr. Aryal paused, giving us time to consider the implications of his story. Could it be that the mythical philosopher's stone, which changes everything to gold, was found in the plant kingdom? Is the power to do such transformations available everywhere?

I continued my work, triturating purified coral powder with rose water under the moon's rays. Earlier in the day we had crushed the chunks of coral in the mortars, then washed it with warm water to remove the sand of the sea and dirt of the marketplace. After the powder had dried in the sun, we wrapped it in cloth and suspended it inside a clay pot filled with a decoction of herbs. This dola yantra was placed over one of the hearths, and the coral boiled for several hours. When completed, it was again washed and dried. The purified powder could now be further processed in two ways, either triturated with aloe vera and calcined to make bhasma, or rubbed with rose water to make pisti. Since it was a full moon, the alchemist chose the latter. When my work was completed, the mortar would sit under the open sky all night, absorbing the moon's cooling influences.

The coral pisti was sweet and alkaline in taste and cold in potency. Dr. Aryal would prescribe it to his patients, alone or mixed with other ingredients, in doses of up to five hundred milligrams twice a day, with honey, milk, or fresh butter. It would act as a digestive stimulant, carminative, and promoter of eyesight, useful for chronic fevers, bronchitis, hemorrhagic fevers, excess sweating, night sweats, and bone diseases. Now the fragrance of fine rose essence wafted from the mortar, enlivening my heart and enhancing the magic of the night.

The conversation paused, and I glanced up into the Kathmandu sky. Rows of shining clouds floated past, the last of the monsoon sailing off the Bengal plains, across the Terai, finally spilling over the western rim of the valley. They drifted through the moonlight, casting beams and shadows across the villages below. On Swayambhu Hill pearl rays illuminated the stupa's spires, and below the Kali ghats the river ran gray and black. In Buranilkanta at the shrine of Sleeping Vishnu, the Lord reclined on His floating bed of serpents, awash in opalescence as He dreamed the universe into existence. I smiled at the thought of His beatific face, and sipped my warm chai. The alchemist was beginning another story.

"Another time my guru and I were residing in a mountainous area," the doctor said. "A man approached us and asked for teachings on making gold. My guru instructed him in a method using one of the local herbs, called eclabir. Before the man left my guru told him that if he had success he must contact him.

"Setting out, the man went to his brothers and together they made preparations for this work. After some time they had success, and produced five tolas [fifty grams]. The brothers were overjoyed. They decided they would build a secret laboratory where they would use this method to produce large amounts of the precious metal. They invested all their wealth into this project and began their work.

"After months of work, however, they had failed to produce any gold, although their formula was the same. The man came back to my guru and told him what had happened. My guru sent him away, telling him that his failure was his own fault, because he had not followed his instructions and contacted him after his initial success. 'Your success was due to my blessings,' he said. 'You could not succeed because you proceeded without further guidance.' After this the man returned to his brothers and lived a life of poverty."

Many Ayurvedic doctors admit the possibility of changing mercury into gold, on scientific as well as historically documented grounds. Some of the elder doctors I studied with said they had seen it done by others, or participated in the process; others said they had heard of it being done in their family lineages within the last few generations, but had not personally witnessed it. All of them had recipes for accomplishing this work.

Dr. Uprenda Thakur is a conservative, highly trained intellectual, who served for years as the chief of Ayurvedic medicine in the Nepali government. When I asked for his perspective on gold transmutation, he replied that preparations for the process were being carried out at that moment at the institute he supervised.

"Doesn't this work require siddhis, some kind of special powers?" I asked Dr. Ram Brikhya Sahu, another physician of the Ayurvedic college at Tribuvan University in Kathmandu.

"No," he replied. "It can be done purely by following electrochemical laws."

The opinions of these doctors were similar to those of other Ayurvedic physicians, who were certain that the alchemical approach to releasing mercury's extra electron was a reality. Dr. Narendra Tiwari, Nepal's foremost expert in Ayurvedic pharmacology and botany, concurred. "There is only one electron difference between the mercury atom and the gold atom," he said. "Mercury has one more electron than gold, and if that is released, mercury may be converted to gold. This can be done using modern technology, and there are many labs that can do this, but the cost is higher than the value of the gold itself."

Dr. Tiwari then described a recent recorded transmutation. "If you visit the Vishunath Temple at Benares Hindu University, there is a monument commemorating a historical event of making gold with mercury. In the Indian Congress movement, when the party was suffering from a lack of money, a yogi from Hardwar prepared some kilos of gold with the help of mercury and donated it to the Congress. The Indian Congress is not more than one hundred years old, so this is a very recent example of making gold from mercury."

There are other inscriptions in different temples attesting to alchemical events that have transpired before an audience of respectable persons. Behind the Lakshmi Narayana Temple in Delhi are two marble plaques on the walls of the fire altar. One of these testifies that on May 27, 1941, a practitioner of Rasa Shastra demonstrated a technique he had learned from a saint by the name of Narayan Swami. The details of this procedure included placing the mercury inside a type of fruit, mixing it with herb powders, covering the fruit with mud, and incinerating it. This process produced twelve grams of pure gold, which was only slightly less than the amount of mercury used, and was witnessed by several high-ranking government and business people. The other plaque describes how in March 1942 an alchemist from Rishikesh demonstrated to a group of people, including the secretary of Mahatma Gandhi and other notables, the preparation of over a kilo and a half of gold from mercury.

According to the atomic theory of the Indian alchemists, every atom is composed of the pancha mahabhutas, the five universal elements, in various admixtures. Metals are predominantly the earth element, ruled by the property of cohesion, while the elements of space, air, fire, and water are present as secondary components. Mercury and gold, however, share the unique characteristic of being dominated by the radiance of the fire element, with the earth element being one of the secondary properties. Without the technology of modern physics, the ancient alchemists understood the close atomic similarity between mercury and gold. This affinity, in conjunction with the use of fire in alchemical processes, makes it possible for the two metals to interact in unusual ways.

Rasa Shastra describes every atom and infra-atomic particle as being in a state of rotational, whirling vibration. This motion is particularly evident in mercury, as seen in its unstable, liquid properties. Mercury is used for medicine and alchemy because it is less cohesive than other metals, and its elemental properties are easily changed. For alchemical purposes, mercury's mutable nature is believed to make it amenable to changes at the atomic and subatomic levels; this allows it to penetrate into the elemental composition of other metals, transforming them into new compounds. Mercury is unable to perform either rasayanic rejuvenation or alchemical transmutation in its metallic state, but through advanced processing, the quantum energies of its atomic particles are released, effecting changes in other metals.

In order to accomplish this liberation of energy, Rasa Shastra uses rudimentary yet powerful methods and ingredients. Mercury is triturated with numerous kinds of herbal juices and fermented liquids, which put its molecules in contact with fats, oils, and acids. Fire is used to bring about changes within mercury's atomic structure. The metal is rubbed in a mortar with a pestle for prolonged periods of time, subjecting it to mechanical pressure and repeated impact. Mercury is put through countless other procedures during the stages of purification. It is made into pastes with herbs and salts, boiled in vinegars, cooked repeatedly in sealed crucibles, evaporated and recrystallized in distilling pots, aged with salts in clay pots buried in the earth, and smelted with other metals and minerals. One process alone may be repeated a hundred times, each time requiring several days of labor.

According to Rasa Shastra, eighteen levels of purification are necessary to produce superior-grade mercury, which is capable of causing true rejuvenation of the body and transmutation of other metals into gold. These stages are described metaphorically, such as making the metal "sweat" (cleansing it of its impurities); making it "faint" (altering its natural chemical properties); "reviving" (restoring its lost potency); "feeding," "chewing," "digesting," and "assimilating" (adding other metals to the mercury); and "penetrating" (bringing the metal to a state where it can enter the atomic structure of other metals). Indian alchemy is unique in that it provides detailed instructions and actual recipes for accomplishing these stages, unlike the purely symbolic allegories or cryptic codes contemplated by alchemists of old Europe.

One of the final stages of alchemical work comes when the mercury has been induced to "open its mouth," making it capable of absorbing other metals. The evidence that the metal can successfully chew, digest, and assimilate other elements is that it does not gain weight. Dr. Aryal claimed to have witnessed this remarkable event, unexplainable by ordinary laws of physics, along with an audience of others. Basuki Brahmachari was an alchemist-yogi living in Pashupati, who had success in causing mercury to open its mouth. He placed the "hungry" mercury in a pot and poured a large amount of milk onto it, which the mercury consumed. I asked Dr. Aryal how this was possible. He replied that he had some degree of understanding but didn't really know.

Gopal's understanding of mercury "opening its mouth" was that it brought one "face to face with God." "If a man can 'open the mouth' of parada, he can give devotion directly to Shiva, because this is Shiva Himself. When mercury opens its mouth, we can give it gifts of gold, sandalwood, eaglewood, camphor, and saffron, and it will never change size or weight. This is a very true puja, which gives direct communication with God; you can pray to any god or goddess and they will appear in front of you. With this devotion many great powers will come."

In the minds of the old alchemists, the transformations of mercury represent the Creator's ultimate miraculous secrets, events that unlock all possible accomplishments in this life and the next. If one can solidify mercury, open its mouth, kill it, then bring it back to life, he can release its atomic energies, use it to create gold out of base metals, and do anything he wishes in this world. The texts of Rasa Shastra and the firelit evenings of the Himalayan alchemists are filled with such wonders. Using rasayanic mercury, alchemists can destroy diseases and stabilize life to prevent aging. By perfecting these practices, the rishis of the past could perform miracles. A successful alchemist can experience internal freedom from all attachments and suffering.

Midnight was approaching. I put the mortar on a high shelf to bathe in the full moon's rays, the white pisti inside fragrant with roses from Indian gardens.

"The Nepali name for mercury is paro," Gopal said after some time. "Par means 'outside,' and paro means 'that which takes one outside of this realm.' Paro has great powers when it is successfully treated. It gives the yogi supernatural abilities and siddhis. One may see long distances, fly in the sky, and walk on water when the power of paro is activated. Is this not true, Guruji?" Gopal asked.

"These are minor powers for paro," Dr. Aryal replied. "It has the ability to completely protect one from all harm and lead one to unimaginable success, even beyond this lifetime."

"These powers do not come from the work of our own hand," Gopal continued. "Our hands do the work, but it is God who gives us the gifts. All we have to do is remain pure, and everything will be done for us. Even death will have to ask if we want to go. If we want, we can do this work for hundreds of years.

"These ways are very ancient, and very secret," Gopal concluded. "I have not seen them, but I am very interested and always talk about them. My vision and intention in this life is to worship Shiva in the mercury. All the faces of God are there."

Overhead, alabaster clouds drifted like mercurial thoughts through the indigo sky.

"If you dedicate your whole life, you can see God in everything, not just paro," Dr. Aryal said.

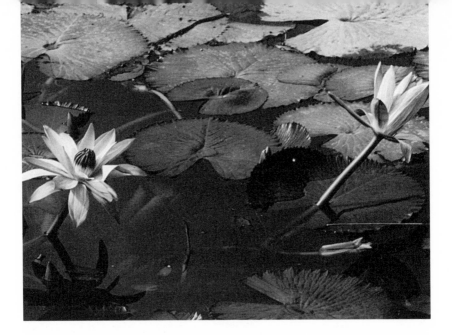

V.

SOMA

Flow, Soma, in a most sweet and exhilarating stream. Give us brightness, give us heaven, give us all good things. Shower upon us wealth abundant for both worlds, and make us happy.

NINTH MANDALA,
RIG VEDA

For those in search of medicines, gold, and jiva mukti, Rasa Shastra and its mercuric sciences offer remedies that heal sickness like soothing balms, and rasayanic elixirs that bestow extraordinarily long life. Adepts who reach the culmination of the alchemical journey by completely purifying and perfecting mercury are rewarded with the philosopher's stone, the seed of atomic energy capable of igniting the golden spiritual light of base metals and releasing the soul from the illusions of existence.

The subterranean labyrinth of the Nagas is not the only realm that has provided this Stone of the Wise. Just as the sperm of Shiva was the object of veneration for those seeking jiva mukti in the transmutational effects of precious metals, minerals, and gems, supremely powerful po-tions from the plant kingdom have also captured the imagination of people since the beginning of time. For alchemists, yogis, physicians, and seekers of health, wisdom, and transcendence, the greenery of the world's vegetation has yielded wondrous mysteries, tantalizing myths, and gyan, profound knowledge and science.

In the primeval jungles and uncharted forests of the past grew dibir bhuti, divine herbs with magical characteristics. Dibir herbs can change their shape and disappear, an ability they use to hide from ordinary people. Only the good-hearted can find dibir bhuti; after purification and respectful prayer, the plants will appear, indicating their pleasure by bending toward you.

The most famous of the dibir plants was Soma, the mythical inebriant of the Brahmin priests. This mysterious being, visible to only the pure, was the source of a golden elixir of immortality, so legendary that it was spoken of throughout the alchemical world.

Soma ranks third in order of importance among the Vedic gods. One hundred twenty of the Rig Veda's 1,028 hymns are devoted to Soma, who is adored as a divinity along with Agni (solar fire) and Indra (king of the gods). After reading the description of Soma's effects in the ancient texts of medicine and religion, who would not want to imbibe this nectar of deathlessness? Its action was calming, strengthening, and rejuvenating; it was said to reverse the aging process and to transport one to visionary states of consciousness. "This Soma is a god," proclaims one of the hymns to the deity. "He cures the sharpest ills that man endures. He heals the sick, the sad he cheers; he nerves the weak, dispels their fears. The soul from earth to heaven he lifts, so great and wondrous are his gifts. We've drunk the Soma bright and are immortal grown; we've entered into light, that all the gods have known."

The search for Soma has preoccupied mystics, herbalists, priests, and scholars for millennia; many theories have been proposed, yet to this day Soma remains an ancient mystery. Was it a god in the form of a plant who bestowed life and inspiration; the juice squeezed from a divine herb that cured all evils by linking humanity with heaven; an ambrosia that gave victory over death; a psychedelic mushroom; an alchemical process; or a moon deity whose essence could be extracted from dibir bhuti?

Some scholars believe that the Aryan priests prepared the *Amanita muscaria* mushroom into a hallucinogenic liquor. Several other botanical possibilities have been suggested, including *Psilocybe*, *Ephedra*, and ginseng; some herbalists believe that Soma may be an unidentified type of fern, fungus, or orchid. Other researchers postulate that Soma was not a plant at all, and that the hymns in the Rig Veda are codified allegorical information describing procedures to purify gold ores. Whether any of these ideas are true or not, one thing is certain: an abundance of alchemical symbology surrounds Soma and its rituals.

The ninth book of the Rig Veda consists mainly of incantations sung over Soma as it is being prepared for ceremonial use. From these verses we learn that Soma dwells in the mountains, flourishes during the rainy season, and is strengthened by rain clouds. The part used is a stalk or shoot, which is pressed, filtered, and offered to the gods. The invocations allegorically describe the stages of extraction and purification. As Soma is "milked" from the shoots, it becomes a "wave" or a "stream," which accumulates in the pot as an "ocean of nectar" and bindu, "bright drops." Different scholars have suggested that the iconography of Hindu and Buddhist mythology derives from the legacy of alchemical work involving Soma. The origin of the vajra, the thunderbolt of Indra, has been traced to implements used to crush Soma stalks.

The cult of Soma is thought to have played a major role in stimulating experimentation with botanical species across Asia as people sought the plant that bestowed freedom from death. Some writers have postulated that the Soma cult was the impetus for an era of botanical research among Taoist hermits and healers of China, which laid the foundations for what is now practiced as Traditional Chinese Medicine throughout the world. It is a fascinating possibility that the current use of Asian herbal medicines by millions of people originally stemmed from the search for an intoxicating liquor of immortality, and that Hinduism is rooted in alchemical extractions of a dibir herb.

Like other deities of Vedic mythology, Soma has found its way into the terminology of Ayurveda and yoga, where it is used to describe alchemical aspects of physiological functions. Pranayama, the science of yogic breathing, teaches that the flow of breath circulates through three primary nadis, or meridians of subtle energy. These channels have been depicted for centuries in Tibetan and Ayurvedic medical diagrams, threads of Tantra and alchemy that have been integrated into the healing traditions as a kind of esoteric physiology. The left nostril opens into the passage called ida, and the right enters pingala; like snakes entwined around the spinal cord, these channels form the shape of a caduceus, the symbol of the medical profession. Ida and pingala have a natural circadian rhythm which causes them to alternate in strength every hour. As the breath moves from one side to the other and back, there is a brief period when they become balanced; at this time it is said that the prana enters sushumna, the central channel associated with the spinal cord.

"True, true. Without doubt," start the words of Hermes Trismegistus, who inscribed the most famous of alchemical dictums on tablets of emerald. "The below is as the above, and the above as the below, to perfect the wonders of the One." Yogic physiology links the microcosm of the body to the celestial macrocosm by attributing the flow of ida to the moon, and the flow of pingala to the sun. In this way, the body becomes an alembic filled with continual interchange between the cool, liquid, nourishing, yin aspects of Soma (lunar waters) and the warm, dry, energetic, yang aspects of Agni (solar fire). When these are in a state of equilibrium, prana enters the central conduit of sushumna, which is described as having the nature of air; as this current rises it carries consciousness upward along the spinal column, through the intersecting points where ida and pingala entwine around the nerve plexi of the chakras, and finally into the infinite space of samadhi, universal awareness.

In medical language it can be said that the circulation of Soma through ida relates to the activity of the parasympathetic nervous system, which produces relaxation, rest, calmness, and flow of blood to the internal organs. The circulation of Agni through pingala can be correlated to the sympathetic nervous system, which produces stimulation, increased metabolism, heightened reflexes, and flow of blood to the muscles. Kundalini, the upward rising energy within sushumna, might be described as the awakening of the dormant capacity of the central nervous system, bringing into activity the largely unused parts of the brain.

In Ayurvedic terminology, Soma is linked to rasa and ojas. The term *rasa* has other connotations besides its references to mercury; it is also used to denote "juices," or the "essence of flavors." Rasa is found as sap within plants, and in the blending of tastes and smells which comprise the life force of food. Physiologically, rasa refers to chyle, the liquid mixture produced during the early stages of digestion; this aspect of rasa also constitutes the first of seven tissue levels formed from food. The word *rasayana*, rejuvenation therapy, means "the path of rasa," which alludes to how nutrient essences are fed to the freshly cleansed tissues and organs following pancha karma treatment. As the intoxicating liquor of the Vedas, Soma is also referred to as rasa.

The influences of Soma can be found in the creation of ojas, nutritional essence. From the raw juices in the stomach to final cellular metabolism, step by step through the body's complex enzymatic transformations, the rasa of food is gradually refined into ojas, a golden yellow and white nectar of sunrays and moonbeams extracted from the plants of our diet.

Ojas is said to be derived from the purified nutrients produced by all the organs and tissues, especially marrow and reproductive fluids, like nectar gathered from flowers. Similar in nature to cerebrospinal fluid, ojas supports the brain, functions as the foundation of consciousness, and shines in the sparkle of the eyes. Classical physiology claims that eight drops of the most refined part of ojas are stored in the subtle psychic nerves of the heart, while two handfuls of the less refined part circulate throughout the body. If ojas were to be correlated with bio-chemical substances, it would be closest to hemoglobin and the anti-bodies of the immune system; it strengthens immunity and resistance against disease.

The luminosity of ojas is closely related to the reproductive fluids, and is depleted by excessive sexual activity and preoccupation. Con-serving and increasing this nutrient essence to feed the heart and central nervous system is one of the reasons some meditators renounce sexual relations and practice celibacy. Preserving ojas is thought to be the best way to promote longevity, strengthen the body, and increase wisdom.

As the breath becomes quiet and its whirling flows enter the deep river of sushumna, the mind returns to its true home—tranquil absorp-tion. Nourished by herbal and mineral rasayanic essences and the inner light of virtuous restraint, the brain responds by secreting hormones of bliss. This is the innermost level of Soma, the nectar of meditation that feeds the deities and lights the path toward immortality. It is the heav-enly elixir never tasted by ordinary beings, for as the Rig Veda says, "One thinks they have drunk Soma after crushing the herbs, but the Soma the Brahmins know is never drunk. No earthly one eats You."

When the mind is energized with prana and nourished by Soma, it effortlessly wills its universal creative forces into existence, and one finds oneself in the realm of the devas and deities. Like the Medicine Buddha, we discover that in the palm of our hand rests the bowl of nec-tar most sweet, which lifts all beings out of illness, poverty, death, and decay, into the eternal fulfillment beyond all craving. "All the water and drink you have consumed through beginningless time until now has failed to slake your thirst or bring you contentment," sang Milarepa. "Drink therefore this stream of enlightened mind, fortunate ones."

Nepal has always been a land of rich and varied botanical life. The geography of the country extends from the low-lying jungles of the Terai to the world's highest mountains; because of these altitudinal variations, there is a great diversity of climates and vegetation. At least seven thousand types of flowering species grow in Nepal's valleys, jungles, and mountains. The emphasis on herbal remedies in the classical traditions reflects the profusion of plants in the environment, and for centuries this verdant region has been regarded as a treasure-house of Ayurvedic medicines.

The Himalayan cultures that once lived close to nature's elements fostered the evolution of Ayurveda. Much of the botanical knowledge used in classical medicine was derived from the experiences of indigenous people, who had daily interaction with the numerous plant species that surrounded them. "A wise physician should learn about the drugs from tribals, cowherds, and others residing in forests and living on rhizomes, roots, and fruits," wrote Todaramalla, the minister of the sixteenth-century Moghul king Akbar, in his encyclopedic works on Ayurveda.

Ayurveda is now being disseminated throughout the world, where it is welcomed by many who are seeking healing; in the green valleys of its origin, however, the traditions that gave birth to this medical system are in a state of decline. The identities of many plants described in the Ayurvedic and Tibetan literature have been lost, because the rural people who knew their uses have left their homes to spend more time in the cities. At the same time many medicines that are known and available are not being utilized, and a wealth of ancient manuscripts preserving a vast collection of medical information lies neglected and unused. Classical doctors and herbalists have always relied on their students to keep these practices alive; as they transmit less of their wisdom, family secrets, and techniques, either because of social disturbances or a lack of interested students, this information vanishes into history.

According to surveys conducted by organizations dedicated to preserving this cultural and medical heritage, if Ayurveda's millennia-old lineages continue vanishing at the current rate, they will be extinct in Nepal within two generations. Comprehensive documentation of these traditions is an immense undertaking which realistically cannot be fully realized. A few dedicated individuals, however, are attempting to save a small portion of their country's valuable legacy. Dr. Lokendra Singh and Dr. Narendra Tiwari are Nepal's foremost experts in Ayurveda and its herbal treasures. Together they have formed the Himalayan Ayurvedic Research Association, which is working to preserve Nepal's vanishing plants and ethnobotanical knowledge.

Dr. Singh is the father of modern Ayurveda in Nepal. Working against widespread political apathy and resistance, he established the Ayurvedic college at Tribuvan University in Kathmandu. Two generations of practitioners from Nepal owe their good fortune of being able to study Ayurveda to the struggle of this brilliant, humorous, and sensitive physician.

Originally from Bhaktapur, home of Newari people, Dr. Singh received his education in integrated medicine from Benares Hindu University, where he studied and practiced both modern surgery and classical Ayurveda. At least three decades of his life have been devoted to intensive scientific research into the effectiveness of Ayurvedic medicines and therapies. When I met Dr. Singh, his twenty-year effort to establish Ayurveda academically in Nepal was finally gaining recognition and appreciation, mostly as a result of interest from the West; decades of economic manipulation by multinational pharmaceutical companies and rejection of cultural traditions by modern Nepalis has left Ayurveda suppressed and neglected in its own homeland.

I found Dr. Singh a wonderful and stimulating teacher. He possessed a unique combination of insightful genius, spiritual irreverence, and sharp wit. Although his primary interest was in the philosophical aspects of Ayurveda, many of our dialogues concerned his efforts, through the Himalayan Ayurvedic Research Association, to convince the government to implement a commonsense solution to the current health care crisis in this poor and remote mountainous country: teaching people how to use the herbs that grow in their local environment. Even though it is a simple, cost-effective, and medically efficient concept, the doctor's vision has not been appreciated by government policy-makers and allopathic physicians. Having to continually cross swords with such adversaries was undoubtedly why the doctor's profound teachings were frequently flavored with a pinch of existential resignation.

Dr. Tiwari was born in Lumbini, the birthplace of Buddha. He grew up surrounded by the jungle's rich vegetation, and from an early age had recurring dreams about his future involvement with Ayurvedic medicine. Dr. Tiwari is now one of Nepal's most knowledgeable herbalists. He holds a Ph.D. in Ayurvedic botany from Benares Hindu University and is a lecturer at the Ayurvedic college in Kathmandu, a consultant for numerous Ayurvedic manufacturing companies, and vice president of the Ethnobotanical Society of Nepal.

Dr. Tiwari has encyclopedic knowledge of plants and their lore. Whether in a garden or a forest, there is no species the botanist is not familiar with; he can identify every weed, bush, tree, vine, grass, and flower growing in the vicinity, describe its morphological characteristics in detail, and expound eloquently on its history and medicinal uses. Even the potted plants in restaurants are a source of ethnobotanical wonder for this gentle and soft-spoken ally of the green kingdom.

The doctor's comprehension of botanical medicine encompasses both ancient and modern viewpoints; he knows the functions of species according to the classical terminology of the Tridosha theory, and is also well versed in modern biochemistry. His expertise in species identification is an invaluable asset to herb companies in Nepal, which rely on his skills for quality control in manufacturing their products. Besides his voluminous plant knowledge, he has an extensive background in the writings of the ancient physicians, has made major contributions to scholarly investigations, and is knowledgeable about contemporary social, political, and environmental issues facing herbal medicine in the Himalayas. He is an herbal activist, deeply committed to the preservation of plants and the traditional knowledge of their uses by indigenous people.

Through the Himalayan Ayurvedic Research Association, Dr. Tiwari and Dr. Singh have conducted surveys of the traditional folk healers in the Gorkha district and the herbs which they use. The geographical distribution of this district is a cross section of all of Nepal's distinct regions, from the lower foothills near Lake Fewa in Pokhara up to the Tibetan border in the high Himalayas. The doctors selected six zones within the Gorkha district, which are home to many different ethnic groups, and investigated how many people were practitioners of traditional medicine and how they acquired their knowledge. They found that only a very small percentage of the younger generation is currently involved with this type of work, and that important lineages of knowledge are not being passed on.

During these studies, Dr. Tiwari collected the plants that are utilized as medicines by local practitioners and compared them to the classical Ayurvedic pharmacopoeias. He found that up to 80 percent are being used for the same purposes described in the medical texts, confirming that the source of much of Ayurveda's herbal information is the oral and written traditions of indigenous people which have been transmitted through the generations.

The work of Dr. Tiwari and Dr. Singh brought to my attention the botanical devastation occurring in the Nepalese hillsides, with many important species of Himalayan herbs becoming rare and extinct. The eastern part of Nepal in particular is one of the ecological "hot spots" of the world, in which a high concentration of biodiversity is under threat.

Although there are no definitive statistics concerning the number of endangered plants in Nepal, it is probably similar to other regions under ecological pressure. Hawaii, for example, has lost 10 percent of its native plants, and another 60 percent are endangered. This is potentially a loss of unimaginable consequences for ourselves and coming generations. As plants disappear, our ability to make medicines, whether as botanical preparations or refined pharmaceuticals, also vanishes. It is not only the future of medicine that rests upon the abundance of the plant kingdom: how will human life continue in an environment where plants cannot survive?

As in most Third World countries, where a growing population is directly dependent on the surrounding countryside for fuel, food, and grazing of animals, Nepal's wilderness areas have shrunk and their condition has deteriorated; only 10 percent of the vast jungles and primeval forests that once covered the country remain. The primary threat to the diversity of plant species in Nepal is human encroachment and the expansion of agricultural areas. Controlling malaria in the low-lying areas of the Terai opened the door to the development of infrastructures such as roads, irrigation canals, and power lines; rapid growth, combined with increased farming and grazing, has had a detrimental impact on the tropical forests. Those forest areas that have not been converted to farming are being stripped of vegetation for fuel and animal fodder by the region's exploding population. The destruction of habitat that accompanies human encroachment leads to the disappearance of plant species that depend on a specific location and terrain for their existence. For example, the habitat of kakad singhi, a type of parasitic gallnut used in treating cough, asthma, infantile diarrhea, and dysentery, is limited to a small area, and the wood it grows on is collected for fuel. The loss of this plant leaves the world with one less highly effective remedy for sick children.

In the alpine and subalpine regions, the primary threat to flora comes less from domestic needs and more from the international pressures of mountaineering and tourism. Supplying trekking and climbing expeditions with fuel has been one of the primary causes of deforestation and subsequent soil erosion; such high-altitude damage has contributed to an increase of serious flooding in lower countries such as Bangladesh. Domestic grazing of animals in high-altitude regions has also changed the composition of the plant populations.

Herb collecting has been a source of income for Himalayan communities for ages. In recent years the phenomenal renaissance of natural medicine, along with the corresponding shift toward more holistic healing paradigms, is helping countless people restore their health and increase their wellbeing. Unfortunately, this resurgence of interest in botanical remedies is also a threat to the plant kingdom and a cause of extinction for many species. The growing worldwide consumption of Ayurvedic and Tibetan medicines has increased the value of Himalayan herbs, which in turn has created a greater economic incentive for more harvesting. The opening of trade with the international herb industry and an astronomical increase in the export of botanical materials for Ayurvedic formulas is exerting tremendous pressure on the flora of Nepal.

Seventy percent of herbs presently used in Ayurveda come from the Terai region and lower foothills. These plants were previously abundant, but due to overcollection and loss of habitat, many are now difficult to find. Improper collecting methods have endangered numerous medicinal species, especially those whose vital life-sustaining parts, such as the roots and bark, are harvested. Many collectors remove entire root systems of plants, hastening their extinction. In the alpine regions many important tubers and roots are endangered as a result of poor collection methods. One of these is *Nardostachys jatamansi*, which has a major role in Ayurvedic formulas as a nervine and sedative; another is *Orchis latifolia*, a nutritive aphrodisiac which belongs to the orchid family. Several kinds of medicinal trees are endangered because of over-harvesting of their bark, such as *Cinnamomum tamala*, the Nepalese cinnamon, and the anti-amoebic remedy *Holarrhena antidysenterica*.

One group of important medicines which has been lost is the "divine drugs" of Ayurveda: plants such as Soma with alleged miraculous powers. At present their identification is controversial and cannot be established. Dr. Tiwari and other researchers are trying to ascertain their identities, but the classical texts lack detailed morphological descriptions. In the past, people who were familiar with the forest did not completely describe the characteristics of many of the documented plants, and recorded only various synonyms. There was no universal language of botanical terminology as there is now, so the same name might have been used for different plants in various regions. This confusion, combined with people moving away from their homes, has made identification of these valuable drugs uncertain.

According to Dr. Tiwari, there was only one type of Soma described in the Vedas, and even at that time it was very rare. In later books after the Vedas, there is mention of the drug adar, which had the same effects. After that, twenty-five types of Soma are described in the *Sushruta Samhita*, which provides various morphological features.

"One characteristic of Soma is that it has fifteen leaves," the herbalist explained. "Each day as the moon increases one leaf comes out, and when the moon is full all fifteen leaves are present. Each day as the moon decreases one leaf falls, and when there is no moon, the leaves are gone. Throughout the entire botanical kingdom, we are not able to find this type of plant at present. It is very sad to say that maybe in those times that plant was available, but at present it may be extinct. In my opinion it is available, but we have lost contact with it."

Mushrooms, ferns, and lichens are the genera that are least known by herbalists and ethnobotanists. These are the untouched and unresearched areas of the plant kingdom, and very important in the search for new medicines. It is Dr. Tiwari's opinion that Soma and the divine drugs are related to this group. "Soma may belong to the mushroom family," Dr. Tiwari continued. "In the *Sushruta Samhita* there is another divine drug called chatra, which means 'umbrella'; mushrooms are the shape of an umbrella. Some species of ferns and mushrooms are very poisonous and must be used only with one hundred percent knowledge of their identity. We know that poisonous drugs act very quickly and can be powerful medicines. The tribes had more knowledge about how to utilize them, because they lived with them. With trials and experiments they learned to identify which were poisonous, which were edible, and which were edible after purification.

"Ethnomedicine has given many new drugs to modern pharmacological science," Dr. Tiwari explained, "including several antibiotics from fungi and algae. I am currently trying to find the Ayurvedic drugs known as astaban. They are described in the *Charaka Samhita* as drugs that increase vitality. Most of them are controversial and not identified properly. I have identified three genera of astaban herbs used by people in high altitudes for energy and strength. I am trying to locate those vitalizers with the help of Tibetan doctors."

In the Himalayan valleys and meadows, as in many parts of the world, important medicinal herbs are becoming rare and endangered, while at the same time unknown numbers of valuable species are waiting to be rediscovered, and ancient formulas that could provide immense benefit to humanity lie buried in forgotten manuscripts.

A winter afternoon finds me traveling through the streets of Kathmandu toward Buranilkanta, on my way to Gopal's new Om Ayurvedic Research Center. The stream of noxious traffic brings the usual sights, self-important men chauffeured by gaunt drivers, the homeless lying on sidewalks, women doing chores, idle young men in front of shops. I am weary of breathing the smoke and dust that fill the air, fatigued by the chronic respiratory infections that everyone shares, and increasingly vulnerable to the misery and despair that confronts me. I can't help wondering what karma binds me to this land of poverty and pollution, this troubling vision of what the world is becoming. The causes of this destiny elude me, but I know what keeps me here and brings me back whenever I leave: it is the small things filled with magic, like Gopal's innocent attempts to restore classical Ayurveda on his little plot of terraced land outside of town.

I turn down a narrow dirt lane filled with streams of sewage, and come face to face with staring children and women gathered at a water fountain. The women look into my eyes, their gaze filled with an intensity of complex feelings. In a moment I am gone, an instant of someone from another world passing through their lives, a man who has never had to perform the exhausting village chores that never end. My mind lingers on these mysteries of fate, until the road becomes steep and muddy with a cliff falling away inches from the tires. Across the valley the view of the mountains is spectacular, toward Gunje where Gopal and I gave away medicines.

I arrive at the entrance to Gopal's dream. He greets me in his humble, charming, amusing way, looking very Muslim with a full beard and scarf turban on his head. He pulls a rope hanging at the gate, and far up the hill a gong speaks softly from a thicket of bamboo. "Welcome, God," he says with hands pressed together; I return his Namaste.

It is good to see Gopal again, and he is happy to have a guest. Much work has been done since my last visit, which my friend is eager to show me. I follow him to a bamboo grove at the western edge of his property, where the land drops off into a hidden valley. "The air is so fine here," Gopal says reverently, "and the effects of inhaling and exhaling it are so beneficial for the mind. The bamboo makes different kinds of music at night," he continues with characteristic wonder, then describes how he will build a meditation hut on this spot overlooking Mt. Nagarjuna.

We walk back across the open field as Gopi shares his visions. "The hillside is beautiful when the moon is full," he says; "soon all-night outdoor ceremonies will take place to get closer to her lunar rays." He takes me to a pagoda built for traditional fire pujas, to the shrine where visiting gurus will receive guests, past the beginnings of a lotus pond, and on to the herbal preparation shed. Inside, Gopal's assistants are chopping and boiling fresh *Adhatoda vasaka*, a great friend of Ayurvedic doctors and their patients. The men pour a cup of the slimy green decoction from an earthen pot on the fireplace and encourage me to drink it for my lungs; it is good, bitter medicine that goes to work immediately.

We move on to the building where the bakery will be. Gopi shows me his antique hand press for extracting vegetable oils, and tells me his plans for different types of herbal breads made to order for patients' individual needs. Wide-eyed with sincerity, my friend claims that in this place, where the currents of pure life force stream down from Shivapuri and Nagarjuna peaks, a person's digestive power is much better than in the city. I notice that the turgid brew in my stomach, combined with the pranic forces of the mountains, is definitely stimulating my appetite.

"How much do you pay for this land?" I ask. It appears to be about five acres of usable property, bordered by a steep hillside on three sides. The view from all directions is magnificent.

"Twenty-five thousand rupees per year," Gopal replies, about five hundred dollars. A year ago, he signed a ten-year lease and began building. It is a big commitment, I imagine, especially since he has no money or income. Gopi laughs and describes his father's response when he asked him for financial assistance. "'What are you doing building a center on land you'll just have to leave in ten years?' my father asked. I told him, 'We have to leave everything. We even have to pay rent to live in this body. If we don't give it food, we have to leave. Everything is like that.'" Apparently, his father was convinced by the simplicity of his son's logic.

Children are singing in the valley below, and a crescent moon hangs over Mt. Nagarjuna. Gopi takes me to see the storehouse, which is filled with sacks of grains and legumes. Reaching into one of the bags, he pulls out a handful of soybeans. "These are very organic," he explains, then tells me about a guru who will come to teach about the healing powers of natural foods. He scoops out a type of lentil, offers to make soup for my health, and suggests different treatments for my chest congestion, such as fresh ginger baths and herbal steam. I smile at my good-hearted, generous, and eccentric friend, and tell him to fix good medicine.

Night comes, and we retire to the open veranda of the main house for dinner. My host's assistants are at work, building a small fire in a clay dish in the middle of the room and preparing dinner down the hall. We sit on woven mats laid over a smooth red earth floor, surrounded by firelight reflecting off mud walls. The view of the sky is blocked by bamboo poles and thatch, but open to the east. Across the valley, lights in cottage windows sparkle against the blackness; dogs bark in the road below. Gopal sprinkles guggul on the coals for incense, and we bless ourselves with its smoke.

The men bring out the feast and graciously serve us course after course of fragrant and nutritious Ayurvedic cuisine prepared from forest foods and the harvest of local farms. There are soups of legumes and roots high in protein, porridges made from grains and seeds, soft basmati rice moistened with ghee, and steaming wild greens rich in iron and other minerals. Everything has been simmered in exotic spices to kindle the digestive power and enhance assimilation, then garnished with slimy sweet pickles of tingling fruits and fiery peppers. Gopi explains the health-promoting benefits of each ingredient and condiment as we savor the exquisite country fare, feeling the evening chill flee as our bellies and hearts are warmed.

The uncultivated bounty of the land was the original food of humans. Once a major part of every diet, consumption of wild food in Nepal is now limited to the remote tribal people. Many of the nutritious, medicinally valuable, and, as my host was proving, delicious foods from the Himalayas are increasingly neglected. Processed foods from the West are culturally appealing, while eating weeds and roots is associated with poverty and lack of sophistication.

In order to survive in their natural settings, wild plants must be hardy and have strong immunity and intense vitality; this gives them superior food value and medicinal qualities. The inclusion of some of these plants as potherbs in the diets of the past was how our robust ancestors got their concentrated vitamins and other essential nutrients. Typically, potherbs were those local and seasonal ingredients that were not substantial enough to be a staple food and not medicinal enough to be a major drug. Some examples known throughout the world are fennel, malva, nettle, milk thistle, dandelion, mustard, plantain, seaweed, borage, grape leaves, and watercress, as well as aromatic culinary herbs such as basil, sage, parsley, tarragon, and hyssop. Although our modern urban diets no longer contain the rich diversity of such delights from the garden and forest, thousands of plants of this type wait in traditional marketplaces and in the countryside, to be rediscovered and enjoyed.

Until the isolation of bitter alkaloid constituents from plants in the 1800s and the subsequent appearance of modern pharmaceutical companies, the concepts of what constituted "food" and what was "medicine" were not distinctly separate. Foods were regarded as having healing powers, and medicines provided nutritional vitality. Asian medical traditions have a wealth of delicious recipes using herbs as part of everyday cooking; some of these, such as dong quai chicken and congees (gruel) made with fresh herbs and greens, are now routinely prescribed by Caucasian doctors of Chinese medicine to their Western patients. Even the simple use of potherbs from local environments can play a major role in bringing preventive and curative plants into people's dietary routines. This bringing together of food and medicine is one of the simplest and most efficient ways to improve the health of society.

Nowadays, unless families make a deliberate effort to find and utilize organic and natural foods, most typical diets contain a high percentage of ingredients that are overly refined by-products of excessively hybridized and artificially sustained plants and animals. The more devitalized these foods become, the less they are able to nourish the body and the more they obstruct its channels with undigested waste. Our modern eating habits are among the most basic causes of sickness in the world; many degenerative diseases, such as diabetes and cancer, appear within one generation after refined foods have been introduced into a culture's diet. Many of the remedies used by herbalists to counteract these illnesses were at one time a regular part of people's meals, and can become so again.

Most of the species listed in books on the wild edible plants of Nepal are also used as medicines by Ayurvedic doctors. For example, varahica, one of the many types of *Dioscorea*, wild yam, is prescribed as a tonic; tribal people boil it, prepare flour from the tubers, and make breads. *Dioscorea* is a widespread genus which has had a major place in traditional Asian medicines and diets for centuries. In old Chinese pharmacopoeias there are descriptions of villages where people were extraordinarily healthy, apparently because of their cultivation and use of different yam species as staple foods.

An important wild food that is available in many parts of the world is stinging nettle. This valuable plant, which I now savored as part of Gopal's collection of Ayurvedic delicacies, is consumed as a highly nutritious vegetable in the Himalayan hills; its stinging formic acid, the chemical secreted by ants when angry, is removed by boiling. Nettle is also an important medicinal herb; it contains many essential minerals and vitamins, is one of the best sources of iron for anemic women, and can be safely consumed during pregnancy to strengthen the fetus. It is a good antidiabetic herb, a valuable remedy for allergies, hay fever, and skin disorders, and high in fiber.

Some toxic plants, such as many mushrooms and ferns, are also used as foods and medicines. Indigenous people have utilized these for centuries, and know from observation and experimentation which are toxic, which are not, and the techniques to detoxify those that are poisonous. Numerous methods are used to render them safe for consumption, such as various cooking procedures and mixing with other herbs. *Solanum nigrum*, the black nightshade of the tomato family, is consumed as a vegetable and also utilized by Ayurvedic physicians as a liver tonic. If eaten fresh it may be toxic, but when it is boiled its toxic alkaloid, solanine, is neutralized. Although some people would be hesitant to eat a plant like the black nightshade, it is widely cultivated and consumed in parts of Africa.

Besides their everyday use and ethnobotanical value, the foods of the forest have played an important role in the spiritual history of the Himalayas. The abundance of wild edibles enabled yogis and hermits to escape from civilization, nourishing their bodies and minds with greens, roots, and fruits growing in the proximity of their huts and caves. These wild foods sustained the contemplatives of the mountains and jungles, who composed joyful poetry and songs describing the freedom they enjoyed beyond the constraints of society, liberated from the responsibilities of having to earn a living in order to eat. Milarepa lived for extended periods of time on nettles; it is said his body turned green from a diet of such concentrated chlorophyll. The herbal knowledge and meditative insights of classical medicine are partly based on the botanical experiences and experiments of the mystics.

Wild foods are a precious resource for the world. By rediscovering their traditional uses, we can reduce our dependency on the overly hybridized, genetically manipulated, and environmentally vulnerable crops created by biological industries. By reintroducing the potent flavors of wild foods into our diets, we narrow the artificial gap that has been created between foods and medicines, and benefit from their curative and revitalizing properties. Discovering old and new uses of these ancient foods makes new cultivation projects economically viable for herb growers; this in turn supports sustainable nontoxic agriculture and leads to a cleaner, healthier environment.

"This is kubindu melon, *Benincasa*, with honeysuckle flowers," Gopal says. The men are clearing the low tables and bringing servings of herbal sweets and digestive teas made from aromatic spices, as we recline in utter luxurious contentment. I savor the melon's unctuous consistency and mildly sharp aftertaste, and wonder if it is related to the famous bitter melon of Chinese medicine. I am well acquainted with honeysuckle flowers, having given them to thousands of patients in formulas for bacterial and viral infections and a host of inflammatory conditions.

Sipping the spicy after-dinner tea, I think of all the wild foods I have studied and harvested back home in California. A profusion of nutritious plants grows in the hills around Los Angeles: dark-green milk thistle leaves that detoxify the liver and improve the quality and quantity of milk in nursing mothers; sweet fennel with its soft anise-flavored fronds, excellent for helping digestion, treating respiratory conditions, and improving eyesight; pungent hot nasturtiums announcing their peppery flavors with fiery orange flowers; bitter dandelion greens, so beneficial for cleansing the liver and kidneys. Farther north, in the misty valleys of the Big Sur coast, more succulent treasures await: crisp, watery miner's lettuce; sweet cisely; sour wood sorrel that cools bladder inflammation; malva, high in mucilaginous properties and valuable nutrients. In the high Mojave Desert, yucca roots and flowers were carefully harvested by indigenous people as a staple food, augmented by delicious nuts of piñon pine and the rich, buttery flour ground from tiny silken chia seeds.

All across California, the most important wild food of the original ancestors was acorns. The great oak forests were meticulously cared for with controlled fires, each family depending on its own stand of grand and ancient trees. So valuable was acorn flour that life revolved around the seasonal cycles of the oaks, which provided not only nourishment but also a natural antibiotic grown on acorn-paste mold. Throughout the Sierra Nevada range, mortar holes in granite boulders sit empty and silent where women once gathered in meadows and by beautiful waterfalls to prepare the flour that fed their tribes.

After dinner Gopal and I walk back to the bamboo grove, and sit listening to the whispering reeds. Inside them, in maybe one out of every five hundred, lies a small crystal. This is the vamsa lochana of Ayurvedic medicine; it is exceedingly rare and highly esteemed. An exudate of silica found only in the females, it is a precious remedy for high fevers in children, and an effective expectorant in phlegmatic chest infections. In the earth at the bamboo's base, young shoots push their way upward; these are also medicine to be boiled and eaten, specifically for leukorrhea. The leaves rustling in the darkness have curative powers as well; they are used extensively in Chinese medicine for febrile conditions of the lungs and liver.

We sit in the cold winter air with Mt. Nagarjuna's dark presence on the horizon, and I appreciate Gopal's ability to be silent. Meditation arises naturally, and we enter the stream of concentrationless concentration, infuse our senses with an effortless flow of undistracted awareness, and permeate the universe with loving-kindness born of inner stillness. The bamboo sings and murmurs.

Much of the night is gone when we rise and make our way down the treacherous stairs to the car. Gopal has made arrangements for classes with several Ayurvedic gurus, and I will return tomorrow for studies. I am tired and chilled as I drive through the dark winter streets, which are empty except for an occasional smoky fire warming the cold bones of the homeless; I wonder again why I have come to this city filled with so much sickness and hardship. It is the small, magical things that bring me here, I remind myself, like Gopal's devotion to restoring Ayurveda that keeps him working tirelessly with no resources except his vision, the help of his faithful assistants, and an occasional gift from his father. "I am creating a center of classical medicine which is close to nature," he had said over dinner. Reflecting on my friend's words, I realize that as modern drugs and medical systems fail to bring us health and wellbeing, people will seek solutions in the wisdom of antiquity. The ancient cures will become the medicines of the future.

I am floating, lost among the sky's reflections somewhere on Lake Fewa. Machupuchare's snow-draped peak is close, the fertility goddess watching over us, looking down as my tiny boat glides across the water. Waves of ferns fall from the mountainsides above, reaching the water's edge to brush against my outstretched hand. Dragonflies with fragile wings of painted velvet hang from heart-shaped creepers, and butterflies navigate invisible air currents.

Along the water, herbs are growing in abundance. Climbers and shrubs compete for space, weaving leaves of yellows and greens into layers of living colors, starburst flowers hiding in their shade. Dr. Tiwari would know them all, of course, having documented them here in the Gorkha district. I hear echoes of his voice as he happily recites their Latin, Nepali, and common names.

In the old cultures, plants were regarded as sacred beings from higher realms, gifts of the gods placed on earth, and embodiments of divine attributes. The seers of Ayurveda taught the people to care for the botanical kingdom, by describing various species in religious and mythical language. They understood that when a society does not respect the consciousness of plants, it will awaken to discover they have vanished, taking their life-sustaining gifts with them.

"Many plants originated from amrita, the nectar of the gods," I remember Dr. Tiwari saying. "One story in our ancient books says the devas and asuras [gods and titans] churned the sea, and from that came amrita. They fought over the nectar, so Indra took it and flew away. During the flight some drops from the pot fell to earth and became drugs. One of the them is guduchi [*Tinospora cordifolia*], another is haritaki [*Terminalia chebula*], and another is garlic. In my view, these stories emphasize the properties of the drugs and their specific actions."

The mythical qualities attributed to important herbs help convey their value to humanity. For example, one of the synonyms of myrobalan is amrita, which emphasizes how this fruit never causes any toxicity or harm to the body. It is also known as patya, meaning it is always beneficial to the body's channels, and rasayan, because it acts as a rejuvenator. To a person whose illness has been removed by the myrobalan, this remarkable herb would seem like a drop of nectar from heaven.

I drift through the shadows of overhanging branches, listening to the trees. They whisper simple gratitude, speaking for all of us who have forgotten the importance of the soil, sun, water, and air. How precious and sacred are the plants of this world, and the elements that nurture them! No life will exist when they are destroyed. Will we listen, remember, and give thanks for their healing powers before they are gone, or will our fate be that of the forests and animals dying of thirst and disease around us? The stones speak silently, reminding us of how soft and fragile our bodies are. Even a butterfly blown by the wind understands this.

"There is an innate respect for all living beings in the Vedas," Dr. Singh once said. "In the Hindu pantheon, so many plants are the incarnation of God Himself. Once you come to the point where you realize they are also living beings, that they have equal rights to be on this planet, I think that particular feeling will give you respect, and you will not harm them or take them for granted.

"The ancients have said 'Aham Brahmasmi,' 'I am the universe.' That was not a delusion; they really experienced totality. Those seers understood that all of life has evolved originally from consciousness, and therefore everything has consciousness, and has been created for a purpose. If we are destroying something, it is because of our narrow-mindedness."

Hindu religious texts contain numerous references regarding the importance of plants. In the *Bhagavad Gita*, Lord Krishna says, "I am present in the plants in the form of aswat. If you want to worship me, worship the aswat." Aswat is the *Ficus religiosa*, the Bodhi tree under which Buddha reached nirvana. Many Hindus worship this tree, offer it water, and avoid cutting its wood. Within this religious sentiment is an important ecological reason to protect this species: it releases more oxygen than other trees.

Another tree that is worshipped and given offerings is the *Ficus benghalensis*, the banyan tree. This species produces aerial roots that become new trunks, thereby perpetuating its life indefinitely. There is one tree in Calcutta which covers an area of about four acres; its main trunk is unknown. This tree also has an important ecological function: it is very good for binding the soil and preventing erosion.

Religious stories describing plants as divine encourage us to preserve precious natural resources, and help bring the sacred into our everyday lives. The earth-based spiritual wisdom found in Ayurveda and other traditional cultures opens our eyes to the sanctity of life; this is crucial not only for health and happiness, but for our survival. Believing that God dwells in trees is not an abstract philosophical concept, pagan superstition, or a quaint Hindu custom: as we destroy the plant kingdom, we decrease the oxygen of the atmosphere. Anyone with asthma or emphysema knows that oxygen is life, and without the presence of pneuma, spirit in the form of breath, the body will suffocate. Perhaps in the future the *Ficus religiosa*, Buddha's tree of enlightenment, and all its relatives, will play a role in restoring the earth's atmosphere. If that day comes, those suffering from respiratory illness will find healing and solace in fragrant groves filled with luxurious air.

"In the Terai region people marry plants together," I hear Dr. Tiwari saying. "We hold a marriage ceremony for the *Ficus religiosa* and *Ficus benghalensis*, just like a marriage ceremony for people. When our children get married, we marry the plants on the same occasion. It is done at the crossroads, and is quite common. This is how we show affection to the plants. There is no scientific reason to do this, but these ceremonies remind us of the great importance of our natural resources." In many places throughout the countryside of Nepal, these two varieties of trees have grown together in marriage for hundreds of years.

"We use many plants in our routine ceremonies," the herbalist went on. "Some people make a ring with the grass *Imperita serendrica* and wear it when making offerings. The Brahmin community make a holy thread from *Sacharum munja* and wear it at the upanayam ceremony, when the Gayatri mantra is introduced to the child. We use sesame oil for altar lamps; it is the best among all vegetable oils, and said to originate from the sweat of Lord Vishnu. The wood of *Butea monospermum* is used for fire in ceremonies, because it is regarded as sacred to Agni, god of fire.

"Aromatic herbs are used in offerings, like *Cedrus deodaria* (Himalayan cedar bark), *Nardostachys jatamansi* (Indian spikenard), *Valeriana wallichiana* (valerian), and neem. We burn these plants and chant to purify or disinfect the atmosphere. We plant tulsi, holy basil, and go to it early in the morning and pray; it is antiviral and antibacterial, and keeps away mosquitoes. People worship the neem tree, and use it during epidemics of measles. They put neem leaves in the patient's bed and use them to fumigate the room and to purify water for baths. In the past people were not familiar with terms like *antibacterial* and *antiviral*, but they knew this tree was effective in preventing infection and stopping the spread of disease. Even today neem is used for treating measles in many villages.

"These things show that at one time people knew the utility of different species. If you know plants are important, you won't disturb them, and this will prevent their extinction or loss. In the past the use of plants in daily worship linked culture and religion together. Now people are abandoning these customs."

"Why are they rejecting these things?" I wondered.

"Because they lack understanding of why they are necessary, and don't know the scientific reasons," my teacher replied. "We are also not communicating this knowledge to our coming generation."

The earth remembers what we have forgotten. Before cars, before freeways, we walked, our feet touching the soil. We knew its fertility by seeing it giving birth to creatures and plants. Before we withdrew into insulated existences, we felt the ground awakening in the springtime sun and saw how it slept in the depth of winter. We knew the coming and going of the wondrous forms of life, the habits of the animals, the flowering and dying of the plants, the turning of the constellations in the night sky.

Soft breezes move along the shore, the breath of the Goddess playing on the vegetation like strings of a formless instrument, evoking murmurs of music in response to Her passing. How blissful to recline all day, listening to these gentle voices, untouched by the anxieties and discord elsewhere in the world. Eagles soar in choreographed perfection, effortlessly embracing the wind; white cranes leave effervescent trails through pastel skies.

All beings are born from, suckled, raised, and eventually reclaimed by the Universal Mother. As the moon, clouds, and rain, she nourishes the plants with her juices. In dark forests and silvery meadows, the queen of the night moves among the leaves, releasing infinite chemical transmutations as she excites the flavors and smells circulating in the veins of her vegetal subjects. The Mother blesses us with foods and medicines; her blood, breath, bones, and warmth are the true nourishment carried within the plants and animals who have sacrificed themselves for the continuation of our lives. All that we eat and drink are forms of her milk, the sweet Soma flowing from the breast of the earth.

Our bodies are sustained by the sun's rays, rain, and nutrients from the soil. Yet we cannot eat sunlight or soil directly. In order to survive, we depend on plants to photosynthesize, to bond the solar energy into the constituents of earth and water present in their green bodies. Could adoration of this divine process, upon which our lives rest, perhaps be the secret of Soma's ancient alchemical cult?

I hear Dr. Tiwari's voice melodically reciting an ancient Vedic invocation to the plants, asking the blessings of Soma's nutriment to come forth. "Those that are dark and that are bright, the red and the spotted, the brown and the black herbs, all of them do we address. Let them save this man from disease sent by the gods. The plants whose father is heaven, earth the mother, ocean the roots, what power is yours, ye powerful ones, what heroism and strength is yours, herewith, o herbs, free this man from sickness. Now I make a remedy. Let the thoughtful ones come hither, allies of my spell, that we may make this man pass forth out of difficulty. Let the powerful plants that are praised save this village, cow, horse, man, and beast. Rich in sweets the root, rich in sweets the tip of them, rich in sweets the middle of the plants, rich in sweets the leaf, rich in sweets the lower of them. Partaking of sweet, a drink of nectar, let them milk out ghee and food, with milk as chief. However many may be these herbs upon the earth, let them, thousand-leafed, free me from death, from distress.

"I want to discuss one word here," my teacher had said when finished. "It is madhu, the sweet taste. In the old days there was a branch of science known as madhu vidya. It was the science of increasing the life span, giving freedom from the aging process, stress, desires, and lust. This prayer belongs to those used for potentizing drugs. *Rich in sweets* means the person takes the plant and prays, 'O God, you enrich the root, you enrich the leaf, you enrich the stem, you enrich the flower, the seeds.' It means you activate these parts of the plants for medicinal purposes and elimination of disease."

As the wind dies down and the heat of the day recedes from the oncoming coolness of evening, the lake's surface becomes a silky skin, moist with impressionistic reflections. The insects of the forest begin their chant. They unite in one voice, spinning wheels within wheels of hypnotic droning. Quietly at first, then louder, pulsing in rhythms of secret entomological meaning, the trees resonate with an otherworldly chorus of primitive sound.

A voice is coming from somewhere in the vine-covered bluffs above. Could there be someone in a cave, hidden among the stony turrets?

Now it's gone, and only the breeze streams through the forest and across the water. Again the song comes, in an alien yet familiar tongue. The voice is distinctly feminine, but still unseen in the heights. Now a woman appears, standing somehow against the vertical face of the cliff. She is working, either harvesting herbs or cutting wood, standing on sheer ledges hundreds of feet above the treetops, singing fearlessly. I watch, amazed, waiting for her next song, her next prayer, to drift down to the lake. But she is gone, leaving only the sound of water against the boat's wooden hull.

The sun departs with regal farewells, painting another noble Himalayan sunset with lavender, orange, violet, and rose. High above, the clouds become weightless worlds of opalescent landscapes. Slowly, imperceptibly, the vision changes to shining bronze, dies down to flaming orange, then fades into the gray tones of approaching night. The peaks around Machupuchare recede in fading gray hues, disappearing into the approaching evening. The invisible veil between inner and outer, earth, sky, and water, vanishes in the stillness. Unknowingly, I have drifted into samadhi, suspended in open expanses of evening light. I float silently through space, among clouds reflected deep in the lake.

All of Creation is breathing together in this moment. We are asleep to its movement, but our bodies remember. The breath flows in to give another moment of life, and then back to its source in a continual prayer, expressing the innermost thoughts of the heart. Echoes of voices are floating in the wind, spoken, chanted, and sung since beginningless time with the same air that now enters my chest. I remember Dr. Tiwari's wisdom, and pray that others may also hear it: "All life on earth is based on plants. Without them we cannot survive. Without plants, there will be no prana vayu, life-sustaining air."

Nighttime has come again. Looking at the sky, I remember a time when we knew the stars intimately, when their presence was close, when their rays danced in the liquid of our wondering eyes. Before our minds were captivated by technology, we saw the world as a magical place. In the depths of our sleep move the dreams our ancestors dreamed as they lay upon the peaceful earth.

I am floating, somewhere between worlds. Outside, the crickets and fireflies are still awake, while inside, my dreams are coming to life. The stars begin to speak in ancient voices, words of light older than this world, roaring suns filling the firmament with quiet wonder. The winds breathe secret languages, inhaling and exhaling the perfumes of the seasons; they have been everywhere, and know everything. Womblike caves enclose the space of contemplative emptiness, mouths agape with the mountain's call to hear the silence of all-knowing. Playful flowers open the iris of their single chakra, giving birth to realms of color and fragrance; anemones and seashells lie in sensual pools of liquid mandalas.

I wander, enchanted, through the invisible landscapes of sleep. Goddess Moon unwraps her silk cloud-kimono, revealing her milky radiance; sighs of poetry rise on coiling incense dragons as she undulates the currents of the night.

Far back in the boulder-strewn canyons of California's high Mojave grow secret gardens of wild medicines. They are protected by a long day's hike in the blazing heat, along streambeds where water flows in the cool of the night and disappears during the day. There are guardians along the way, copper rattlesnakes coiled in unseen places, red-tailed hawks watching every movement in the landscape from the heights. Where there is no trail, nature's finest remedies are close by.

I hiked past granite walls and flowered grottoes, pushed through tangles of cottonwood, climbed through a thicket of willow, and entered a clearing. The stream emerged from overhanging branches, funneled through chutes and pools of smooth rock, then turned to ripple across a sandy bed at the base of a cliff. In the sun lay a moist embankment awash with white flowers, a small stand of precious herbs, a fine collection of native yerba mansa.

My first impression of this beautiful wild garden was that of a feminine, yin quality. Tender shades of green, the wet creek soil, and delicate petals dancing in the breeze gave the place a vulnerable, pristine feeling, as if bending a single leaf or making any imprint upon nature's innocence would be a violation of its quiet harmony.

I sat, meditated, and prayed, then began my work. As I started digging I discovered that beneath the landscape's soft exterior lay a tenacious foundation of strength. The sandy soil on top covered a deeper layer of dense, firm, and impenetrable clay. As I labored to extricate the first plant, it became obvious that these were creatures who would not be easily removed from their home.

Here was a tightly knit family. The larger plants stood proudly over younger ones, who eagerly spread their leaves in anticipation of the time when they, too, could boast a tall stem topped with white. Long bundles of roots reached deep into the compact soil, intertwined like arms linked in companionship. Strong, stubborn, and succulent, the stalks snapped easily in my hand, leaving the taproot intact in the earth. Even if I took their upper parts, this community was here to stay.

All around the herbs was a bedding of mulch which had accumulated from dried grasses and fallen leaves. This, too, was a community, I discovered. At the first disturbance of their home, swarms of ladybugs emerged, awakened from their afternoon siesta. They began running up the stalks of grass and yerba mansa, groping in space with tiny hands and feelers, then turning around to run down or taking flight if the way was blocked by newcomers. They climbed over one another, swiveling from the top and bottom sides of overhanging leaves, getting pushed off to fall back into the soft bedding.

I worked through the afternoon, slowly gathering a few well-entrenched roots. It was good to be close to the earth in this quiet place, gently digging, scraping, pulling, and prodding, wishing I had magical powers of love that could coax these beings to release themselves willingly into my waiting hands. I thought of Dr. Tiwari, the most knowledgeable of herbalists, and some of the words of wisdom he had imparted to me in my studies.

"Most plant functions are also in our body," he had said, describing how similar and closely related the human form is to the botanical realm. "We can say the bark is the skin, the xylem is like our blood vessels. The roots are the main source of absorption, so we can say they are the oral cavity and intestine, where everything we eat is absorbed. The heartwood is like bone. Plants absorb and release gases, which we can correlate with our respiratory system; they vaporize water, which is like our sweat, and also have hairs.

"There are metabolic systems in both plants and humans. They biotransform solar energy, and we consume that energy as food and drugs. They have defense mechanisms, such as releasing aromatics from leaves or chemical toxins from the roots. Cacti in the barren deserts transform their leaves into waxy layers to avoid evaporation of water.

"Plants are alive, so they have prana, like our bodies. They die and are reborn; according to Ayurved, we also take rebirth. Plants have ojas and produce seeds, which grow the next year. They try to continue their race, which is the main activity of living things."

And what are the differences between the vegetal world and human life?

"The only difference between plants and humans is that we can express our views and feelings in words," my teacher explained. "Plants are beings, and because of the karma of their past actions, they have been reborn in the botanical kingdom. They have a specific kind of consciousness known as antas cheta, internal senses. They feel pleasure, pain, desire, and worry, and express themselves in symptoms. Maybe they use words, but we don't understand them. They have minds."

"Plants have minds?" I wondered.

"Yes. If you have no consciousness, you can't feel pleasure or pain. There are many yogis who have powers, so they don't feel pain. The mind is present, but they control it and cut the feelings. Plants can't do this; they always feel."

"Worry means thinking of the future, and desire is based on memory," I observed.

"Yes. Plants have memory. There are studies which have shown that they can remember individual people."

"How do plants communicate?" I inquired.

"In some form of signals," Dr. Tiwari replied. "If you are able to catch that signal, you can know what they are saying. One study showed there are some species that like music very much, and that it increases their growth. It is difficult to say what is the mode of action or mechanism, but observation shows that they have consciousness and they communicate."

"Have you heard of people who can communicate with plants?" I asked.

"I think that is at the mental level, in the form of feelings. There was a hakim in the past, a Muslim Unani doctor named Lukuman. When he went into the forest the herbs would say to him, 'I am useful for this type of disease,' and when he needed to he would go and get them."

How wonderful to have that gift! I reflected, thinking of other stories I had heard about herbalists who could hear those languages. No need for the burdens of scholarly academic training in biochemistry, no debates about the flavors, temperatures, and modes of action, no uncertainties about the side effects possible in every clinical application; just simple, direct knowing from listening deeply enough to the voices from the earth.

And what would happen, I wondered, if we all woke one morning and our ears could hear the subtle messages spoken by the plants? Would we still be able to cut down trees, spray poisons on our crops, and slash and burn the jungles? Or would we suddenly realize that our lives depend on the wisdom and power of these sentient beings, and that only by caring for them and providing them what they require will we survive?

"According to Ayurveda," my mentor continued, "when we collect plants, we first pray and invite them by saying, 'I want to use you as a medicine.' We worship them, then dig. This means you recognize them as a living being, not just an herb. Those types of drugs are more effective."

"How does praying increase their potency?" I asked.

"We know plants have consciousness and can feel internally. When you pray, you show them your soft nature. They become delighted, knowing that they are going to serve others."

I stood to stretch and breathe. As I gazed at the land around me, a renewed appreciation of the herbs began to dawn. Here was the work of the Creator's hand, lovingly sculpted with fingers of fire, wind, water, earth, and sky. How could the plants not be sacred food? Across the stream directly facing the wild garden, marbled granite slabs rose like stacked pyramids, skin smooth and cracked by the fierce sun. Veins of textures and patterns of lichen wove a quilt of color across their surfaces. From the cracks hung small bushes and shrubs, and in larger crevasses an occasional piñon had made itself at home. In the other direction huge boulders rose on yucca-dotted hills to the highest ridge. Every place I looked was shimmering with dry heat, heat which sucked the moist vapors from living things. This green embankment was a jewel island of moisture in a dry sea of blazing stone. All the vegetation around was toughened like tortoiseshell and lizard skin, protecting the core of vulnerable life from the sky's exhausting rays. Yet here stood this yerba mansa, soft and playful in the harsh environment, embodying the vitality of the desert.

"And what is the effect of mantra and puja on the preparations of medicines?" I had asked the botanist.

"According to Ayurveda, mantras and pujas make medicines more efficacious," he answered. "You are using your inner energy to potentize the drug. The biochemistry of this is unknown.

"Sanyasins and saddhus just give the ash of their fireplace to patients, and many people claim they have been cured. Maybe those saddhus somehow put their own energy into the ash, and that is how it cured the disease. Some people use mantras for treating illness, generally in psychic conditions. They read some prayers, put some drugs in the fire and fumigate the patients, and after some time they will recover. When we recite mantric verses, the words change into energy, and that may decrease the doshas. When we pronounce sacred syllables, the pitch, tone, and wavelength vary, so maybe these are responsible for changing the enzymes and hormones in the brain, which could give relief. This is the science of sound."

I tasted a small piece of yerba mansa root; my tongue told me it had captured the healing powers of fire and water, the desert heat and the soothing stream. It was pink, succulent, and slightly fibrous, and crunched as I chewed it. Immediately a sharp pungency sent a fiery sensation through my mouth, like tasting the intensity of long Mojave days. As the flavor decreased and my saliva mixed with the plant's juices, a sweet, clean aftertaste began to emerge. It was the water element, the ripples of the stream in the cattails, the shade of the willows, the coming of evening.

"Sun and moon are responsible for drug efficacy and action," Dr. Tiwari had said. "We know that the moon is soft in nature, and the sun sharp. Drugs that grow in areas where daytime is longer are hotter in nature, quick-acting, and sharp. On that basis we classify our drugs into Agni (solar fire), and Soma (lunar liquids). Drugs which are responsible for increasing pitta are related to the sun, and drugs which are responsible for increasing the body weight, the semen, bone, and fat are related to the moon."

"How does Ayurveda understand photosynthesis?" I asked, curious about the classical understanding of the relationship between vegetation and the solar current.

"The terminology is different," the botanist replied. "In the Hindu tradition we worship the sun, and know that it is responsible for all growth, creation, and energy on the earth."

"Never dig herbs at night," he explained. "Always dig them in the presence of the sun, and that drug will be more effective. Due to sunlight many biochemical transformations take place, and specific chemical constituents are present. There are many studies that have proven that in specific seasons and times of day, the concentration of chemical constituents is higher or lower."

I chewed the root, trying to taste my memories of how this yerba mansa cured illness. The Native Americans thought highly of it, and used it as a general tonic. Its pungency spread upward from my stomach, and I could feel it enlivening the prana of my lungs and opening my breathing. It was a renowned restorative of the mucous membranes. This influence would resolve phlegm, ease coughing, and strengthen digestion. As I assimilated the plant I felt the curative powers of the wilderness enter my body.

The remedy was very potent, like the uncompromising desert. It demanded respect and caution, mindfulness and care, so as to not cause harm. I instinctively knew that a small piece was quite sufficient for now. I returned to digging and soon felt the second phase of digestion sending waves of heat rising through my upper body. A pungent aroma from the opened soil perfumed the late afternoon air.

A golden glow descended as the sun withdrew toward the hilltops. Orange light retreated up the boulders to the piñon tops, and shadows covered the garden. Harvesting proceeded slowly as I reached deeper into the soil, meticulously excavating around the bundles of rootlets. When each plant emerged I touched its leaves to my face, smelling its perfume, listening to what it might tell me. Thinking of it as an offering,

I imagined its journey into a world of ailing people, and its noble purpose of healing sickness. My hands respectfully held each one, as if to make them feel calmer. Once, I sensed communication. *Put us in the stream and we will be happy,* they said without words.

When the day was gone I lay on the grass across the stream from the precious herbs. The desert night found me lost in contemplation about all I had seen, heard, and felt that day. There were the stones decorated with lichens, which had their own curative virtues, the willows with theirs, the wild nourishing foods given by the cattails, oaks, and piñons, the potent essential oils of the pines and junipers, the mysterious forgotten powers of the cacti. Along the water were many beneficial flowers and shrubs, mosses, molds, and fungi that I had no knowledge of. The rattlesnakes had their own powers, and the hawks and other birds that had gone to rest had theirs. The ladybugs played their role, as did the tadpoles in the stream.

"We only think of those species which are directly useful for us," Dr. Tiwari had said, "but so many things in nature are responsible for our existence. Frogs control mosquitoes, snakes control rats, turtles purify water. Earthworms digest leaves and increase soil, birds are responsible for the propagation and survival of plants. Microbes decompose waste and convert it into other forms.

"These things are always helping us indirectly, and are necessary for our survival. This is why spiritual teachings say that everything is created by God, and the things created by God are very important. They say: Do not destroy those things, but live with them in harmony; don't show your supremacy and think you are the rulers of those species.

"We are always taking rebirth, going in a circular movement, and we will not necessarily be born in a human body. With that kind of thinking, we become very conscious about nature."

That night the harvested yerba mansa slept piled together in a bundle, their roots bathed in cool water. One last time their leaves drank the light of the desert moon.

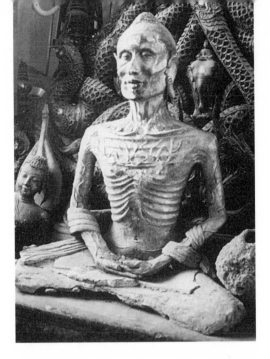

VI.

DESIRE AND EMANCIPATION

In our Hindu culture, there are many austerities which are practiced. Some yogis

take only one meal a day, some sit naked in the cold, or under the hot sun without

protection. Since the age of thirteen I have given up all the tastes; I returned to the

first food, that which we ate when we were children. For me, this was a kind of

penance.

In this world there are two kinds of knowledge—material and spiritual.

Through this austerity of living on milk alone, I have gained spiritual knowledge.

I have become free of desire. Nobody can be entirely free of desire, of course, because then we would be only a corpse. But I have no wrongful desires, like those that fill the minds of people in this Kali Yuga. I have only the simplest of desires: for meditation, and milk. In this way I have gained much understanding, and can now give many people good counsel.

THE "MILK BABA" OF PASHUPATINATH

Dr. Chopel opened his text of the *Root Tantra*. We were beginning studies of the "branch of root causes of disease." He adjusted his glasses and looked up to make sure he had my full attention.

"The path of the healer leads to knowing that even the complete cure of a disease is only symptomatic treatment," the physician-monk said. Even after years of considering my teacher's pithy statement, I would find new levels of meaning in his words. What he was saying, I realize now, was that medicine eventually brings one to the realm of spirituality.

"This branch of medical knowledge has three leaves, which represent the three 'root obscurations' of desire, anger, and ignorance," Amchi-la explained. "These are known as the three 'mind poisons.' Because of their presence in the body, they develop into Air, Bile, and Phlegm humors." On the Tree of Knowledge, the leaf of desire depicts a couple in sexual intercourse under a blanket; the leaf of anger shows two men fighting with swords; and the leaf of ignorance, or mental dullness, shows a man lying asleep.

"Human beings are born due to karmic forces," Dr. Chopel went on. "Once this form is taken, the three biological humors are present within us. These are called the three 'foundations,' the 'preservers,' or 'pillars of life,' because they give us good health and strength when they are balanced. They are also called the 'destroyers' or the 'punishments,' because when they are out of balance they cause disease and death. Therefore, all physical wellbeing or suffering is dependent on the three humors. Typically, Air, Bile, and Phlegm are governed by the three mental poisons."

I knew from earlier lessons that the humors had both physical and mental characteristics, which functioned inseparably. Now, Amchi-la was clarifying that the ripening of past actions is the cause of the body's creation, and once consciousness is embodied, its "three obscurations" affect health by influencing the activities of the biological humors. Craving is the primary force which activates Air, the nerve currents; anger aggravates Bile, the acids of digestion; and mental torpor increases Phlegm, the body's mucous secretions.

"Desire, anger, and stupidity all come from one cause," the doctor said. "This is marigpa, spiritual ignorance. Since all non-virtuous thoughts and actions come from marigpa, it is very important to understand what it is. Marigpa can be compared to blindness: it is non-seeing, non-understanding, and non-recognizing. Every person, having been born from a womb, identifies with his or her body, and has the feeling of 'I' and 'my.' This egocentric thinking, along with the natural greediness it produces, is marigpa."

I remembered Kalu Rinpoche explaining how consciousness becomes obscured by the limitations of the body. The mind in its natural state is inherently pure, he had said. It has no form, no center or cir-cumference, and resides in no particular location. From the time of birth onward, this universal field of awareness is distorted by the flow of self-oriented thoughts, feelings, and perceptions, as the attention of the in-dividual becomes preoccupied with the body. The stream of discursive thinking flows continually through waking hours and into sleep, creat-ing the dualistic experience of self and others, inside and outside, dreamer and dreaming. This continues throughout one's lifetime, and does not end with the death of the physical body; the experiences and visions which occur in the afterlife are similar to the dream state.

Dr. Chopel continued. "The consciousness of each of the senses per-ceives the various sense objects, then judges what it perceives. If a sight, sound, taste, smell, or feeling is perceived as pleasing, then desire and attachment arise; if consciousness perceives things as ugly or bad, then anger and aversion arise. This is marigpa operating within the sense or-gans.

"When the three humors are well balanced, they act as preservers of the body, but when they are decreased, increased, or conflicting, they become pathological factors, and diseases arise. Under the influence of marigpa, sense consciousness continuously pushes the three humors toward imbalances. In order to have equilibrium among the humors, one must control marigpa, the ultimate cause of imbalances. Since marigpa is at the root of all sickness, and ultimately all suffering, it can be seen that there is one cause to the numerous diseases, rather than many."

Marigpa is the loss of pristine awareness that occurs as subjective consciousness interprets sensory experiences within each mental mo-ment. In the instant following every sensation, there are gross and sub-tle reactions of grasping and aversion, seeking gratification and avoiding discomfort, which cloud our otherwise pure perception. In turn, the proliferation of likes and dislikes sets in motion the karmas of habitual behavior, and the cumulative effects of these actions become, as this branch of the *Tsa Gyu* revealed, the root causes of diseases.

"Like a moth attracted to a flame," Amchi-la said, "each sense organ can be the cause of diseases, and lead to destruction. In Kham [eastern Tibet] hunters use flutes to attract deer, who are deceived by their attraction to the melodious sound. The smell of fat attracts the fox; fish are attracted to the taste of the worm on a hook; and the elephant is attracted to the sensation of rolling in the soft leaves laid over the trap."

The old doctor paused and smiled. "It is easy to understand these things in medical practice," he said. "Look how many people eat themselves to death because of their attraction to the sense of taste. We can find many examples of diseases that are caused in this way."

As Dr. Chopel observed, mentally clinging to sensory pleasures is one of the primary ways people destroy their health. Whether due to grossly destructive addictions such as alcohol, tobacco, and drug abuse, or subtle and insidious hungers for stimulation, power, and wealth, most illness can ultimately be linked to marigpa. Under the influence of the mind poisons, we crave that which is harmful, have aversion to that which is beneficial, and are bewildered about how to care for ourselves. This primordial ignorance is not only the root of individual illness, but the ultimate cause of collective suffering for communities and nations as well. Marigpa's spiritual darkness creates greed, hatred, and fear; these in turn give birth to war, poverty, and environmental degradation of soil, water, and air, resulting in famine and epidemics.

Ayurvedic and Tibetan medicines provide a complete and systematic understanding of how lifestyle, diet, and psychological states affect individuals, and what therapeutic regimens can be used as antidotes to imbalances caused by the three mental poisons. Knowing how marigpa affects us, and how to remove its detrimental impact by using specific healing protocols, helps cure and prevent diseases and improve the quality of life. If applied by enough people, the methods prescribed by classical Tibetan and Ayurvedc medicine for achieving wellbeing can become the basis for healthy communities, nations, and the natural environment, thereby eliminating the need for many medical treatments.

Yet, as Dr. Chopel had stated, even curative medicines and treatments are ultimately only symptomatic relief. As long as marigpa remains, individually and collectively, emotionality arising from attachment to the body will be the seed of future unhappiness and disease.

"A healthy person also has marigpa," Amchi-la went on. "Balance of the three humors gives good health, and there appears to be no affliction. However, like a bird flying high in the sky whose shadow cannot be seen, marigpa still exists, and the potential for suffering is still present. In order to remove a poisonous tree, it must be taken out by the roots; if the branches are cut, they will simply grow back. Likewise, if medicines are given, they will help the disease, but will not remove marigpa, the original cause."

If good health alone is not enough to eliminate the seeds of marigpa, how are we to remove the veil of spiritual ignorance that covers the senses, and resolve suffering at its root?

"Wisdom is the opposite of ignorance," Dr. Chopel explained. "Wisdom leads to understanding, and ignorance obscures wisdom. Ignorance gives rise to various forms of craving and aversion, and from this come the multitudes of sufferings. When wisdom is obscured, we lack a clear understanding of the true nature of how things are. Because of ignorance, we cannot understand true happiness; we are like a person trying to choose between precious and non-precious metals with eyes closed. The cause of diseases, suffering, and unhappiness is the mind poisons; these obscurations should be abandoned, and one should seek the everlasting happiness of enlightenment.

"In order to stop marigpa, we must cultivate the 'wisdom of not possessing.' Our body is the primary source of attachment and aversion, but any phenomenon can be their cause. Knowing how the senses can lead to destruction, we contemplate how the body and all things are impermanent, and examine whether they provide lasting happiness or not. By recognizing the impermanence of both external objects and oneself, we can clearly understand the true nature of phenomena. Thinking in this way develops the 'wisdom of not possessing'; this controls marigpa, overcomes the three obscurations of consciousness, prevents attachment and aversion before they cause harm, and pacifies disease."

According to Ayurveda, even if the biological elements are balanced, a person is not healthy unless the mind, senses, and spirit are happy. As long as primordial ignorance obscures consciousness, it is impossible to find the inner peace that nourishes physiological harmony. Under the influence of marigpa, our attention is disturbed by endless distractions, which cause the mind to fluctuate between restless agitation and fatigued oblivion. Seeking relief from the pain of inner turmoil, unhappy memories, self-judgments, unconscious habits, and destructive ambitions, we take refuge in material comforts, social diversions, and sensory pleasures, only to find them becoming toxic addictions. Blinded by marigpa, we fail to perceive the ungraspable nature of sensory experiences and how every feeling dissolves the moment it arises. Cravings for transient sensations of pleasure are ultimately impossible to satisfy; instead, they tend to cause dissipation of life force, accelerated aging, and illness.

Dr. Chopel continued. "When we perceive something as beautiful and attractive, it is the creation of the mind. When we analyze the object of our attraction and attachment, we find only the elements that constitute that object. For example, when a man sees the face of a beautiful woman, attraction arises within his mind. If we analyze what the face is actually composed of, we find such things as the pores and oils of the skin, the bodily secretions such as tears, saliva and mucus, teeth, hair, and so forth. Even the individual parts can be seen as being subject to impermanence and decay. Outwardly the body appears as beautiful, but inwardly it is filled with impurities. If we examine the objects of our attraction in this manner, we ultimately find there is nothing to become attached to."

Amchi-la's discourse presented a formidable challenge: to see the illusory, ungraspable, and dissatisfactory nature of what we are most

attracted to. Why would we want to think of ourselves and others as re-
pulsive bags of bodily wastes, I wondered, when making the body desir-
able and attractive has been one of the primary goals of human life? The
doctor's words came directly from Buddha's first noble truth: all realms
of samsara are permeated with suffering. Even the most blissful sexual
embrace or the highest pleasures of the gods are tinged with subtle dis-
comforts, and always end. The most handsome men and beautiful women
grow old, their attractiveness evaporates, and the body becomes plagued
with the miseries of aging and illness.

Dr. Chopel's teaching also expressed the second noble truth: that
the dissatisfaction inherent in existence has a cause, marigpa, the spiritual blindness preventing insight into the nature of what we crave or
wish to avoid. His words also contained the third noble truth: that there
is an end to this cycle of unhappiness, nirvana, the cessation of craving.
The way to this goal was the fourth noble truth: the Path. In Amchi-la's
teaching, this was the "wisdom of not possessing," recognizing that
everything we grasp and cling to is impermanent.

Amchi-la's terse and concise comments on the "branch of root causes
of disease" were pure Buddhist Dharma. Using the language of Tibetan
medicine, he succinctly described how equanimity and detachment born
of insight into reality liberate us from the poisons of desire, anger, and
ignorance, freeing us from disease and suffering. Lasting happiness cannot be found through any activity motivated by the three mental poisons. To achieve happiness, the mind must be purified of its poisons, so
its inherent spiritual qualities can become manifest. A peaceful mind
promotes equilibrium of the biological humors, restores health, and infuses the body with the light of inner happiness.

"Marigpa is depicted on the Tibetan wheel of life as an old blind
woman walking with a cane," Dr. Chopel concluded. "This is because
marigpa eliminates the wisdom of seeing. Although one may have intelligent wisdom, marigpa in the body obscures and veils it. There are said
to be 84,000 types of emotional conflicts, the root of which is marigpa;

because sentient beings have marigpa, they wander in the world of suffering.

"By understanding marigpa and the mental poisons, we can close the door to all diseases arising. Trying to comprehend marigpa right now doesn't mean we will become free from suffering immediately. However, from now on, we can begin to realize its meaning and to lighten the weight of suffering. Simply lighting a full butter lamp will not burn all its fuel at once; the flame will slowly consume the butter, and eventually it will burn out. Likewise, as we slowly learn to understand marigpa and how to become free of its negative effects, we attain enlightenment."

It is dawn in Kathmandu. Fog lies on the valley, a thick shroud of penetrating cold that seeps into one's marrow. As the sky brightens, the outline of the surrounding mountains slowly emerges, like ancient figures from a distant world reclining against the horizon. Huge houses dominate the misty skyline of my neighborhood in Balwatar, multistoried structures of layered rooftops and balconies, draped with vines, flowers, and laundry. The brick and concrete of the homes absorb the dampness of winter, and every house, no matter how affluent, is permeated with a mildewed atmosphere.

Every morning my neighbors stand on their terraces, making incense offerings of guggul and camphor to the sky, throwing pinches of grains to the devas in their celestial abodes, as pigeons watch eagerly. A woman next door brushes her long, luxurious black hair, while the sky changes from steel gray to faint translucent turquoise. The sound of drums and horns comes from the distance, and a pujari drones a stream of verses.

Flocks of crows wing toward the east, their rasping calls mingling with a chorus of dogs barking in the alleys below. One of the birds alights on the railing of my roof, momentarily becoming a black silhouette against the aquamarine light of morning. For an instant the creature is transformed into Kag Basundi, the immortal crow god, who knows many languages and the lore of herbs. To learn the secrets of plant medicines, the yogis of the forest say, watch the ways of animals. The bird stares in my direction, the last ray of Venus fading above its head.

As the sun rises through prayer flags hanging across rooftops, I find myself mentally repeating the Gayatri mantra, the Vedic invocation to the Creator of earth, space, and heavens. The mantra is a salutation to the light of the Supreme Self, visibly manifest as the dynamic energy of the rising sun. The solar face of God looks upon the world with dazzling golden eyes and speaks with a flashing golden tongue. His arms of sunlight reach out to embrace the cosmos in loving benediction, as He rides a chariot drawn by the glittering steeds of a new day. It is His life force that awakens all beings from the small death of sleep, and greets them when they return from the deep sleep of death.

The sun's magnificence is the object of daily veneration by Brahmins; their lineages of praise, hymns, and rituals greeting the morning light have been passed down from father to son through the millennia, since the days of the early Aryan nomads. They stand and greet the rising face, reciting the most sacred of prayers descended from the glorious ages of Vedic fire-worship. "Let us worship and adore the wondrous spirit of Divinity," they chant in Sanskrit. "May its light inspire our minds with divine qualities."

As another day begins, the women of Kathmandu start their cooking fires. Agni, the personification of fire, is also worshipped by the Brahmins, as the visible and tangible presence of God. Every morning, in every town and village across Nepal, Agni leaps to life in the hearth, his altar, ravenously devouring the wood that gave him birth. He is the guest of every home, watching with flickering eyes over those who bring offerings of fuel, sending rays of light from his restless body as he consumes the oblations with golden teeth.

Agni is the creator of the sun, and the one who fills the night with stars. He appears as lightning flashing through the sky, phosphorescence in dark ocean waters, the bubbling lava of volcanoes, nuclear fire within atoms, the electrical current illuminating modern homes. Agni is the inner animating warmth residing within all creatures. At death he consumes the empty corpse on the pyre, revives the soul for its journey into the afterlife, and then lovingly nourishes the embryonic seed of a new incarnation in another womb. Everything and everyone has entered and emerged from Agni many times in the transmigration through cyclical existence; he knows all intimately, yet they know him not.

The god of fire plays a central role in the medicine of the Vedas. Agni is the universal thermogenic power that catalyzes matter from one state to another; Agni functions physiologically as the enzymatic and cellular fire that releases the light, energy, and warmth stored within food and leaves residual wastes for elimination. These two processes, which cover the scope of all metabolic activities, are the basis of health; when they are disordered, they become the two primary roots of disease: decreased vitality and increased toxicity. Our health is entirely dependent on Agni's harmonious functioning. All illnesses, especially those that affect the abdomen, are associated with disturbances in Agni's activity.

Classical Asian medical philosophies use the cooking fire of the hearth as an analogy for the digestive process. Ayurveda describes Agni as the fire of digestion, the god in our bellies to whom we make offerings every meal. Agni resides throughout the body but is concentrated in the stomach and intestines; a simple correlation can be made between Agni as understood by Ayurveda, and the secretion of bile, digestive acids, and enzymes known to modern physiology. Agni's primary function in the digestive tract is to separate pure nutrients from impure by-products and to detoxify wastes in the gut. Agni's fiery appetite releases the essences derived from the soil and sunlight and stored in the plants of our diet, making them available to nourish the body, leaving behind the residue of ash to be carried away by the bowels.

Using the metaphoric language of natural phenomena, Ayurveda describes the physiological events that occur when Agni loses equilibrium. When Agni becomes too hot, it produces symptoms of hyperactive metabolism. Food is digested rapidly; there is frequent hunger and thirst, and an increase of pitta, Bile humor. When Agni is decreased, it produces symptoms of hypoactive metabolism and phlegmatic conditions of kapha humor. Digestion of food is slow and nutrients are poorly assimilated; metabolic processes become sluggish and blocked by fluid stagnation. When Agni is erratic it is said to be affected by vata, the Air humor. Sometimes the appetite is high with rapid digestion, sometimes it is low and digestion is weak; the bowels tend to be loose, and peristalsis uneven.

When Agni is balanced, digestion proceeds smoothly and comfortably. There is no gas, distension, burning, belching, reflux, pain, or stagnation. The movement of the intestinal tract is regular, nutrients are efficiently extracted and utilized by the body, and waste products are easily eliminated. The body temperature remains steady, the complexion has a healthy glow, the light of the eyes is bright, the mind is clear. One feels a natural happiness arising from the comfort of good health.

All around Kathmandu, from the simple gardens of its neighborhoods to the thick jungles of the far mountainsides, the plants are adoring the king of warmth and light as he rises into a new morning. Their sprouting seeds push up through the soil, branches multiplying like arms outstretched in worship, leaves unfurling in joyous devotion, and flowers bursting with nectared offerings of colors and fragrance. All day the vegetal kingdom drinks the shimmering rays from the sky, transforming them into the nutritive basis of life on earth. Agni ripens the rice in the terraces, the yellow mustard dancing in the fields, the fruits of the orchard and vegetables of the farm.

Agni has many appearances, both beneficent and terrible. He awakens the diverse forms of life, then lives within them as the continuous appetite they must appease. When the stomach hungers, it is Agni who wishes to eat, and from the first suckling to the final meal, it is his blessings that satisfy us. Two thousand years ago the fire god's scorching fingers altered the Indian landscape forever, as Aryan tribes burned away the virgin jungles, opening the way for agriculture, livestock, villages, and empires. Now the air of Kathmandu is a heavy brown as its energy-hungry population consumes precious wood from what remains of the vanishing forests. Without trees the sweet Soma of the rainy season's moisture will not come, and Agni changes from a loving god to a fierce demon who mercilessly lays the earth to waste with drought.

Whether it burns within an individual or inflames an entire planet, fever, says Ayurveda, is Agni's way of purifying the toxins created by life that is out of balance, the fire sent by Shiva to afflict those who do not live by the laws of nature. "In this dark age of the Kali Yuga," Dr. Chopel once said, "less virtuous beings are attacked by different kinds of fevers. These fevers are similar in nature but also changeable, so the doctor can be easily mistaken. There are fevers that are hard to identify, and those that are hard to cure. The rapid flourishing of fever is also very common; in the Kali Yuga some types of diseases will be fatal even within a few moments of exposure. When a fever is combined with infection, it can also develop into mysterious diseases, such as various forms of cancer."

Cars honk on the Ring Road in the distance; they are lined up for blocks, waiting to get to the petrol pumps, closed due to a strike against a new gas tax. The police watch the angry drivers, as the deep and volatile frustrations of poverty and hardship threaten to ignite into violence and upheaval. Desire and anger are also forms of fire, said the mystics through the ages, whose minds flowed with Soma's cooling equanimity. The more we incite the flames of aggressive passions, the darker grows the future, as the spreading fires of war poison the fragile skies. High in the Himalayan snow ranges where Shiva and Shakti dwell, armies fight suicidal battles in the name of religious hatred and imaginary boundaries, tempting the Creator's wrath. Devoid of compassion, the marriage of science to the military has given birth to the sacrilegious alchemy of transforming nature's vital energy into atomic incineration; India, in its nationalistic pride, has christened its nuclear child "Agni." Will the beautiful history of this spiritual homeland end in radioactive annihilation, Agni's retribution for our desecration of life's sanctity?

Or will we dispel the coming darkness by opening our hearts to universal wisdom, so eloquently expounded by the ancient seers? Agni, they proclaimed, lives within us as the light of the mind, heart, and soul. Agni's transmutations purify us at every level, from cellular metabolism, through the mental assimilation of thoughts and ideas, to the innermost radiance that cleanses the spirit and sets it free of karmic seeds embedded within layers of habitual cravings. Agni is the capacity to discriminate between truth and illusion, and the flame of attention which illuminates reality and dispels the shadows of confusion. It is the brightness of intelligence and understanding that nourish the mind and help us accomplish our goals, whether they be worldly attainments or the highest emancipation from all suffering. Humanity is blessed with Agni's powers, yet lives in ignorance of its divine presence; we hold the key to our future existences, whether they be nuclear hell-realms or ages of enlightened culture.

Deep in the heart, the center of our being, where Agni burns with pure love and unclouded perception, is the true alchemical gold, the "gold of the wise," which renders metallic gold worthless. Compared to Agni's spiritual effulgence, the sun of our world is a black orb, illuminating maya's shadows of delusion. Blazing with the beauty of its ancient fire, the pearl of supreme consciousness lies waiting, calling us from the slumber we mistake for wakefulness. Its wonders unfold around us in every moment, yet we do not see them; the path to emancipation is open before us at all times, yet we choose not to follow it. How long will we resist the nectar of freedom?

The sun is climbing across the Nepalese sky. The dew has evaporated from the jungle leaves, the mists have dissolved into the browns of another smoggy Kathmandu day. The streets are full of people and ve-

hicles moving under the watchful eye and outstretched arms of the solar deity, burning since time immemorial. His beams are streaming down
on the vegetation of the earth, nourishing our bodies with life-sustaining
warmth, flowing through our blood, shining from our eyes. It is an instant
within the eternal cycle of light.

Agni is proclaiming his presence in my belly, reminding me that a
good physician gives attention to regulating the temperature of the digestive heat. It is time for porridge.

"I will now teach you about incense therapy," Dr. Aryal said. Gopal and
I sat in the alchemist's room, ready for another day of study and work.
The doctor reached into a cabinet and removed an old text and a bag of
brown powder; he put the book down so we could examine its elaborate
miniature calligraphy, and opened the bag of powder. "This is called
Graha Shanti Dhoop, meaning 'Peaceful Planet Incense,'" he said, sprinkling some on the coals in the censer. The room was filled with a soothing, sweet, mildly floral and spicy fragrance.

Wonderful healing powers are found in the art and science of aromas, one of the oldest forms of medicine in the world. Wafting through
the olfactory channels into the recesses of our ancestral brains, the mysteriously subtle and richly complex smells of essential oils secreted by
plants awaken memories, trigger positive alterations in mood, and stimulate immunity. Fragrance is the bridge connecting the colorfully scented
plant realms, the human heart and soul, and the spheres of the gods.

"This formula makes the ancestors happy," the guru explained. "It
pleases the gods and goddesses, removes negative astrological influences, and guarantees success in one's endeavors. It cures restlessness
and insomnia, and helps the mind become peaceful." The smoke swirled
through shafts of sunlight penetrating the shadows, producing an atmosphere of mellow tranquillity.

Since the dawn of human history, fragrance has accompanied utterances of prayer; incense offerings made to Agni's tongues flickering in altars fill the sky with clouds of pleasant aromas, a feast for the etheric devas dwelling in celestial abodes. This ancient alchemy has always been practiced in temples and shrines, which were the original centers for healing body and mind. When floral nectars cast their spell, the spirit is uplifted, the deities are happy to grace the earth with auspicious events, and magic begins to manifest.

"The most important of the incense formulas is called Siddha Chintamani," our teacher went on. "This means 'What one thinks, manifests,' or more simply, 'Wish-Fulfilling Gem Incense.' It is made from the various herbs you purchased yesterday, which are combined with honey and blessed with mantra. It should be used in a sacred way, because it has great powers."

The alchemist began reading the ingredients from his book. "Take white eaglewood (*Aquillaria*), bark of the cedar tree (*Cedrus deodaria*), white sandalwood (*Santalum album*), kuth (*Saussurea lappa*), nach (*Helix ashera*), nagkesar (*Messua ferra*), and saffron (*Crocus sativus*), in equal parts. Grind them to powder and mix with pure honey."

A long and fascinating botanical history was contained in this simple mixture of flowers, bark, roots, and heartwoods. For centuries, aquillaria, sandalwood, and saffron have been highly esteemed by Tibetan and Ayurvedic doctors, who utilize them as ingredients in oral medications and for fumigation therapy in the treatment of psychiatric conditions. Eaglewood exerts an extraordinary therapeutic influence upon the mind and nervous system by virtue of its sweet, pungent, and warming essential oil, known as "oil of oud." The effects of this rare and exquisite perfume on consciousness are so potent that it is used to open the doors between this world and the next, allowing the dying to pass peacefully into the afterlife. From the sandalwood tree comes a rich oil that is regarded as the most sacred, devotional, and meditative of all fragrances. Sandalwood produces a soothing, calming, and harmonizing effect on the mental atmosphere, helping restore tranquillity lost in the turbulence of worldly distractions; it is said to be the scent emitted by enlightened beings, who have gone beyond cares of the self. Saffron is a medicine for the heart which strengthens faith and devotion and induces compassionate feelings.

These three ingredients were valuable items of commerce along the ancient trade routes of Asia and the Mediterranean countries, finding their way into medicinal formulas of physicians and ceremonial preparations used by shamans, priests, and yogis. Sandalwood and eaglewood trees were once abundant, but centuries of demand for their precious oils have decimated the original forests; their fragrance is not only food of the gods and medicine of the mind, but also a potion that awakens erotic passion, desired by all who enjoy sensual pleasures.

"This formula is more than a thousand years old," Dr. Aryal commented, "and perhaps from another age. The individual ingredients are simple, but their interconnectedness is profound. The ritual use of this compound benefits any kind of work. It brings good luck and good fortune to all endeavors. It is good for one's business, for influencing kings and other important people. It increases the power of magnetism and attraction and helps develop psychic powers. It also drives away snakes if they are troubling your house."

The doctor put down his book. "I have given this to many people and have seen that its powers are effective. One man came to me recently who was seriously troubled by poverty. He had nothing, and was suffering terribly. I gave him this incense and instructed him to offer it to the gods. He started doing this and soon began to attract good fortune and wealth. Now he owns a house and a car."

Siddha Chintamani, the Wish-Fulfilling Jewel, is also the name of White Mahakala, one of the wrathful deities in the Tibetan pantheon of "Dharma protectors." Siddha Chintamani Mahakala dances in a mass of flames upon a fiery sun-disc, red beard and hair flowing upward around his three eyes. With six mighty arms representing the transcendent perfections, he makes gestures of power, scaring away demons with frightful weapons, the sound of his mantra resounding like thunder. A drop of supernaturally pure mercury floats in the center of his heart, while retinues of goddesses remove obstacles and bestow abundance. Pouring priceless gems from a crystal vase, he fills the skies with resplendence and showers the earth with prosperity. His world is a mandala of treasures: the sun is iridescent gold, and the moon polished silver; diamond stars burn in the translucent aquamarine sky; opal clouds float over oceans of liquid turquoise; ruby flowers grow among emerald trees and jade grasses.

White Mahakala is Buddhistic compassion embodied as dynamic energy which liberates from limitations. His form expresses the intense concentration, undistracted presence, unbending will, and joyful detachment needed for manifesting both mundane and extraordinary attainments. Attracting worldly wealth to relieve the suffering of poverty is the most superficial of this deity's powers; his deeper purpose is to provide the spiritual and material resources necessary for Dharma practice by removing self-created obstacles to enlightenment. Like all deities of the Tantric path, Mahakala's immaterial body reveals the supreme accomplishment of overcoming existential ignorance through insight into the inherent insubstantiality of all phenomena. The confused and unenlightened mind is impoverished by ego-clinging, endlessly preoccupied with needs and wants, but in ultimate reality we are wealthy beyond the ability of our conditioned consciousness to imagine. This insight releases the vitality of the spontaneously creative, prosperous, and generous heart.

The day before, Gopal had purchased the herbal ingredients required for Siddha Chintamani incense and had them ground at a local mill. The guru now instructed us to open the bags we had brought, and began measuring the ingredients of the formula, weighing them against old silver coins in his handheld scale. As he added each new powder to the mix, he sprinkled a sample on his censer for us to smell. The room filled with clouds of exotic aromas, and our mood changed to cheerful and talkative. When all the herbs had been measured, Dr. Aryal began mixing honey into the powders.

"Health is not just for man," the alchemist said, meticulously squeezing the sticky mass through his hands. "It is for all—people, animals, and plants. Everything needs health."

Emancipation from the pain of sickness is one of the deepest human desires. As disease sinks its claws into the body, the priorities of one's life are dramatically altered. When it becomes impossible to breathe without a gasping struggle, and discomfort continuously racks the body and agitates the mind, performing work becomes impossible, and ordinary activities are overwhelming. If food cannot be digested and sleep is impossible, all enjoyment vanishes. Without the comfort of health, accomplishing even the smallest task is difficult, and wealth becomes meaningless.

All beings wish to be free from the sorrows of illness. And how intimately interdependent is their wellbeing, I reflected, like the organs of a single body. If the plant kingdom is diseased, humans and animals become sick; if the water, soil, and sky are poisoned, civilization will perish.

"There are many homeless and helpless people suffering from diseases," the doctor went on. "It is very difficult for poor people to go to doctors; one course of modern medicine costs three thousand rupees. But disease affects everybody, those with nothing and those with a lot of money. A doctor should do the best he can for everyone's health, and not look for rich people only. Medicine is for everybody."

When Dharmic generosity and the healing arts are combined, as taught in classical medicines such as Ayurveda, a sublime path of spiritual merit and refinement of virtue is created. For those who are ill and bereft of resources, finding a compassionate physician who practices medicine primarily for the joys of generosity and the wellbeing of others is like discovering a wish-fulfilling gem. "A physician who desires wealth for his own happiness, in lieu of the auspicious fruits that accrue to him as a result of the gift of life," say the Ayurvedic writings of To-daramalla, "is like a person who has given up his gold and gone to a high mountain with great difficulty to search for mud."

Dr. Aryal continued. "People become tired of doctors, because the disease is not relieved. In the end, if there is nowhere to go, they come to Ayurveda, like this clinic. I use fifteen to thirty doses of medicine, and those people are satisfied. The lady who was just here had a serious disease and thought she was going to die. After the first treatment, half of it was removed. She gave me only a little money, but I am happy."

How many times have I seen this in my own clinic? I wondered. If classical remedies are able to cure diseases unresponsive to modern medicine, why not use them as the first treatment, instead of the last resort? It would be so much easier for both the patient, who would not have to go through the miseries of side effects and economic distress, and for the doctor as well, who would not have to face iatrogenic symptoms complicating the original condition.

Surely, karmic debts are created when physicians, without making any significant contribution to the betterment of their patients, enrich themselves from those who are sick and financially burdened. "A drunkard can get salvation," declares Todaramalla, "and a criminal who killed a Brahmin may also get salvation. But a physician has no salvation if he takes money from the patient but does not endow him with the requisite benefits."

More and more people are finding themselves with no medical recourse except the ancient wisdom of the classical healing philosophies; even the wealthy frequently cannot find healing, even with the best medical care money can buy. When doctors have failed in their efforts, and technology's genius appears an empty promise, the patient's hope and faith often return to the eldest healers of humanity, the plants that have been with us all along. For those whose illness is unresponsive to modern treatments, the beings of the green world are wish-fulfilling gems who selflessly give their own bodies so we may attain our desires of life and happiness. The practice of herbal medicine is filled with profound gratitude for the earth's compassionate powers, as patients and physicians alike rejoice in the banishing of sickness and restoration of vitality.

The alchemist continued his work, slowly mixing the herbs and honey. After an hour he declared that the formula was ready.

The guru lifted his censer onto his desk. "These coals have been burning since I performed puja at dawn," he said. He sprinkled some of the finished formula onto the embers and lifted the bowl of herbs into the cloud of smoke. As the incense burned he chanted an invocation, melodious holy words that conferred blessings and protection upon those who would use it. Then he looked up and smiled. "Siddha Chintamani is now finished," he said. "I have recited the mantra of Shankar, which purifies the world."

The doctor pointed to a large picture of Shiva in his incarnation as the king of Himalayan yogis. He sits wearing a beatific smile of samadhi, cobras dangling around his neck. "This place is not mine, it is Shankar's; I am just the keeper. Shankar has told me to work with you in this way, so I do. You are now also part of Shankar's family. 'Shankar has three eyes,'" Dr. Aryal chanted in Sanskrit. "'He has a good heart and looks after all people. Shankar is the Lord of the whole universe.'"

The alchemist poured the magic incense into a bag. "Store this medicine in a clean jar, in a sacred place," he said. "Use it with a religious mind, offering it to God."

"This is Guruji's last cycle of teaching," Gopal said quietly. "Soon he will close his books and become a baba. We are very fortunate that we can learn from him now. After this period of his life is finished, his work with alchemy will be over."

"Life has come from the Ancient Power," our teacher continued as he cleared his desk. "It made the 840,000 forms of life on earth, and left something in the soul of everything. Man came in the end, with more power. Before, we were in a place where whatever we thought happened. Now we have come to this earth, only to travel through."

Dr. Aryal reached under his desk, lifted up a shining silver bead of solidified mercury on a black string, and motioned for me to come forward. "This will protect you from all diseases and harmful influences," the alchemist said as he tied the cord around my neck. "It will increase your success and give you the power to manifest what you wish. It functions as a great magnet, increasing whatever energies you are sending out. Be careful! It will increase the power of your negative thoughts as well as the positive! This parada loves the Dharma, and will give you much support in those endeavors."

"It is hard to find a good student," the doctor concluded. "I am old, and need the support of people like you so this tradition can flourish."

I thanked him sincerely, affirming that I would work hard for the success of Ayurveda.

Bidding Dr. Aryal farewell, Gopal and I stepped from the cool shade of his simple clinic into the hot Kathmandu afternoon. Nothing could be more precious, I thought as we walked quietly through the backstreets of Sanepa, than a bag of wish-fulfilling incense and a Dharma-enhancing drop of Shiva's essence. What priceless treasures they were, especially when I knew that the old guru might never share them again. The smooth bead of mercury was a tiny mirror of mindfulness, and the fragrant herbs spoke of wondrous prayers waiting to be answered.

Tibetans call Bodhgaya Dorje Den, the "diamond seat" in the navel of the world. They say it is where every Buddha of the past has become enlightened, and every Buddha of the future will, for it is the only place on earth that can withstand the power of such an awakening. The garden around the sacred Bodhi tree is filled with images of Sakyamuni, the Buddha of this eon, standing, meditating, teaching, reclining, carved in stone, cast in metal, and painted on cloth. Inside the Mahabodhi Temple, faithful from around the world shower his golden feet with flowers, find happiness gazing upon his beatific smile, and add their prayers to the echoes of the ages.

To the east of the village rises the rocky mountain where Gautama meditated, emaciated from seven years of ascetic living. Leaving his retreat, he came to the river and collapsed from weakness. That river still flows, 2,500 years later, across the same sands where he lay until revived by a young woman's offering of boiled milk. Now, dark-skinned villagers carry huge baskets on their heads to market, women wash saris in the muddy river, and children gather the dung of white Brahma bulls for fuel.

The prince of the Sakya clan came to rest under the graceful ficus, its heart-shaped leaves rustling in the evening breeze. When night arrived and the stars came out, he began his final vigil. Now, monks of many nationalities scurry in and out of their monasteries, old saddhus wrapped in thin shawls huddle in courtyards, and rickshaw drivers retire as cold fog rises from the ground. The monk who tends the Burmese inn sits in the dark and smokes Bidhis, discussing the Dharma with his evening guests. The late-rising moon shines on weary dreamers.

It was under such a moon that I found an old Tibetan nun, lying among her few possessions in the back entrance of a Bodhgaya monastery. She was in great pain, her body consumed by a fever that had raged for days. Her eyes were bloodshot and protruding, her face gaunt, and her skin hung loosely from her skeleton. Her abdomen was bloated and hard, she was unable to urinate, and she exuded a strong rancid odor. As I listened to the forceful, rapid pounding of her pulse, she told me in a rasping voice that she was dying.

It was the nun's wish to be taken to the Tibetan monastery where Kalu Rinpoche was staying, so she could be close to her teacher. The short ride by rickshaw was nearly fatal; by the time we arrived her labored breath was rattling in her chest. She was unconcerned about receiving medical care, and none was available. After finding a bed in an empty room and making her as comfortable as possible, I made my way back through the village to my room at the Burmese Vihar.

I sat alone on the balcony under a dim bulb, the drone of an occasional mosquito accentuating the stillness of the night. Overhead, Orion was shining in the depths. According to Tantric cosmologies, triquilio-cosms of universes were evolving, galaxies and solar systems unfolding their ages and epochs in response to the karmic propensities of myriad beings, their thirst for existence forming planetary worlds from empty space as vessels for future incarnations.

My thoughts drifted across the village to where the nun rested, and I wondered what dreams might be passing through her mind. Amchi-la's words echoed softly in the silence, admonishing me about the fragility of life. "We don't know which will come first, tomorrow or the next world. I have seen how true this is. A man might be drinking a cup of tea one minute, then lie down and die the next."

Soon, the old nun's pain would cease; she would exhale for the last time, and her lifeless body would go into the fire. "Even when life is nothing but hard work, suffering, and disease, no one wants to leave it," Gopal once mused, gazing into the hypnotic flames on one of the ghats of Pashupatinath, as another human being met inescapable destiny. I thought of Buddhist monks sitting beside pyres, contemplating the transitory nature of existence, and yogis who live among the dead in charnel grounds. For those whose minds are possessed by the "corpse-guarding demon" of attachment to the body, such practices are morbid and terrifying; those who live in the flow of impermanence attain fearless freedom.

Indra's shining net of constellations glistened like multifaceted jewels cast across a firmament of black velvet above Bodhgaya. Soon, dawn would arrive, the same brightening of the sky that brought Buddhistic awakening to Gautama. In the last watch of a night such as this, Mara, the king of devas who bewilders the mind with illusions, rose against

Gautama's meditation, seeking to turn him from final liberation. In response, Gautama serenely touched the earth, the witness of his lives; defeated, Mara and his armies of sensual enticements evaporated into nothing. Crossing the ocean of existence born of craving, Buddha reached the shores of nirvana, the cessation of thirst, the beginning of freedom without end.

Now, another morning has come to timeless India, another day of plowing fields, hauling water, raising children, burning the dead. Beggars sit with bloodshot eyes, matted hair, and gaunt bellies, hands and feet withered and deformed, breathing the oily soot of the streets. They appear crazed, anguished, and despairing, or impartial, proud, and serene, offering the teachings of their existence, asking for generosity. Crimson lotuses float in translucent ponds, and pilgrims from the four corners of the world pray in the shade of the venerable Bodhi tree. They have come with restless minds, peaceful minds, exhausted bodies, euphoric bodies, karma-ripening bodies, to listen to the holy Dharma and be uplifted again by its compassionate truth.

The nun had slept during the night, but at dawn her lungs began filling with fluid. I sat with the old woman through the morning, getting water to moisten her parched lips, helping her sit up, lie down, then sit again. She was patient and tolerant as I listened to her pulses, feeling the life force fading beneath my fingers. The rapid, taut, and forceful pulsations of the night before were now the feeble and unsteady "death pulses." "The prognosis for life, karma, and spiritual fortunes are read at the 'life nerve,' located at the ulnar artery at the wrist," Dr. Chopel had instructed. "It should be read several times before diagnosing. In general, if the beat is irregular or uneven, it is considered a bad sign."

Sometime in midmorning, Kalu Rinpoche's regent, Bokar Rinpoche, arrived with an attending monk; he had come to perform a mo, a Tibetan divination. The lama sat facing the nun, smooth mala beads passing slowly through his fingers. He began to chant, invoking beams of streaming sunlight that illuminated his shaved head. After a while, the

Rinpoche touched the nun in different places with the prayer beads, then quietly sat back. Eventually he spoke.

He told the old woman how all beings are impermanent. Because she was a nun who had maintained her vows, he said, she could expect to go to Dewachen, the Buddhist land of great happiness. He told her it was time to remember the instructions in Powa, the art of transferring one's consciousness out of the body at the time of death. Reviewing these instructions, he explained how the central channel passes like a hollow tube upward through the core of the body. The dying person imagines his or her consciousness in the form of a radiant seed, vibrating in the channel where it passes through the heart. Amitabha, the Buddha of infinite light, is visualized resting on the crown of the head. As the final breath of life is exhaled, the seed of consciousness rises, and is expelled from the top of the head into the heart of the Buddha. Those adept at this practice are said to attain instantaneous rebirth in one of the pure realms, eternally freed of all suffering, and set upon the direct path to enlightenment. When Bokar Rinpoche was finished he rose and left the room, followed by his attendant.

About an hour later a Tibetan shaman arrived. He wore ragged clothes and had a rough manner. The nun seemed pleased to see him. He listened briefly to her pulse, then gently laid her wrist back down. Reaching into a small pouch, he drew out a chunk of ink, an inkstone, and some woodblocks. He untied the nun's robes so her belly would be exposed, and proceeded to mix the ink. When it was prepared, he stamped the talismans on different parts of her body. As soon as the ink had dried, he left.

"When life, karma, and spiritual fortunes have reached their end, no one can stop death," Amchi-la had said, commenting on the "exhaustion of the three factors which sustain life," from the *Root Tantra.* "If only one is exhausted but the others remain, life can be prolonged. If karma is finished, one can prolong life by doing virtuous actions, such as visiting holy places and receiving the blessings of spiritual teachers. If spiritual fortune is exhausted, one can reaccumulate it by giving alms to beggars, making offerings to the gods, and other such actions. If all three are exhausted, it is like a sky exhausted of clouds at the end of the monsoon. No one can help, and there is no method to save yourself."

Late morning found the nun in a state of great agitation. Her breathing had worsened, and she was unable to get comfortable, extremely thirsty, unable to speak clearly, and in overwhelming pain. The night before, I had asked if she wanted painkillers, but she refused because they had previously sickened her. Her pain was so intense at this point, however, that she requested something. The nun wished to be alone, so I walked into the village in search of morphine. When I returned she was dead.

The residents from other rooms stood peering into the doorway. The nun was frozen in a half-sitting position, one arm reaching out as if trying to raise herself. Her eyes were half closed, her dry lips pulled tight over her teeth. I sat quietly on the opposite bed while others came, looked, then left. The abbot of the monastery, Bairo Kyentse Rinpoche, arrived. When the Tibetans saw him coming, they ran out and stood in line to receive his blessings. He was obviously displeased, and I soon found out why. It is considered inauspicious if someone dies in an unconsecrated monastery; this monastery had yet to be completed and had not been consecrated. The nun's body was taken immediately to the bank of the river and cremated.

I wandered away, reflecting on the old woman's demise. It seemed to me that she had died in auspicious circumstances: at the most sacred place in the Buddhist world, near her beloved teacher. She had received profound instructions for spiritual emancipation in her final hour, so difficult to practice during the last stages of suffering. Now, her ashes lay on the sands where Gautama had walked before and after his awakening.

Here in Bodhgaya, when it was only a grove of trees, Gautama saw the truth of existence. He saw the pain of birth, aging, sickness, and death; of change, uncertainty, and certain impermanence; of bewildered mind and karma's infallible law; and of endless rebirth. Sitting on the diamond seat at the navel of the world, he conquered Mara's enticements with tranquillity born of insight, shook the heavens with his awakening, and pierced the veil of ignorance so all beings could find their way home.

Dawn finds me luxuriating between sleep and wakefulness, in the place where dreams continue unfolding even as the outside senses call. Are both worlds not ephemeral? To our dreaming self, this waking state is but an illusive memory. How blissful it is to leisurely stretch the limbs, inhale the fresh breath of life, then sit in quiet absorption and enjoy the clarity of an unfettered mind as the first rays brighten the sky. My heart gives thanks for being reborn into another day.

I walk into the forest and find the ideal meditation place. A small stream splashes through a shady grotto below my seat, sparkles beneath the alders, then disappears into the rice terraces. The face of the rock beside me is adorned with grasses, herbs, and moss, where butterflies come dancing down from the heat and play unconcerned among treacherously hung webs. The air is lightly accented with sounds of insects and the occasional grunt of a water buffalo; eagles are nesting in the gorge below. I watch them preen, then lean lazily into the drafts, letting their flight draw my eyes toward the shimmering sunlight on the far shores of Lake Fewa.

My meditation seat is perfect. With a small flat area conducive to proper posture, high, steep, and narrow enough to keep me awake, it is an excellent support for practicing physical stillness and undistracted attention. Breath and mind flow seamless and smooth as I sit, mingling my awareness with empty space, like a child returning to its mother. Thoughts effortlessly dissolve of their own accord, so what need is there for the endless activities of grasping? Absorbed in the truth of our own presence, we find comfort and ease.

Contentment is medicine. It soothes the body like a healing salve, calming the currents agitated by mind's turbulence, restoring the peace lost in whirlpools of preoccupation. Contentment loosens the knots of muscular constriction, relaxing and softening layers of tension, bringing lightness to the body. It is an elixir for long life which protects from disease, giving potency to the immune system by harmonizing the physiological functions. From the flowing stillness of deep contentment come the rejuvenating powers of life force, restoring equilibrium to the humors and organ systems. The heart becomes calm, the circulation of fluids and essences smooth, and the breathing open; habitual thought patterns slow down. We remember a time before our lives became filled with worries and concerns.

Tranquillity is potent medicine for all illnesses, and the antidote for samsara's troubling complexities. It is the pearl of great price, the flower of serenity, found hidden within the depths of perception where time's movement slows. Time's motionless river now spreads like a rich nutrient through my blood, unhurried in the gentle undulation of quiet breathing. I absorb this feast of spiritual nourishment, as life unfolds before my undistracted senses. There is renewal in this ancient yoga of non-action, so empty and uncluttered; overflowing contentment liberates from hungers and need. What a joy to be released from all cares and burdens of the self!

I remember a faraway place, Los Angeles, where time is a precious commodity. Time has evaporated like the plentiful springs and creeks that once nourished the Southern California desert. Lost in the relentless rush of continual anxieties and overwork, pushed out of our lives by the demands of complex ambitions, consumed by the repetitious routines that maintain technology's frail comforts, time has become harder to find than food.

The streets are on fire, blazing with the hot exhaust of 10 million cars painting a smoggy still life of perpetual motion. Pulled by the tides of hope and fear, the traffic swells as the sun rises and sets, waves of faces framed by tinted glass and steering wheels, faces filled with financial worries, with aspirations to riches and power, with the desire for simple gratification in this complicated world, with boredom and preoccupation.

The breath of contentment courses through my quiescent body.

I think of people I know, sick from lack of time. No time to prepare food, to eat without pressure, to digest without something disturbing the mind. Lacking time to rest, with bodies wearing down, they are sinking deeper into exhaustion and depletion. In the race against the clock, stimulants become routine, then sedatives to counteract them; toxic saturation is inevitable. We have trapped ourselves in the nets of our hungers, and are quickly exhausting the forces of life.

"What is the most important thing you have learned?" I once asked the saddhu Narayan Giri. He was a man who knew the hearts of others, so I listened to his words, and have thought about them through the passing years.

"The most important thing to know is who and what we are, where we come from, and where we are going," he had replied, as the sounds of the monsoon-swollen Kali Gandhaki river swirled softly below, and the smell of moist greenery hung in the mists floating through the forest. "What is this body?" Narayan asked, pointing to his brown belly; his smooth skin, warm eyes, and gentle movements revealed how years of yogic solitude in the jungles of India had brought the comfort of royal ease. "It is only the pancha mahabhutas that are dancing ceaselessly. We are born into this form, but it is always changing, and then we pass away. Everything is impermanent. This world is a dream. Knowing this is Self-Realization."

"And why is there so much suffering in this world?" I asked, as clouds descended around the tiny village of Devkot, God's Place.

"It is because people have forgotten Self-Realization," the saddhu replied. "It is because their minds are on fire, because they are attached to the things of this world, because they thirst."

The dark sky opened and rain fell on the oasis of quiet, where elders come to retire from the "world of illusion." "With more devotion, peace will increase," Narayan had said, smiling, as the flowering plants lifted their open lips to receive the blessings from heaven.

Now, afternoon radiance warms my meditation garden, so beautifully enfolded within the forested cliffs above Lake Fewa.

There have been ages in the past when people's minds were more pure. They were free of strong attachments, the cravings of self-cherishing, conflicting emotions. Before the world was troubled by the disturbances of collective ignorance, those who received meditation instruction easily entered the fathomless current, remaining undisturbed for days, weeks, and even months. "Now," Kalu Rinpoche once said, "even if a person practices all day, he will only experience a few moments of meditative absorption." How inestimably precious are contemplation's joys.

Far away, in the whirling vortex of the roaring city, people are moving here and there in repetitive gestures, producing this and manufacturing that, generating sales and increasing profits; those unwilling or unable to participate struggle to survive. Lines wind through stores, gas stations, bars and restaurants and theaters, hospitals, courts, jails, and churches feeding the destitute. Machines whir in thoughtful tones as they monitor our consumption; computerized corporate eyes and electronic mouths inform us of our balance due. A siren screams the pain of this existence, another wails as a life comes to an end somewhere. My heart murmurs ancient words of blessing and protection.

I sit, letting my thoughts unfold across the surface of consciousness, like the waves on Lake Fewa. "As every thought arises, let it effortlessly fall away," Tulku Urgyen instructed me years ago. The old Rinpoche sat in his meditation box in a room full of shadows and incense, fingering his mala and looking out the window of Nagi Gompa. The monastery floated on the horizon of another world, surrounded by waterfalls and wildflowers high above the crowded streets of Kathmandu. Sitting straight up, the Tulku had looked at me intently through wizened Tibetan eyes and asked, "If you see the moon in the sky, and you see it reflected in pools of water, which is in reality the moon?" Taken aback by the simplicity of the question, I answered, "The moon in the sky." "Correct," Rinpoche had said. "So it is with the mind and thoughts."

Tulku Urgyen then told me to place my consciousness in the back of my head, look directly into my mind, and let thoughts fall away without grasping. Holding up his mala, he let it drop into his lap. "Like this," he said, repeating his gesture. "Look into the space between thoughts." We meditated in the silence of Shivapuri mountain, while hermits practiced their devotions in caves in the vine-covered cliffs above us.

The *Flower Ornament Scripture* describes suffering as a web of fancified conceptualizing, habitual emotional attachment, grasping, and wishing. We chase every thought and passing fantasy as if they were inherently real, like the moon above, and fail to see how they arise from nothing, abide nowhere, and return to nothing, like pictures drawn with our finger in water, the trail of a bird's flight through the air, or the moon's reflection. All our actions follow this empty play of nothingness, our attachments leading us into endless repetitive behavior and its subsequent consequences. "Discursive thoughts are the chains that bind us to suffering," Amchi-la once said. "As soon as we become attached to a thought, it leads to another, then another, and soon they spread into the myriad emotional conflicts and karmas of cyclical existence."

Kalu Rinpoche's spiritual forefather, Milarepa, sang of his liberation from the illusory chains of the mind. "He who is enslaved by his desires, insatiable and always longing, is ever sad. He who renounces all worldly things, free from worry and consideration, is ever joyful. A yogi who discards all ties, realizing everything is magic and illusion, is ever joyful. He who diverts himself, taxing his body and mind with sensuality, is ever sad. Do not bestir yourself and think too much. Put your mind at ease in a state of naturalness, and make no effort whatsoever."

And what happens when we sit and let each thought fall away, like

Urgyen Rinpoche's mala falling softly into the folds of his robes? What do we see when we look into the space between each passing idea, concept, and fantasy? "I have realized that flowing thoughts are phantom-like projections," the yogini Sahle Aui sang to her guru, Milarepa. "As waves rise from the sea they will vanish into it again. All doubts, errors, and temptations in the world are thus wiped out!"

The extinction of suffering lies in cutting off compulsive mental activity. With nothing to practice, resting in non-fabrication, non-doing, and non-striving, we discover tranquillity, equanimity, and peace.

I think of Tulku Urgyen sitting quietly in his room, wrapped in blankets in his meditation box, casually fingering his mala like a rosary of forgotten worries. He was gazing out the window when I left him, across the Kathmandu Valley with its crowded and busy streets far below, so much like any other city. Everywhere, people are chasing after something, driven by hopes, fears, and needs through days of routines. It is rare in this age of confusion for one to dwell in the open expanse of mental freedom, contemplating the clear space of ungraspable quietude. Liberation is a joyful path, I imagine; maybe it is also a lonely place, where the great masters find themselves awake in a world of dreamers enslaved by the empty reflections of their minds.

Eagles soar through the afternoon sun, rain gathers on the eastern horizon, and evening spreads up the green canyons around Lake Fewa. In the mirror of my mind, I see sunset over Los Angeles. The freeways crawl like stagnant vaporous sewers, their inhabitants sitting transfixed with fatigue or impatiently accelerating their vehicles against the immobile mass. Above, the sky is the color of feverish blood, while below, the homeless gradually slip away from their unbearable reality into the strange realms of madness. The chemical slime of the city seeps through the storm drains into canals where the poor wash and drink, then to the ocean where children at the beach laugh and imagine the sea creatures that their ancestors once saw. I count the cycles of my breath on fragrant sandalwood beads brought from sacred Bodhgaya, inhaling the sadness of these hardships, and exhaling tranquillity.

What have I accomplished today? No working hours have dragged by, changing minutes into dollars. I've made no business deals, attended no meetings of great importance. No material progress has occurred, and I have gained no delightful acquisitions to distract myself and impress others. Fame and fortune have not come my way while I rested in simple awareness, free of all such concerns. No worldly attainments, no socially redeeming productivity, no heroic deeds.

A bird begins to sing in the approaching darkness. It has a message, and I am listening. It sings for the sky, it sings for the trees, it sings for the animals, and it sings for the children. It sings gratitude for my doing nothing.

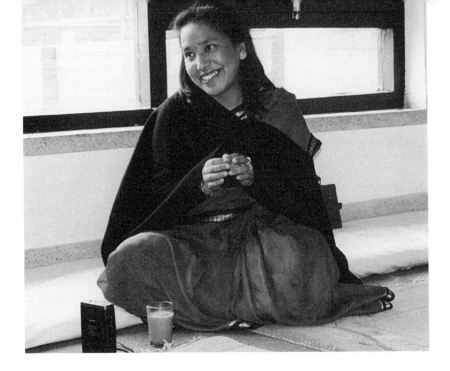

VII.

THE

FORGOTTEN GODDESS

Where women are worshipped,

divine souls dwell.

VEDIC PROVERB

In my search for healing medicines I found what I was seeking—far beyond what I had ever imagined—but the discoveries were not simple. The value and goodness of these medical teachings did not come as refined gems; they came as threads woven into the fabric of societies that are at once wonderful and terrible, sophisticated and degenerate, magical and dysfunctional, goddess-worshipping and chauvinistic. Classical Asian medicines offer great hope for healing of individuals, society, and the natural environment, yet ironically their philosophies are embedded within religious and cultural sentiments that contribute to sickness and suffering. They are rich with inherent truth, but their interpretation can also perpetuate injustice, social malaise, and spiritual confusion. Nowhere is this more evident than in the deeply ingrained attitudes about women that pervade Hindu and Buddhist cultures.

Although Ayurveda offers many benefits for both men and women, there is no branch of this medical system devoted exclusively to gynecology and women's health. Reflecting their role and status in Hindu culture, women in Ayurveda are considered a secondary subject, important only in relation to the child they are expected to produce. The branch of medicine that deals with the health of women and children is called kaumar bhritya, meaning "care of the child." Women are included in Ayurvedic medicine as the soil from which the child is born and nourished; the specific subject of gynecology is included in the broader field of pediatrics, since the health of the child is dependent on the health of the mother.

While containing medical knowledge of great value for women, the classical Ayurvedic writings on gynecology and their view of female anatomy and physiology are deficient and burdened with erroneous information. For example, one text gives complex rules for menstruating women, complete with descriptions of the dire consequences if not followed: if the woman uses mascara, her future child will be blind; if she receives oil massage, the child will contract leprosy; if she laughs, the child will be born with black teeth; if she brushes her hair, the child will be bald. Rather than providing useful medical information, these commentaries are a poignant reflection of social customs of the times. Most of these customs would be ridiculous and irrelevant to modern women, but some beneficial ones gave women of the past freedom to rest from their otherwise grueling chores.

In the Samhitas of Sushruta and Charaka, the 2,500-year-old encyclopedic writings of India's two greatest physicians, the descriptions of gynecology, obstetrics, and embryology are poorly developed and incomplete. Of the two doctors, Sushruta performed more detailed research and briefly described surgical procedures such as cesarean delivery for obstructed labor, laparotomy, and hysterectomy. Kashyap, who was a contemporary of Sushruta and Charaka, wrote more extensively about kaumar bhritya in his Samhita, but most of the manuscript has been lost through the ages. The first serious development of gynecology in Ayurveda came in the eighteenth century from Pandit Hemraj Sarma, who reconstructed the *Kashyap Samhita* from remnants of manuscripts found in the archives of Nepal, and from Pandit Gananatha Sen, who developed the specialty of obstetrics during the nineteenth century.

The reasons for early Ayurveda's neglect of gynecology can be found in the cultural status assigned to women by Hindu philosophy, and the role of Ayurveda within society. Most of the ancient physicians were men; since women were generally denied formal education, they were unable to pursue academic achievements and become doctors. The men, in turn, were unable to develop a complete understanding of female anatomy and physiology because of taboos against examining women's bodies. Without modern methods of visualizing the interior of the living body, knowledge of embryology and obstetrics was gathered mostly through empirical observations, such as examining a fetus after a miscarriage. Laws against abortion prevented in-depth medical examination of the various stages of embryological development. In spite of these restrictions, a high level of theoretical understanding about women's health evolved, which reflected the astute powers of observation, deduction, and intuitive insight of the ancient doctors.

Another reason why gynecology was poorly developed in Ayurveda can be found in the reproductive role of women in Hindu society. In the view of orthodox Hindus, females are merely a biological adjunct to the procreative powers of the male, whose primary purpose is to reproduce himself for the continuation of his lineage; a woman produces the child, but man is the Creator. This belief is reflected in kaumar bhritya, which was developed in societies governed by monarchies and supported by the kings who ruled the various regions of India and Nepal. The primary concern of medicine in this environment was the health of the king, and the production of male offspring for the preservation of his lineage.

Although Ayurvedic gynecology was male-dominated, academic, and oriented to the continuation of monarchies, women in traditional societies were not without health care. Folk medicine, which is the basis of much of Ayurveda's herbal knowledge, has always been primarily in the hands of women. The knowledge of how to treat women's health problems was passed from mother and grandmother to daughters in an experiential tradition, requiring no academic education or formal medical knowledge. These traditions of home health care continue into the present day in almost every household in Nepali society; in many parts of the Himalayas, it is the only form of medicine available to women. In spite of Ayurveda's patriarchal orientation, it is women who continue to provide the primary form of medicine within the family structure.

Over time I learned that religious dogma, derived originally from Vedic philosophy, is the root cause of the perpetuation of much of the suffering and sickness of women in Nepal and India. This is not the fault of the Vedas, but of their interpretation and application by men, for men. During my years of studying in Nepal, I had ten teachers; nine of them were men. The views of these highly educated individuals concerning women were naturally more informed than those of the average Nepalese farmer or Tibetan nomad. Nonetheless, their sentiments ranged from socially conservative and religiously orthodox to radically unconventional. Their comments were often permeated, either subtly or overtly, with the chauvinistic views of their culture—views that, when put into daily practice, affect the health and happiness of millions of women, children, and men alike, as well as the natural environment.

The failure of family planning programs is one of the best examples of how the imposition of religious orthodoxy causes health problems for women. Birth control is rejected, especially in the Brahmin and Chetri castes in the villages, where cultural interpretation of Vedic philosophy dictates early marriage, desire for male children, multiple marriages if male children are not produced, and laws against abortion. Religious beliefs also contribute to malnutrition by teaching women that they are not good wives unless they feed the husband and children before themselves. In the conditions of poverty which prevail in rural areas, this practice leads to widespread illness.

Many of the health issues facing women are related to ignorance about healthy sexuality. Sexuality is a closed subject in Nepali Hindu culture, and there is little discussion about it within society, in families, or between couples. Even though Ayurvedic gynecology deals with women's reproductive health, it does not discuss sexuality. Kaumar bhritya includes treatments for painful intercourse and similar conditions, but there is no discussion about sexual physiology or topics related to erotic enjoyment, pleasure, and satisfaction. Ratri charya, the branch of Ayurveda that deals with the "duties of the night," is discussed briefly in the Samhitas of Sushruta and Bagwat. It provides recipes for herbal and mineral preparations, and teaches methods of enhancing the enjoyment of marital life. Sexual pleasure as an art and science is traditionally taught in the Kama Shastras, such as the *Kama Sutra*. Although these teachings are part of Hindu culture, they are not widely accepted or practiced. Without sexual education for couples, there is difficulty achieving intimacy in relationships, and intercourse is often reduced to mere gratification for the male. This lack of communication about women's bodies supports exploitation by men, who control not only the sexual activity of the marriage, but the decisions about conceiving children as well.

These deeply ingrained and infrequently questioned attitudes about the female body have serious negative impacts on women's health. Women are taught to repress their emotions, deny the needs of the body, and avoid communication about their desires. Most women in Nepal are shy and inhibited about their bodies; many will simply run away from a physical examination by doctors or wait until a disease becomes acute before seeking help. As a result, many women suffer unnecessarily with health problems that can be easily prevented and treated.

While the Hindu interpretation of Vedic philosophy has had unhealthy effects on women, Ayurvedic philosophy supports women's health and wellbeing. Ayurveda suggests that the optimum age for marriage for women is twenty-two; Hindu culture, on the other hand, encourages marriage much earlier. Pregnancy in girls whose bodies are not fully developed can lead to gynecological, obstetric, and pediatric problems, as well as deprive girls of opportunities for education, thus perpetuating the cycle of illiteracy and suppression. When girls enter into marriage, they are expected to assume heavy household responsibilities. But if the health principles of Ayurveda were followed, young women would have increased opportunity for education, self-improvement, proper physical development, less burden of multiple pregnancies, and more self-determination in the family structure.

Vedic philosophy as practiced in everyday life encourages women to accept frequent pregnancies as the gift of God. Because of the manpower needs of an agrarian society, women are taught that having numerous children is beneficial. The man is considered the king and ruler of the family, while the woman has little power to decide how many children she will have, and when; it is common for Nepali village women to conceive every year and a half. The result is serious health problems for both mothers and children as a result of multiple deliveries under poor medical conditions, and the ravages of overpopulation which affect the entire society and environment. Ayurveda, however, recommends that a woman conceive not more than once every three to seven years. Observance of this principle would reduce the suffering of mothers from too many childbirths, decrease infant mortality rates, and stabilize Nepal's exploding population level.

Ritu charya is the branch of kaumar bhritya that deals with ovulation and the menstrual cycle. It clearly explains the rules of conduct for couples who wish either to conceive or not conceive, by accurately describing the cycle of fertility. It has thus described the rhythm method of birth control for at least 2,500 years. In order for the rhythm method to be effective, the woman must have a healthy menstrual cycle, and the man must be willing to practice abstinence for part of the month. Both of these requirements are addressed in Ayurveda. Din charya is the branch of Ayurveda that describes the daily conduct that leads to good health; observing its prescriptions, along with using herbal medicines for balancing and strengthening the reproductive system, gives a woman greater awareness of when she is fertile. For the male, Ayurveda promotes sexual moderation as a path to good health and longevity. If this knowledge were practiced, the quality of life would improve for men and women alike.

Ayurvedic obstetrics has described month-by-month dietary and behavioral regimens to enhance a woman's health during pregnancy and prevent problems such as miscarriages. For example, dairy products such as ghee, butter, curd, and milk are prescribed throughout the pregnancy, along with foods and herbs such as honey, brahmi (*Centella asiatica*), lotus root, saffron, asparagus root, and ashwaghanda (*Withania somnifera*). During the third month the use of gokshur (*Tribullis terrestris*) is considered especially important; it is also used during the sixth month to reduce edema during the later stages of pregnancy. A pregnant woman, according to Ayurveda, is as sensitive as a pot filled with oil; she should avoid strenuous work, especially in the early and late phases of pregnancy, because the slightest disturbance will spill the contents of the womb. Unfortunately, these various regimes are difficult for most village women, who typically work throughout the duration of their pregnancy, doing hard labor both outdoors and indoors during every kind of weather, neglecting their dietary needs.

Ayurveda elucidates the natural laws of healthy life. The wisdom of the Science of Life teaches us how to live in such a way that disease can be both prevented and treated. It provides many valuable guidelines that, if applied, can reduce the suffering of women, children, and men alike.

"In this human life we are blessed with a body, speech, and mind. We have the choice to use them virtuously to attain happiness and enlightenment, or to use them non-virtuously, which brings us suffering. Most of the time we are engaged in using them non-virtuously." This was Dr. Chopel's assessment of humanity's condition in this age. His view was that of a classically trained Tibetan monk, a man who had lived in a remote monastery for much of his life, a celibate Buddhist scholar and physician. Many of Dr. Chopel's pithy teachings, flavored with moral precepts, described the effects of virtue and non-virtue on our present and future life. His comments presented ample opportunities for me to examine my own beliefs and to untangle the relevant and meaningful from the biased and unacceptable elements of Tibetan medicine.

Dr. Chopel's attitudes about life were understandably different from those of most people today. As he saw it, the world is a transient place filled with the ripening consequences of one's own thoughts and actions. It is a brief existence, a temporary fortunate condition in which to practice the teachings of Buddha in order to achieve liberation from suffering. After a lifetime of maintaining full monastic vows, Dr. Chopel no longer found the world a place to become attached to as if it were permanent and ultimately real. He taught that the senses and the mind are to be carefully guarded through discipline so that entanglement in samsara, the whirlpool of mundane existence, can be avoided. It is through desire, the old monk instructed, that we fall into states of torment and misfortune. The right use of this human incarnation is to purify ourselves and become free of our karmic bondage. This philosophy naturally had a strong influence on the doctor's comments regarding women, sex, birth control, and abortion.

Dr. Chopel's views concerning sex reflected the renunciate monastic environment in which he lived. "Sex is a form of non-virtue," he once commented. "Its motivation is selfish desire for pleasure, and the result is weakening of the body." This was a challenging statement that I found difficult to accept, and equally difficult to deny.

When introducing his lectures on Tibetan gynecology, Dr. Chopel stated the conviction held by men and women alike in Tibetan and Indian society that being female was the result of inferior karma. His explanation for this was that the female possessed "the three defects" of breasts, uterus, and menstrual blood. When I asked him why they were considered defects, he replied that they were sources of suffering which men did not have to endure.

As I became more aware of the medical and social problems affecting Himalayan women, I could understand why they would often agree that having a female body was an unpleasant experience. There was certainly truth in Amchi-la's observation about women's suffering, but his comments were inherently dangerous in their applications: the belief that women are "defective" and inferior is what ultimately causes the most detrimental impact on their health.

As the teachings on gynecology continued, our discussions turned to the subjects of birth control and abortions. Tibetan medicine, like that of most other cultures, once had access to numerous herbs which successfully prevented pregnancy. Starting his commentary on these drugs, Dr. Chopel said, "These formulas were given to us by the Medicine Buddha, who foresaw the age when nuns and other women would risk pregnancy because of their desire for sex. Using these formulas for contraception is a form of non-virtue. This is because they encourage more sexual activity, and because they might prevent the birth of a noble being who would help humanity."

Referring to his manual of Tibetan herbal formulas, the doctor said, "This text considers that birth control pills will increase the Dark Age by helping nuns have sex and not get caught. Unless a mother gives birth every year and has a lot of children, it is considered sinful to stop the birth of humans with contraceptive herbs. These medicines were created to help nuns and laypeople by stopping them from killing their babies." Amchi-la then described how poverty sometimes forced people to commit infanticide by throwing newborns into the forest or fields because they could not feed them. "This practice was done in Tibet," he said, "and perhaps even more in Nepal. Contraceptives are therefore considered less sinful than outright killing, and not as serious karmically as having an abortion or abandoning the newborn. The Medicine Buddha has provided these medicines to compassionately reduce the karmic suffering of these times."

With these teachings I found myself unraveling the profound from the absurd. Dr. Chopel's opinion was that birth control drugs facilitate sexual activity and promote desire, but it was difficult to envision old Tibet as a place where chaste, innocent monks were preyed upon by lascivious, promiscuous nuns, who were causing a dark age by indulging in lust. I suspected that rather than being a gift to nuns who would risk pregnancy in the heat of carnal desires, these herbs were probably used by women to protect themselves from the consequences of their husbands' sexual appetites. Even though the text quoted by my teacher was undeniably sexist by contemporary Western standards, it contained an important medical revelation: the Tibetan pharmacopoeia includes herbal contraceptives. The miseries that impoverished women and children endure from multiple pregnancies, such as the infanticide Amchi-la described, illustrate the crucial need for safe anti-fertility medications to be more widely available.

When discussing abortion, Dr. Chopel said, "If the lives of both the mother and the child are in danger, then abortion must be done, since it is better to save one life than to lose two. The following medicines were created by the Medicine Buddha for this situation; their use is considered to be against religion otherwise. One who causes an abortion is said to be trading in the karma of the next life for this one." He then instructed me in the use of different formulas, which included various types of salts, datura, and purified mercury.

When I asked Dr. Chopel to elaborate on the karmic consequences of abortion, he said, "If the mother is preoccupied with emotionality and has no love for the child, then for several future lives she will experience rebirths which are aborted. In this case she is thinking only of herself and not of the future life of the child."

"And what of the father?" I asked.

"The father will also have bad karma, but it is not the same as for the mother. It is the responsibility of the mother to know of the possibility of conception, and so her karma is greater. Karma is greater for those who do not take responsibility for their actions, such as those who engage in promiscuous sex."

I found that many of these statements, from Amchi-la as well as my other teachers, had elements of truth blended with varying degrees of misunderstanding about women. They were sometimes simply blatant sexist hypocrisy.

One afternoon I asked Lobsang Dhonyo, Dr. Chopel's main student, what he had learned about our teacher's attitudes concerning women. The young monk's comments confirmed what I had seen and heard over the years: that the old physician had the classical views of an orthodox Buddhist monk.

"Amchi-la teaches that male and female have attraction all the time," Lobsang said. "He told me that attraction is due to ignorance. Our attraction to other people, our likes and dislikes, liking the beautiful things and disliking the ugly, all depend on ignorance. What appears beautiful is just outward appearance. When we study physiology, we see that inside our body there are blood, pus, and other impurities. This is one of the contemplations that comes directly from Lord Buddha.

"Amchi-la taught us that because of ignorance we can't distinguish between good and bad. Due to this ignorance, we humans are not only attracted to the illusion of beauty, but also have the tendency to look for the faults of others. Because of this there are conflicts between individuals and among nations. All problems in the world arise from this basic ignorance."

And what advice did the old monk give concerning how to relate to women? I wondered.

"He advised me that if a beautiful girl comes in and I have attraction to her, to think about how her beauty is impermanent. He said that if I have relations with women, there could be quarreling any time."

Dr. Chopel's instructions were an echo of the Buddha's words from 2,500 years earlier. When Ananda asked Gautama how monks were to relate to women, he was told that they should avoid them; if they couldn't avoid them, to not talk to them; and if they had to interact with women, to establish mindfulness.

"Are you having success with this practice?" I asked.

"Since we are human beings, our basic nature is to have likes and dislikes," Lobsang replied. "When I remind myself of Amchi-la's advice, it helps reduce the differentiation between human beings.

"When the patient enters the clinic, whether a man or a woman, the outcome depends on the attitude of the doctor. If the doctor has kindness, and thinks 'All human beings may have been my parents in the past or will be in future lives,' and considers the laws of karma and reincarnation, there is no difference between male and female."

I asked Lobsang to explain why Tibetan culture considers women to have inferior karma.

"Usually we consider the female a lower incarnation than the male," he replied. "In terms of the medical system, women suffer from many diseases which are not present in men. The woman has to carry the child for nine months in the womb, she suffers so much pain delivering the child, and afterward it is the mother who cares for the child. The man has problems, but compared to the woman, they are much less."

"From your experiences with Amchi-la, how would you describe his conduct with women?" I asked.

"He treats all people as equals, whether it is men or women, rich or poor. All patients are the same, because all have the same basic ignorance. We were taught to consider everyone's disease as equal."

Although his views concerning women and morality were religiously orthodox and conservative, Dr. Chopel also taught that these issues went far beyond simplistic concepts of right and wrong. He emphasized that in real life these were complex subjects that no one other than a Buddha could fully comprehend. Even though he was a physician working in society, Amchi-la praised the value of retiring from worldly life; living in a hermitage, he would tell me, was the solution to the multitude of attractions and involvement with the objects of desire. But he also claimed that when one has recognized true Reality, this is no longer necessary. "When Dharma practitioners have realized the true nature of desire and phenomena, they can enjoy the pleasures of the senses without causing bad karma," he said. Dr. Chopel then described how advanced meditators are able to maintain mindfulness of the inherent emptiness of apparent reality, its illusory, impermanent nature, and are therefore unattached to the world even while enjoying it.

Ultimately, it was Dr. Chopel's living example, more than the religious precepts inextricably entwined in his medical lessons, that spoke most about the kind of man he was. As I saw him age over the years, the fruit of treasuring morality and religious discipline became more apparent. An aura of calm and loving-kindness infused his old body, which inspired humility and respect in those who were in his presence.

We were two very different people from two very different worlds. The old man provoked my young mind with controversial statements I didn't always understand or agree with, especially about women. I knew that Amchi-la had never faced the challenging complexities of a romantic or marital relationship, and had no experiences with female sexuality.

He admitted that he was not an authority on women's health. I listened to his words with an open mind, and learned about the widely held and deeply rooted beliefs they echoed. I regarded my teacher as highly accomplished in the practice of detachment, and had great respect for the degree of self-control required to maintain a lifetime of celibacy. I watched his interactions with women and saw that he was respectful and impartial—behavior that other men would benefit from emulating.

In my studies I had met many men with much to teach, but had not encountered any women in the field of classical medicine. This was not surprising, for although there are many traditional practitioners of Ayurvedic and Tibetan medicine in Nepal, fewer than one hundred are registered and licensed as doctors, and only four of them are women. When I finally met one of these exceptional healers and learned of the social barriers she had overcome in order to study medicine, I considered myself fortunate. Ayurveda is considered the domain of men, specifically of the Brahmin caste, who claim outright that "it is not for a woman." Ayurvedic education for women in Nepal and India is still in an age in which "religious" men quit school in protest of attendance by female students, university deans discourage girls from pursuing careers, and teachers are grossly abusive. Ayurveda, like Hindu society in general, has been weakened by overlooking the faith, strength, and compassion that women bring to all walks of life, especially the healing arts. What negative karma do men create for themselves in the name of spiritual superiority, I wondered, by their denial of women's self-determination?

I met Dr. Sarita Shrestha on a sunny afternoon at my home in Balwatar. She made time in her busy schedule for an interview after hearing of my interest in meeting a woman who was practicing Ayurveda. Eloquent, knowledgeable, and direct, she expounded astutely and at length on whatever questions I asked, then would laugh at herself cheerfully and wonder if what she said had been useful. I immediately had great admiration for this small dark-haired healer, who was Nepal's first woman Ayurvedic doctor; she in turn seemed genuinely honored by my interest in her work.

Dr. Shrestha had been a general practitioner in rural health posts before deciding to specialize in Ayurvedic gynecology and obstetrics. Now, after a decade of helping the women of Nepal, she was highly respected and had a large following. She held a full-time government position at Naradevi Hospital, and in the early mornings, evenings, and on her day off saw patients at two private clinics. All these places were filled with seriously ill people who came with high expectations of her skills.

Dr. Shrestha's daily work in Kathmandu took her through streets of dust and sewage, down hallways of crowded, filthy hospital wards where physicians despair, into mazes of medical bureaucracies and professional feuds, to homes where patients lay too sick to move, and into the glaring light of publicity in the local media. It was love and concern for her patients, and a deep commitment to Ayurveda, that allowed Dr. Shrestha to maintain such a grueling workload. The conditions of Naradevi Hospital were unimaginably bleak, and the pervasive poverty of the country affected many of her private patients. In order to make treatments and medicines available to those who could not pay, she used her own income. The words of this strong and gentle physician brought to my attention the severity of health problems affecting women in Nepal.

"Reproductive health is a serious issue in this country," Dr. Shrestha said. "It affects the health of the female, the child, and the family. If the female is not healthy, the entire family will be disturbed. She is the one who looks after the family, household, and farm. She is the source of nourishment for the babies, and the primary source of education for the children. If the mother's health suffers, the wellbeing of the children is affected, both physically and psychologically. In Nepal the condition of women's health is very poor, especially during reproductive age."

Dr. Shrestha is a devout Hindu whose life has been shaped in many ways by the religious attitudes that affect all Nepali women. Unlike most, however, she does not remain silent about the social customs that perpetuate women's suffering, but is forthright and uninhibited in expressing her views. During our discussions about family planning she clearly elucidated the influence of religious dogma and the cultural suppression of women on overpopulation and disease.

"The main causes that deteriorate women's health here are early marriages and multiple pregnancies," the doctor explained. "Even though health education is widely available and they know about birth control, the women here get pregnant frequently, because there are factors they cannot control. The woman doesn't have any right to decide whether to conceive or not. There is no discussion or mutual understanding concerning conceiving the baby."

"Two people came to me recently," she said. "The girl was so shy that she was not talking, and her history was explained by an older person. I asked, 'Who are you?' and he said, 'I am her father, and I want her to conceive.' I asked her how old she was. Can you imagine? She was just sixteen, had already been married for two years, and the parents were worried about conceiving. They were worried because of the social impact and the culture. If the wives don't have babies, there is the fear of a second marriage. I said, 'You have to wait at least two or three years, and if she doesn't conceive after that, I will do whatever I can.' I tried to convince the father, because the girl didn't have any right to say anything."

"The women have to accept these things," Dr. Shrestha went on. "People know that having too many children will cause poverty, but when we ask, 'Why are you having so many babies? How will you give them education and good nutrition?' they will say, 'Who will look after our cattle, our babies?' When they go to their field for planting or harvesting, one baby is needed to look after another baby—that is their concept. They have children only for manpower: one to go to the field, one for cooking, one for the cattle. Because of this, family planning programs are not successful."

The pressure on women to procreate is reinforced by the threat of the husband taking a second wife if there is no male offspring. "Unless and until she has a male baby," Dr. Shrestha explained, "the woman will always have the fear of her husband having a second marriage. Because of that fear, she will always be ready for the next conception."

And why is it so necessary to have boys? I wondered, remembering Dr. Jha's special "sex change operation."

"This is the impact of our male-dominated society," Dr. Shrestha replied. "We have a culture where, once the daughter is married, she will leave the house and go live with her husband's family, and only the sons will stay with the parents. The son will look after the parents, so the importance is given to him. When the son gets married, he will bring another woman."

The result of this arrangement is simple: the more sons, the more daughters-in-law to help the parents. In many households the new woman is treated as a servant, or worse. The daughter-in-law's dowry also brings financial benefits to the parents of sons.

"At the marriage ceremony the daughter has to give some gifts, and throughout her life, on every important occasion, her family has to give something. They think the daughter is only for giving, and the son is only to take. This is a selfish society, and everybody likes to take."

The way Dr. Shrestha described them, these customs seemed to be based on insecurity about surviving in old age. They would certainly be to the advantage of parents with many sons. But what of the unfortunate parents who had only daughters and could not afford to buy them husbands? A particularly gruesome photograph on the front page of an Indian newspaper showed two daughters who had hanged themselves to help their despairing elders.

Dr. Shrestha had many stories about the impact that the desire for male babies had on families. "There was a very pretty lady who had pso-riasis," she told me one day. "When I saw the patient, it was shocking. Her whole body was badly infected, there was discharge everywhere, and the smell was terrible. Her urine was scanty and dark red, and she would scratch herself until she bled."

The woman's relatives were upset, but not primarily because of her suffering. "Her in-laws were badly disturbed," Dr. Shrestha said, "be-cause her husband was the only son in his family, and the couple had no children." The couple had tried all types of medicines, without success. Dr. Shrestha's Ayurvedic prescriptions cleared up the psoriasis, and the woman conceived. Her mother-in-law accepted her because she was pregnant, and the family was happy and grateful.

"I think that if it were not for us," Dr. Shrestha concluded, "the fam-ily would have been broken, and it would be a great disaster for that lady."

Besides the financial benefits that the dowry system brings to par-ents with boys, and the security of daughters-in-law to help the house-hold, orthodox Hindu men believe that unless they father a son, they will not be able to enter heaven after this life. This religious conviction, the economic and domestic benefits of having sons, and the production of children for labor are all strong incentives for multiple pregnancies, regardless of whether the woman wants them or can endure the physi-cal trauma of childbirth, or the children can be supported.

"The first answer women will give in their medical history will be that they conceive one baby after another each year, with poor delivery. When I ask, 'How many babies?' they will usually say, 'Five have lived and five have died.'" Dr. Shrestha laughed with amazement. "So many women like that come to the clinic. After conducting deliveries, I just can't imagine how people can think about having eight, nine, or ten children!"

One of the most common problems that brought women to Dr. Shrestha's clinics was prolapsed uterus. She estimated that over 50 percent of the women she treated had varying degrees of this condition, and in some villages almost all the women suffered from it. Every pregnancy and delivery weakens the muscles and connective tissues around the uterus, she explained, especially when delivery services are poor and there is no opportunity for postpartum rest or recovery. As a result, the uterus begins to sink, and may become extroverted from the vagina.

A standard Ayurvedic treatment that Dr. Shrestha frequently prescribed for uterine prolapse includes sitz baths of triphala decoction, followed by application of tampons with dashmool tel (oil of ten roots), or jati tel (a formula based on jasmine leaves). While these are neither expensive nor difficult to administer, many women cannot find the time or resources to treat themselves. As a result, more serious complications develop, such as cervical cancer. The doctor sees many cases of uterine bleeding that are the result of carcinomas.

"With an increased number of pregnancies, the chances are higher of uterine prolapse," Dr. Shrestha explained. "The uterus is hanging down all the time, and the ladies have no time to wash it and keep medicines there. They go on working, the friction starts, it starts bleeding, ulceration begins, and finally it becomes cancerous.

"If we can reduce the frequency of pregnancies, and provide good delivery service, we can prevent these kinds of problems. For that, we have to go to the villages, because they are too busy to come to us. That is why I am conducting Ayurvedic health camps."

In contrast to the practice of most other doctors in Kathmandu, Dr. Shrestha's service to the sick has not been confined to the local valley; mountain trails lead to distant villages, where few physicians venture. She and her assistants regularly trek long distances to remote areas to conduct health camps, which are frequently the only access to professional health care for the women in those places. In the city Dr. Shrestha's work is illuminated by fluorescent lights, in the remote forests by kerosene lamps, cooking fires, and moonlight. In both places she is surrounded by virulent microbes—staph, hepatitis, tuberculosis, typhoid;

in the jungle she is visited by malarial mosquitoes, leeches, and storms. After a typical day in Kathmandu she returns home to delicious cooking and a comfortable bed; in the villages she eats whatever her hosts can provide, and sleeps on earthen floors. To endure this rugged lifestyle, Dr. Shrestha had to cure herself of gastritis and allergies, the result of stress during medical school. Using yogic purification techniques, she trained her body to tolerate even the roughest foods and harshest climates.

To get to Sindhupalchok, Dr. Shrestha and her assistants traveled by bus to its farthest destination, then walked for eight more hours along a narrow ledge high above the Melamchi River. Returning from Bhotechur, the doctor was forced to climb across a treacherous landslide brought down from the steep mountainside by unrelenting monsoon rains, as rocks fell from the heights above. High above the clouds in Sallyan, where the villages touch the sky, she narrowly escaped a terrorist bombing. Everywhere she journeyed there were impassable roads, vehicles broken down at night in remote jungles, rivers with no bridges, and crowds of people waiting for her.

It was not unusual for Dr. Shrestha and her nurse assistants to see over a thousand patients in three days. In Lumbini the air was thick with dust, and the line of patients so long that people were fainting from the heat. When she opened her camp in Sallyan, the local health workers spent the day observing her work, skeptical about the value of Ayurvedic medicine; the next day they brought all the patients from the nearby hospital for her to treat.

Besides prolapsed uterus, the most common gynecological problems Dr. Shrestha encountered in her clinic and camps were dysmenorrhea (painful periods), menorrhagia (excess bleeding during or between the period), and leukorrhea (vaginal discharge). "I have used Ayurvedic medicines for these problems," Dr. Shrestha said, "and have seen excellent results. We don't consider these conditions to be serious medical problems, since we can treat them very easily." Dr. Shrestha's treatments included douches, oral medications, medicinal oils and butters, wines, and fresh juices, all made from herbs.

Ayurvedic medicines are highly effective for a wide range of gynecological problems. Many herbs are locally available in the villages and are therefore cost-effective; they are also relatively nontoxic and have long-lasting effects. Dr. Shrestha's herbal specialty was knowing how to use the simplest, cheapest, and most easily available remedies. Although well trained in the use of more expensive and exotic Ayurvedic preparations, she preferred to teach her patients how to use common spices from their kitchens and easily available herbs growing in their gardens. Ingredients like ginger, turmeric, cloves, and cardamom, she said, can produce excellent results in most common illnesses. The doctor's ability to cure patients using medicines that cost very little or nothing was one of the reasons for her fame.

"Another tragedy of Nepali women is lack of delivery services," Dr. Shrestha continued. "It was recently published that every hour, five women are dying in Nepal due to problems related with delivery. This is because of poor services, lack of knowledge and awareness of health, and the low status of daughters-in-law in the family."

Many pregnant women don't come for medical examination, Dr. Shrestha explained, so they are not able to prepare for complications during delivery. If they are fortunate, a trained midwife will be present at the birth, but frequently only family members are there. As I listened to Dr. Shrestha describe all the forms of trauma that are possible during delivery, I couldn't help considering the words of Dr. Chopel, discussing why the female incarnation is inherently more painful than the male. It was also a reminder of the first noble truth of Buddha, that suffering is part of every stage of life. Just as giving birth is difficult and dangerous for the woman, it is a painful experience for the child as well.

Potentially serious problems can occur when a baby has an abnormal positioning or the birth canal is too narrow. In these cases the attendants must use manipulation and instruments, sometimes with force, and both the mother and child suffer. During an obstructed labor a child may die from oxygen deprivation or suffer mental and physical retardation from injury to the skull. In the villages where Dr. Shrestha worked, there were no facilities for emergencies; she had heard of women who had died trying to give themselves cesarean deliveries using farm instruments. Even when the delivery proceeds smoothly, the mother can be injured when the baby is pulled out. The vagina can be lacerated and ulcerated, sowing the seeds of future problems.

Malnutrition and anemia during pregnancy are widespread in the villages and remote areas of the Himalayas. "We get these cases everywhere in Nepal," Dr. Shrestha said. "The mother will serve the children, husband, and others, and will eat only those things that are left. She is not aware of her health, doesn't know what a balanced diet is, and doesn't know about having food rich in iron or vitamins." Dr. Shrestha's treatment for anemia included dietary prescriptions and the use of mandur bhasma, alchemically prepared iron oxide.

"Seeing the women in Nepal and India makes me feel very sad," Dr. Shrestha said. "After the camps I feel very sorry about the poor condition of Nepali village women; they are really suffering. The women don't know anything, and even if they know, they can't do anything. They don't have time to think or do anything about their health. They will look after the family, the children, the husband, the in-laws, but they won't look after themselves. This is a pitiful thing for the women of Nepal."

Dr. Shrestha's eyes conveyed the sadness of sharing so much pain with other women and facing tragedy on a daily basis, but her smile was full of inner strength.

"There is a lot of feeling of surrender in women," she said. "They won't try to think: Why is this happening, why should I follow this, why shouldn't I break down these rules? Very few women are like that. You see, we women are weak, and men don't want to change themselves.

They want their throne, and to rule by themselves. They don't want to give to others. For that we have to struggle."

Although her male contemporaries in the field of Ayurveda would not give her credit, Dr. Shrestha's progressive thinking was having a major impact on health care reform in Nepal. It was not unusual for a government agency to implement her ideas after she had presented them on radio or television. When she publicly stated, "In order for women's health care to be effective, it must have the involvement of the husband," this concept was immediately promoted as one of the government's novel ideas. "Women should have mental, physical, and emotional support from men," the doctor said, "and respect for their feelings. Women should be treated as equals, and should not be dominated by the male ego."

Chagdol Hill rises above the rice terraces at the western end of the Kathmandu Valley. The view from its homes looks east toward the spires of Swayambhu's temples, southeast toward downtown, south to the green cloud-covered cliffs behind the village of Kirtipur, west to Mt. Nagarjuna and the King's forest preserve, and north to Gunje and the Ganesh Himals. The neighborhood is relatively affluent by Nepali standards, since most of the men work in town as well as farm small plots of land. For the women it is still rural living; water has to be carried in urns from the fountains up long flights of stairs, cows and goats need to be tended, gardens planted and harvested.

Bernard had been living on Chagdol Hill for ten years, in a small red earth house he built for himself. The neighborhood was being invaded by Westerners dealing heroin, he told me, who were smuggling the brown powder from Thailand and selling it to the local youth. Wanting better company, Bernard started inviting his friends to take up residence in the vicinity. I rented a room from a family next door, as an escape from Boudhanath after the monsoons closed the road to Gunje. Gradually, a group of people from around the world began congregating on the hillside. Bernard's cottage became a small salon where an eclectic crowd gathered to share meals cooked over a cow dung fire. French intellectuals, German saddhus, Nepali locals, Swiss Buddhists, and an American herbalist would philosophize late into the night, then walk back to their homes in the quiet darkness of early dawn.

The Nepali family I rented from was friendly and hospitable. They brought fresh milk every morning from their cow, and curries with rice in the evening. During the day the men would go into town to their jobs, the children went to school, and the grandmother worked quietly in the garden. Kamala, the eldest daughter, did chores in the courtyard while her young son played with the neighborhood boys. I studied, meditated, and watched the monsoon clouds floating over the valley. When the children returned, they climbed the steps to my room and practiced their English lessons. Sometimes I would sit in my doorway and talk to Kamala as she spun wool on the balcony. Our conversations were usually about life in Nepal or my life in the West. She was always hesitant to talk about herself, and a shy smile was the only answer I would get about her personal world.

Her father, however, never hesitated to talk about himself. Mr. Acharya would pound on my door at six in the morning, announcing his virtues as a Brahmin who rises with the sun and washes his feet, and tell me of his great God that he worshipped every day. I learned that his God was a Naga, a serpent deity, who lived in a giant rock in the garden. From my window I could watch as he anointed the snake's head with vermilion, gave it flowers and rice, and recited prayers before going to work. When he returned in the afternoon, he would again pound on my door and ask if I had had a nice day, then proceed to the garden for more worship. Despite his devout behavior, though, my new landlord seemed to be a hard-hearted and angry man. Because of some feud, he and his brother, Bernard's landlord, had not spoken for over ten years, even though they lived next door to each other. Mr. Acharya proclaimed his spiritual virtues, but I knew from his face that he was very unhappy.

As I got to know my landlord's family through spending time in their home and listening to Bernard's descriptions of the intrigues on Chagdol Hill, I came to understand more of why Mr. Acharya had so many worries on his mind.

"As you know, Kamala's uncle has badly mishandled his karma," Bernard said one afternoon, referring to his landlord.

I replied that I had no idea what he was talking about.

"You don't know the story? Well, you're not supposed to know. He has a second wife. He is one of these old, archaic Brahmin types that think they are the Lord Creator Himself, and the woman is nothing."

"Where did this thinking come from?" I inquired. Being a sociologist and a long-term resident who knew both Nepali and Sanskrit, Bernard was a rich source of insights into the complexities of Brahmin life. He was an animated philosopher, and it never required much prompting to bring on an erudite discourse concerning the topic of one's choice.

"It is written in the Vedas," Bernard explained. "Some of the gods had several wives, so he has the chauvinistic attitude that he had every right to bring another woman. Of course, his first wife was extremely unhappy. The poor fellow became quite unpopular in his own family, and created a very uncomfortable situation for himself. He had to sell the second wife, then had to share the family land, and the whole affair is still not finished.

"This goes back to the role of Shakti, the Great Goddess," Bernard went on. "If you look for the origin of Shakti in modern Hinduism, it is not so easy to find, because all the main gods of the Vedas, like Brahma, Vishnu, and Shiva, are all male. It seems that the origin of Shakti as a feminine power is to be found in the pre-Aryan civilization in India. She was very prominent then, and her worship was very important; she was God in female form, the Mother, the Earth. We know that this mysterious Indus civilization worshipped the goddess at least as much as the gods, since the number of male and female images extracted from the ruins are quite equal. The goddess was then, and has been throughout history, very popular, very emotional, very appealing to the bhakti, the devotional side of man. But in the Vedas, Shakti was made the wife of the Aryan gods' king, Indra, and given a minor secondary role."

As a result of his emulating the polygamy of the Vedic gods, family life had become extremely difficult for Kamala's uncle. And as I soon learned, the subjugation of the ancient goddess, and the subsequent demise of devotion and respect for the female as her embodiment, had made life intolerable for another member of the family.

Below my little room of mud and wood was a shed where the family kept a large black cow and a small white calf. The youngest son would take the cow to graze on the sweet grass of Swayambhu Hill every morning, while the calf remained tied to a stake in the yard, munching on cuttings from the garden. Whenever I climbed the steps to my room I could peer into the darkness of the shed, but never saw anything other than straw and manure on the floor. One evening as I sat on the steps looking at the night sky, I made a startling discovery. From below came quiet voices, and a dim light illuminated the shed's open door. Walking silently down the stairs, I looked inside.

At the far end of the room was a small bed set above the urine and feces of the animals. On it sat Kamala, reading a book to her son Jagadis by the light of a bare bulb. They looked up and smiled as I entered, then invited me to sit with them. The room was filled with the ammonia stench of the animals, which stood tethered against the wall. We sat silently, not knowing what to say. Finally, I asked Kamala if this was her room. Painfully embarrassed, she replied that it was. We began talking about her life, and how the injustices of traditional beliefs had brought her to this miserable dwelling.

"This Nepali culture is very difficult," Kamala said. "Brahmins marry Brahmins, and marriage between different castes is not respected. I am from a Brahmin family, my husband was a Chetri, and I was his second wife.

"My husband and I met while we were in school. He was already married and living nearby, but he asked me to marry him. I said, 'Why? You are married, you have children. This is very difficult.'

"He said, 'No problem, everybody has two or three wives. I can take care of you, don't worry.' He asked me many times, and I said, 'This is too much of a problem.' His parents and wife also said no to him about this.

"But we got married, and then the baby came. When I told him I was pregnant, he said, 'I won't forget you.' He never helped me, didn't come over, stopped sleeping and eating with me, and was always going other places. During the delivery he went somewhere else.

"I didn't see him for four months after the birth. Six months later I went to my husband's house, and his parents and wife were crying and fighting with me. Then so many problems came. He always gave his money to his parents and other wife. But who will love me and help me live? Who will help me with food and clothes? I have nothing, no money, no food, no clothes. I feel crazy from so many worries, and hate everybody. My father doesn't speak to me. He won't look at my face, and won't help me. He says I can't live at home, and forbids me from entering the house where I was raised."

Kamala and her son had been banished from their home. Her father locked them in the cow shed every night. Kamala would never again have the opportunity for marriage and family. In the eyes of the Brahmins she was reduced to the rank of a prostitute, unworthy of marriage to any man. It was the fate of this young woman to live as an ostracized single mother, working at small jobs whenever possible, with little hope of bettering her situation. Jagadis had been taken out of several schools because of abuse from other children and teachers.

Kamala had been a young beauty, and was only twenty-four, but she looked forty. Her thick black hair was dry and graying, her olive complexion replaced with brown patches and dark circles under her eyes. When I asked about her health, I learned that she lived with the continual misery of parasites, digestive and menstrual disorders, as well as severe depression and a broken heart.

"I am an old woman already," she said. "I am sick from living in this cow house." As we talked, Kamala's mother appeared outside in the courtyard, pacing back and forth. "You should go now," Kamala said. I bid her good night and climbed the stairs to my room. Looking back, I saw Mrs. Acharya locking the door to the shed. Her daughter and grandson would be released in the morning when the family rose.

I lay down on my mat to ponder this sad and disturbing discovery, feeling the weight of spiritual impoverishment afflicting this difficult land. The melodic words of an ancient Sanskrit verse floated through my mind, a remnant of a forgotten era: "Yetra nari pujante, gamante sarwa devataha," "Where women are worshipped, the gods and goddesses abide." In the quiet of the evening I could hear Kamala's voice below, softly reading a bedtime story to Jagadis.

Dr. Shrestha and I met Dr. Singh at one of his offices at the end of New Road, where the plaza stretches from Freak Street to the Hanuman Temple. We arrived before he did and stood watching as he made his way through an acre of low tables covered with bizarre tourist items. Behind him on New Road a crowd had gathered around three traveling fakirs, who played with cobras in the hopes of frightening, fascinating, and coaxing a few rupees from their audience. The doctor walked slowly past the rows of hideous carved masks, skulls inlaid with bulging silver eyes, prayer wheels, strange musical instruments, and ugly jewelry. I could tell he wasn't feeling well.

He had been having diarrhea, he said when he joined us, but insisted that we proceed with our appointment anyway. We followed him up the stairs, past office clerks pretending to be busy, into a tiny room where we were immediately served tea.

"Tell us some stories and forget about your loose bowel movements," I said after we had made ourselves as comfortable as possible on the sagging furniture.

"You have to ask questions," he replied irritably.

"There is no end to my questions. Let's talk about women."

"No comments. I refuse to talk about it. The moment you talk about women, it is very personal. It means you have to expose yourself to the innermost core."

"Then let's talk about famous women in Ayurvedic history."

"No. I refuse to talk about that also. There have not been many famous women in Ayurvedic history. Ayurveda has been somewhat male-dominated."

"Why?"

"Do you know any, Sarita?" Dr. Singh inquired, hoping to shift the conversation.

"In history, no," she replied simply. I could see she was worrying about our teacher.

"Why do you think that is?" I persisted. "Thousands of years of Ayurvedic history . . ."

"There is a lot which is said, and a lot which is practiced," the doctor answered impatiently. "I think this is true in every society, but more so in this subcontinent. We have got goddess temples all over the country, we have the Kumari, the virgin who represents a living goddess, and we worship her in so many different ways. But when it comes down to the practical aspect of how to treat women, I think there is a lot to be desired."

"What's causing that?"

"David, let me tell you very frankly, there are certain things that I don't want to get into," the professor said sharply. "I can't solve those problems. I would like to limit myself to those things that I am competent enough to talk about. I don't think I am competent enough to talk about women in general, or women in Ayurveda, or women in society."

"Of course you are."

"If I am competent enough, it will be strictly my personal views, and it may not reflect the social norms. Sarita would be more competent. I would not like to talk about the condition of women. For me they are very precious. It bothers me to talk about them as a class. Every person is an individual."

'Then let's talk about Sarita. Why in the thousands of years of Ayurvedic history were there no women doctors? She is the first Nepalese woman doctor in Ayurveda. Why?"

"There must have been doctors, but there are no records," the doctor muttered.

"But there are famous men."

"I have not come across any famous women. Society preaches one thing and then practices another. She should be able to tell you that better."

"Has it always been like that in this society?"

"It has been like this in most societies. Don't you think that even in the Bible women are taken as a commodity? It is only different in the most primitive societies. There the women have better rights and a better position. Rape is a disease of civilized society. There is nothing like rape in primitive society.

"I know a tribe in the eastern part of India," he went on, relaxing a little. "They are a matriarchal society, so everything is owned by the women. The child knows the mother, not the father; the father is just the means of procreation, which is how women are being treated here. In that society the women rule, and the men are not even allowed in the house without the permission of the woman, and the moment she has had it, he is turned out. Men here get drunk, they quarrel, and all kinds of violence is common. In that society this is also common; they get drunk, they loaf around, but the moment the woman is there, they behave.

"Let me be very frank," the doctor said. "I have got my own opinion, views, and experiences. But what are you going to do with all these things?"

"This question is of universal importance," I answered. "It is intimately connected to health at all levels: public health, family health, individual health. The relationship between men and women is the most important aspect of society."

The professor sighed. "Since you won't leave me alone, I will tell you. What I will be telling you will not be the typical Nepalese or Hindu tradition. I don't hold to any tradition. I am totally nonconventional.

"The basic problem of society has been that the more civilized you are, the less spontaneous you become. With that loss of spontaneity, problems increase. At one point ancient civilization used to have strict formalities that had to be observed. You had to get up at a certain time, you had to do everything in the proper way, otherwise you were punished. The more developed a society is, the more codified the behaviors become, and the more civilized society thinks itself to be, the less it actually is. In the Victorian age, even in the Vedic age, things were done in such a severe way that society is still bearing the scars. You become an automaton, not a person. It is a negation of the whole human spirit."

Dr. Singh paused for a long moment before continuing. Dr. Shrestha sat wrapped in her shawls, listening quietly and trying to make herself invisible.

"What a woman represents to me is a mother," the doctor said, relaxing more. "She is first of all a mother. I had one of the most beautiful mothers that one can have. My mother was the kind of person who was practically the mother to the whole area. Nobody had any other name for her but Ma. Even the women in the street used to call her Ma. She could talk to the lowest person, sit down, exchange smokes, give them food, irrespective of what level of society they were. I think she represented the best in the woman.

"I think a lot of my behavior toward women has been influenced by that. To me, every woman is a very special person, from any society. For me the woman represents love, affection, all the qualities that make a man human. And here we are, with all these things which are so painful to me. That's why I don't want to talk about it. Within my sphere I try to behave the way I want to behave, but I can't do anything about it in general."

"How has that been forgotten in this society?" I wondered. "Those things are worshipped in temples everywhere, people recognize it spiritually, but they cannot practice it in their everyday life. Why?"

"I don't know. I can't answer that. I think if this world was ruled by women, it would be a better place to live."

We paused, sipped tea, listened to the noise in the streets. Dr. Singh was tired and vulnerable; Dr. Shrestha was absorbed in her own mood.

"What is understood classically about the healing powers of women, and the benefit of women being doctors?" I finally asked.

"The reason women are better, for me, is that their approach is from the heart. They are rational, but they are more likely to be influenced by the emotionality. They can be very cold-blooded, no question, but they become cold-blooded because they hate something, so it arises from the emotions."

"What can men learn from women?"

"They should be nearer to the heart," Dr. Singh said, becoming more inspired. "They should be more right-brain-oriented, rather than left-brain; not so rational, more feeling. I think this is what our ancient system is trying to get across. All these spiritual sciences talk about a state where there is no reason, that is beyond reason. What can that be? You cannot conceptualize it; it can only be felt through the heart. They have emphasized it repeatedly in all the old books. They all say you must commit yourself to God, to surrender yourself to God, you must have faith in God. When they say God they may have meant something specific, but for me it is a state beyond the human framework. You have to admit that not everything is within the scope of human intelligence. And once you admit that there are so many things you don't know, does it not make you humble? What is it that has made such a beautiful world? Are you going to deny the existence of that? Call it by any name, it doesn't matter at all.

"Yehudi Menuhin played in front of Einstein, and then Einstein came to him and said, 'Now I believe there is a God.' He was moved beyond his intellectual framework. You must have noticed that I am very logical and rational, but I don't want to submit myself to it in totality. I would rather submit myself to that totally unconventional thing."

"I'll give you the example of the mother," Dr. Singh said, his face softening. "Does the mother have to think about loving the child? It is totally spontaneous. The same when you fall in love with someone. That is also totally illogical. You don't just decide 'I want to love.' You just fall in love. This is what I appreciate about women. They are very spontaneous. I trust women much more than a calculating man. To me, it is they who make the beauty of this life, they who make this life worthwhile. Even in the jungle, in the most inhospitable place, if you are with somebody in love, that place becomes heaven. Heaven is not a beautiful building, it is where the heart is. If somebody can give you that kind of joy, how are you going to treat her?

"But this civilized society with its rules and regulations has killed all the spontaneity of human relations. That is why I am against codified religion. Every codified religion has its dark aspects. Remember that most of the murders have been done in the name of religion. Even now you can see so many people being killed and maimed. There were the Crusades, the Inquisition, the Hindu and Muslim conflict in this subcontinent, and they were all doing the great job of God. God must be the greatest criminal on earth, if He is really allowing his followers to commit such unthinkable crimes!

"I have lived through a period of history where there was this partition of India. It was a most traumatic period, and you can see the brutality that has been committed. I have met so many women who have been really brutalized in the name of religion. With any disturbance in any society, it is the women who are first brutalized. Are you aware of that? During the Hindu-Muslim riots, it was the women who suffered the most."

The professor sat back, watching me intently. We sat in silence; long minutes passed as the pain of the doctor's words gradually subsided.

"How can the wisdom of Ayurveda help us undo this damage?" I finally asked. "How can we learn a new way of thinking, to appreciate the feminine?"

"We are all obsessed with ourselves," the professor answered. "You are looking at society through your own perception, and what you think is good for you, you think is good for society. We try to impose our views on others, or at least try to preach to people that this is good or bad. Everybody should be an individual, and the ideal would be to tolerate others the way they are, not the way you want them to be. The only provision should be not to harm each other, not to violate the sanctity of others' individuality."

Dusk is falling in Thamel, and another Friday night is approaching. I sit on the curb, my back to one of the Tibetan jewelry shops, waiting for Dr. Shrestha. The shop is closed for the day, its owner perhaps eating momos and drinking chang in his home nearby. The traffic is congested as usual, the tiny alleys blocked and chaos guiding the circus of smoking vehicles in their erratic travels. A dead dog lies on the curb in front of me, probably thrown out of the street after being hit.

Its days of foraging, fighting, barking, and being cold and hungry are finished.

There is a new creature on the streets, one I hadn't seen in my previous visits. Indian-looking girls in tight Western clothes walk past, chewing gum, smoking cigarettes, spitting on the sidewalk, on the way to the local bars with their pimps strolling behind. Sexy, tough, and deeply abused, they try to simultaneously stand out and blend in, watching for both clients and the police. They check me out but refuse eye contact, and I wonder if they know about HIV, or have it.

The government estimates there are currently about 3,000 cases of HIV and 1,200 cases of AIDS in Nepal, but these figures cannot be realistic. The social environment is such that people don't discuss the problem, and men don't want to hear about using condoms. There are few medical facilities for testing, and treatment services are almost nonexistent.

"We don't have exact data for HIV and AIDS, but the number is increasing every year," Dr. Shrestha had said the week before. "The border to India is open, and people are going to the big cities from the villages. They are uneducated and not aware of HIV or this epidemic. It is a big problem, and it will increase."

HIV is being spread into Nepal primarily by men who have had sex with prostitutes in India, or girls returning from working in the brothels of Bombay or Delhi. Dr. Shrestha had been in some of the villages most directly affected by the trade in female flesh. In these places husbands have discovered that their young wives, described so nicely in the marriage negotiations, have infected them with the deadly virus, and wives learn that their husbands have brought the epidemic into their home.

"The village where I went for the last health camp is in Sindhupal-chok, a district that is known for the trafficking of girls," Dr. Shrestha had said. "When a girl reaches the age of twelve, the father or brother will take her to India for prostitution. They don't think that job is sinful. They feel proud, because she will bring money and they can build a house. If a house has a tin roof, it means the girl from that family has gone to India. Sometimes even the husband will take them. This is one bad aspect of our country."

I hadn't seen the sex business in Thamel before, but it has always been here, when the streets are dark and filled with offers of heroin and hashish. Dr. Jha once commented cynically that Nepali men never had enough money for what they needed, but they always had enough for prostitutes.

And there are the children, whose undeveloped bodies are the object of attraction for another kind of man. These men come from all over the world to Kathmandu and other Asian cities, to find homeless boys and girls, take them in, bathe them, feed them, and use them to satisfy their sexual and emotional hungers. The children hope for survival, but there are always new dirty faces in the street, and others vanish without a trace, a name, a family, or a history.

I sit on the steps in front of windows full of Tibetan turquoise, silver, amber, and coral, and pray. I pray to Avalokiteshvara, imagining his thousand compassionate arms embracing these destitute children and setting free the young women brought to sexual slavery, the life-giving lotus of their birth canals desecrated with infected semen so their families can have a tin roof. I see him touch the lonely men with his thousand radiant hands, removing the blindness of primordial ignorance, dissolving the simple confusion between the enticements of sensual pleasure and genuine happiness. With five thousand nectared fingers he blesses the stream of consciousness that once inhabited this dog's body, now wandering in the Bardo seeking a new existence. I pray for myself, that the deity in my heart bestow peaceful coexistence of erotic vitality and dispassionate wisdom.

Thousand-armed Avalokiteshvara first appeared in this world in India. As the Kashmiri princess-nun Gelongma Palmo lay dying of leprosy in a jungle cave, she beheld the countenance of the deity. Pouring crystal-clear water through her body, he instantaneously cured the disease. Now, he shines like the moon from the windows of thangka shops in Thamel's tangle of narrow carpet-lined alleys, glowing with blessings in the darkness of spiritual poverty.

Avalokiteshvara is male yet filled with feminine qualities. The incomparable alchemy of transmuting the pain of the world into loving-kindness infuses the deity with qualities not unlike those of a goddess, and he has appeared in that form to many. His essence is that of Quan Yin, the female bodhisattva whose Dharma blossomed across China. They are both emanations of pure love, showing us the deep path of the heart that carries us across the ocean of suffering to the far shore of emancipation. I visualize Avalokiteshvara, his princely demeanor ornamented with symbols of truth's power and beauty. The deity looks upon us with exquisite lotus-petal eyes, his face shining with splendor. He is draped in soft pastel rainbow silks, the blush of dawn adorning the snowy conch-shell whiteness of his body. He is praying for our release, reaching out to bless us, a thousand eyes in the palms of his tender hands looking upon our plight. He welcomes all with a thousand embracing arms of refuge, yet the stream of hungering humanity in the streets goes about its painful business, unaware of the deity's presence. Our world desperately needs this feminine compassion.

How far the gods and goddesses are from our lives, now that we no longer worship women as embodiments of the divine. At one time the devas lived among us, but now the streets are thick with fears of survival. What is it that man hungers for, that has brought women and children to such utter degradation, their bodies reduced to a feast of disease and sorrow? Can he not hear the woman and child inside him, calling him to wholeness? Man is born as Avalokiteshvara, so gentle, harmless, and soft, but the graceful eloquence of his spiritual masculinity has vanished, leaving only these shreds of broken families struggling in the virulent dust outside my closed eyes.

In my mind the deity is melting from male to female and back, revealing the dance of duality within our being. Surrounded by infinite oceans of atomic space, Shiva and Parvati are moving together in ecstatic union, spreading ripples across the surface of the Void, birthing worlds and their inhabitants from the stillness of equanimity. They are the original Creators, Purusha and Prakruti, primordial emptiness and dynamic manifestation, living inside us as the extension of our own mother's and father's flesh and blood. Our body is a magical alembic containing the seeds of union and polarities of Creation, where endless alchemical refinements of fire and water expand and contract with every breath. Sun and moon circulate through secret channels, like the entwined snakes of a caduceus around our spine, governing the homeostasis of a myriad physiological events. Every human being is biologically and spiritually masculine and feminine, made in the image of Ardha Narishwor, Shiva and Parvati residing together in the same body.

In Rasa Shastra, mercury is considered the sperm of Shiva, and sulfur is the orgasmic vaginal secretions of Parvati. Mercury is never used alone, due to its highly toxic and unstable nature; in order to be valuable for medicines or alchemical purposes, it must be bound to the female molecules of sulfur. Likewise, the sperm of man's body is mercurial in nature, and masculine power without feminine stabilization becomes poisonous to both society and environment. I open my eyes to the passion play of craving, and glimpse the invisible presence of mutated viruses burning slowly in the tender softness of the hardened young women of the streets.

"Unification is the cause of consciousness and creation," Dr. Tiwari once said. "If male and female are united in body, heart, and mind, they can do anything. Whatever problems exist can be solved; whatever negativity is in the world can be eliminated. Working together, men and women can create a very good society." I pray again, that the deep disturbance between the sexes may cease, and that men may gain mastery over the mercurial winged dragon of their sexuality. The ancient wound between male and female has plunged the world into chaos.

The cacophony of the streets comes roaring back to my senses as the night darkens, deepening the fatigue that rests so heavily upon me. Finally, Dr. Shrestha arrives, dodging the cars and tuktuks to cross the street. She is tired and haggard from another exhausting day of service to her patients, another drop of sacrifice swept into Kathmandu's sea of hardship. Conversation is impossible as we flee the churning crowds, pulsating music, honking cars, and begging hands. The luxurious respite of the Yin Yang Restaurant is waiting, where we slowly regain our composure and sense of humor over bowls of spicy tom yam soup.

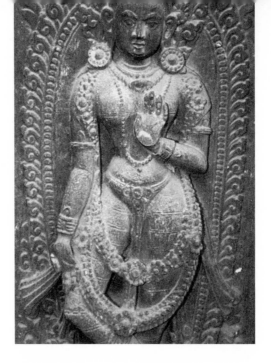

VIII.

INTO THE LOTUS

May all sentient beings attain an adamantine, indefatigable body; may all sentient beings attain an indestructible body that nothing can injure; may all sentient beings attain a phantomlike body, appearing throughout the world without limit; may all sentient beings attain a delightful body, clean, beautiful, strong, and healthy; may all sentient beings attain a body born of the realm of reality, same as the enlightened, depending on nothing; may all sentient beings attain a body like the radiance of beautiful jewels, which no worldly people can outshine; may all sentient beings attain a body which is a treasury of knowledge, and realize

freedom in the realm of immortality; may all sentient beings attain a body of an

ocean of jewels which is unfailingly beneficial to all who see it; may all sentient be-

ings attain the body of space, which none of the troubles of the world can affect.

AVATAMSAKA SUTRA
(FLOWER ORNAMENT SCRIPTURE)

The study of human embryology is a deep contemplation on the origin of life. From where do we come? How did we gain this precious human incarnation, in a body that surpasses all other forms in its potential for achieving enlightenment? What universal laws can we find unfolding during conception and gestation, and what do they reveal about what lies ahead in the cycle of existence, as it reaches its completion and subsequent renewal? Where else but in the flowing together of the seed tides does so much mystery surround Creation? The wisdom of the classical Tibetan and Ayurvedic doctors again provides us ample nourishment of gyan, the knowledge of higher truths with profound meaning.

Early physicians observed that in order for a plant to grow, four factors must be present: seeds with power to germinate, soil for them to grow in, water for nourishment, and a season conducive to their growth. For a human being to take birth, physicians reasoned, these conditions must also be present; sperm and ovum are the seeds, the womb is the soil, the nutritive fluids of the mother are the water, and the cycle of fertility is the season. Using an inferential and intuitive approach to research based on astute observation of natural phenomena, doctors of the distant past were able to comprehend the processes of conception and stages of fetal development in a way that was both medically insightful and spiritually sophisticated. Working without the advanced technology of microbiology, they described the week-by-week growth of the embryo with remarkable accuracy, provided specific diagnostic and treatment parameters for reproductive disorders, and elucidated a conceptual model that anticipated later discoveries of genetics.

The spiritual sophistication of early Asian embryology lies in the integration of medicine with the sciences of Tantra, the doctrines of karma and reincarnation, and Sankya's elemental model of the universe. Using the language and concepts of these integrated philosophies, the seers extrapolated what consciousness undergoes after leaving the old body, before entering a new one, and as it begins residing in the form growing in the womb. Their descriptions of the complete cycle of life have provided people through the ages with reasonable hypotheses, plausible answers, and—most important—experiential access to these great mysteries, which normally lie buried in the unconscious layers of the mind. These teachings have led to the development of meditative and yogic methodologies to guide seekers of transcendence out of the wheel of endless rebirths, while their application to the field of medicine has created therapies such as punshavan karma, the science of conceiving healthy children.

Ancient embryology is the study of cosmological principles within the microscopic realms. While the medical focus is specifically concerned with conception and gestation of a human being, the laws defined by this science extend to all forms of life, and ultimately to the formation of the universe. We find in Ayurvedic embryology a bridge from the individual seed and egg to the archetypal forces of Purusha, who as Shiva is the formless, motionless Father of Creation, and Prakruti, who as Shakti is the Mother of all forms and movement. These Creators of the infinitude of existences are none other than our own flesh-and-blood parents, who provided us with the bodily constituents necessary for birth; they live on within us as deities in union, the polarities of spirit and matter, sun and moon. Ayurvedic and Tibetan embryology therefore reflect the creation philosophies of their cultures, which assert that consciousness is the ultimate cause of the phenomenal world. The same forces that move an individual mind-stream to seek rebirth cause new galaxies and world systems to coalesce in the womb of empty space, to become the body of innumerable consciousnesses.

Birth and prenatal events are among the most formative and influential experiences that affect soma and psyche, yet our memory of them has vanished into the mists at the dawn of time. Only a few short years ago we each had an embryological form that was indistinguishable from that of other humans, even other animals; in both physical characteristics and utter dependency on the nourishing Mother, our similarities transcended all superficial differences. The study of embryology reminds us of our common ancestral heritage; it is the contemplation of our emergence from the shared womb of origination. Reawakening this memory restores respect for all of life, and helps us comprehend what the seers proclaimed as the ultimate solution to the suffering we are creating in the world: "The whole universe is a family."

The study of classical embryology begins with teachings concerning the health of the parents, specifically as reflected in the vitality of their reproductive juices. Using the terminology of the Tridosha theory, this science describes the physiological processes that form the sperm and ovum, and the various disturbances that can interfere with fertilization, gestation, and the long-term health of a child. The practical applications of this medical information can be found in the associated practices of vajikarana (sexual rejuvenation) and punshavan karma (conceiving gifted and healthy children). Some of these methods are culturally irrelevant and too esoteric for most of the modern world, but many valuable aspects remain, especially botanical therapeutics, such as the use of nutritive herbs for overcoming impotence or developing the strength of the placenta. The vision inherent in this knowledge is that of a world populated by healthy people, the result of parents who purified their bodies for the benefit of future generations.

I found Dr. Chopel at the Gelugpa Monastery at the base of Swayambhu Hill. He sat on a low couch in a small room, wrapped in heavy maroon robes to ward off the morning chill. It had been a year since my last journey to Kathmandu, and Amchi-la had aged noticeably since I last saw him. The old doctor's head was freshly shaved, revealing all the weathered contours of his striking features. The bony sculpture of his skull was more prominent, his face more emaciated beneath the wrinkles of brown Tibetan skin, but his eyes were as clear, penetrating, and expressive as ever. When he spoke I could hear the advancing age in his voice. It was higher-pitched and hoarser than before, but with a brevity that left no doubt about the authority of his words.

I was pleased to see the venerable doctor again, and he seemed happy to know that I would travel halfway around the world to listen to his words. Unfortunately, he was in the midst of monastic activities. "I have brought the Shelkar monks here for Dharma teachings," he said. "There will be very little time to give you medical instruction. A high abbot will be arriving soon to give empowerments, and there are many preparations we must make. However, if you come early in the morning we can meet for a few hours every day." I gratefully accepted the offer.

Each morning I rose at dawn and drove through misty fields to the foot of Swayambhu Hill. At the monastery the monks were busy hoisting poles of prayer flags, laying down rolls of colorful Tibetan carpets, assembling a brocade-covered throne where the Rinpoche would sit. While they worked and played outside, I sat with Dr. Chopel in a small room upstairs, as he gave teachings on whatever subjects I requested.

One of his first lectures concerned conception and formation of the human body. Bright beams of morning light filled the cold room, illuminating the doctor's robes and smooth ochre skin. A young monk repeatedly refilled our cups with steaming sweet tea as Dr. Chopel consulted his medical texts. Illustrating his ideas with graceful movements of his hands, my teacher explained and commented on the Tibetan medical view of embryology.

"To have a human birth, there are many links that must come together," Amchi-la began. His teachings were from the *She Gyu,* or *Explanatory Tantra.* Like the other three Tantras of Tibetan medicine, this knowledge was first articulated by the sage Rigpe Yeshe, the Medicine Buddha's emanation.

"There are four requirements for the formation and development of the fetus. The first is the pure essences of the parents. The second is the five universal elements of earth, air, fire, water, and space. The third is the three biological humors: they are Phlegm, which is composed of earth and water elements; Bile, which is composed of water and fire elements; and Air, which is composed of air and space elements. When these elements and energies are provided by the parents, then development of the fetus begins. The fourth link is the karmic and emotional conditions within the mind seeking rebirth, which lead to attraction toward the parents."

The Tibetan understanding of conception is derived from a synthesis of Ayurvedic medical theory and Buddhist philosophy. The basis of conception at the physical level is the harmonious balance of elements and humors within the parents. On a spiritual level, it is the consciousness undergoing the process of incarnation, and its karmic relationship with its new parents.

"For a child to be conceived, the uterine blood of the mother and the sperm of the father must be pure. Whatever we eat is ultimately refined into menstrual blood or sperm. Due to the activities of the bodily elements, the blood becomes red and the sperm becomes white. When these are united, then consciousness arises."

Amchi-la's simple words contained a wealth of knowledge. Many earlier lectures had been devoted to explaining the physiological processes that occur as the body refines the raw nutrients of diet into the reproductive fluids. From the most coarse level of juices in the stomach, step by step through the enzymatic transformations within the organs and tissues, the doctor had described the understanding of metabolism in Ayurvedic and Tibetan medicine. The end result of this alchemical purification is ojas, luminosity of the body.

Like ojas, semen is regarded in Ayurveda as a fluid which pervades the body, rather than being stored specifically in the reproductive glands. It is compared to the juice in sugarcane, butter in milk, and oil in sesame seeds. When the semen is stimulated by the heat of passion, it flows from everywhere in the body to the testicles, and from there outside the body. It is described as being like ghee, which melts from the fire of desire.

The reproductive essences of the parents are the first link in the process of conception. From the father comes white kua, or sap, which is sperm and seminal fluids, and from the mother comes red kua, the ovum and nutrient blood in the uterus. Both of these living fluids must be healthy and contain the proper proportions of earth, water, fire, air, and space elements; this is the second requirement for conception. These five universal elements are the basis of the three biological humors of the parents' bodies, which are the third necessity. Through these three factors the child's constitution is created.

The purity of the kua is crucial for healthy conception and growth of the child. Being the end result of the refinement of nutrients, kua contains the cream of all the bodily constituents. If the biological humors of the parents are imbalanced, the constituents of the reproductive fluids will be affected. Using the Tridosha theory, Dr. Chopel proceeded to elaborate on the specific corrupting influences of aggravated humors. His traditional concepts described a diagnostic system that can be directly applied to understanding and treating modern conditions of infertility and sterility.

"If the uterine blood and sperm are affected by unbalanced Air humor, they become dry and lose their color. Air diseases cause the menstrual blood to become rough and black. If the blood and sperm are affected by a disease of the Bile humor, they become yellow, sour, and smell bad. If they are affected by a disease of the Phlegm humor, they become white, sweet, cold, and sticky. When Bile and Air are combined, the blood and sperm become dry. If Air and Phlegm humors are combined, the blood and sperm disintegrate. When Phlegm and Bile are combined, the blood and sperm congeal. When all three humors are corrupted, the blood and sperm become putrid, and conception cannot occur. For a healthy conception to occur, these elements must be pure."

Dr. Chopel was using classical terminology to describe common medical conditions of the reproductive system. Air affecting the reproductive fluids can be seen in cases where people suffer from high stress and poor diet; the dark blood discharged during some cases of endometriosis is an example. The yellow color of Bile humor is evident in bacterial conditions, such as discharges from gonorrhea and prostatitis. Phlegm humor disorders can be correlated with mucogenic conditions, such as yeast and fungal infections.

"If the baby has good karma, its parents will be healthy," Amchi-la stated. He sat cross-legged on his cushions in the rich light of the Himalayan morning, looking dignified with age. The turquoise cover of the *Gyu Shi* lay open in the maroon and saffron folds of the doctor's robes as he consulted its writings. "If the essences and elements from the parents are all pure and the karma of the child is good, then a child will be conceived. If not, the body will not form. The blood of the mother should be clear, like the water of the ocean, and like the blood of the rabbit, crimson and light. The sperm of the father should be pure, a little white, abundant, and heavy."

According to Dr. Chopel, being born with a healthy body into a healthy family is the fruition of positive karma, while being born with an unhealthy body into an unhealthy family is the fruition of negative karma. Every generation is formed from the concentrated cumulative influences of the previous one; the health of the parents directly impacts the coming generations. Individuals may be indifferent or apathetic about their own health, but health consciousness is a basic requirement for conceiving and raising children. Reproductive responsibility includes having the foresight to provide children with good karmic circumstances.

A healthy child is an asset to the family and society; a child who is chronically unwell as a result of a weakened constitution may become a heavy burden. Poor diet, drugs, chemical poisons, and stress all find their way into the seeds which create children. If we pollute our bodies, the "sap" of regeneration will be weakened and contaminated with toxins. This will become an increasingly crucial issue as environmental pollution increases, the long-term transgenerational effects of pharmaceutical drugs emerge, and pediatric health declines.

Dr. Chopel's teachings revealed an important source of healing for humanity. If their implications were applied to farsighted preventive medicine, it would be possible through purification of the body to create a more balanced and refined kua for future generations. The more pure the fluid essences become, the stronger children's physical constitutions will be, and the more evolved their potential for intelligence.

Ayurvedic and Tibetan medicines recognize the possibility of consciously conceiving gifted and healthy children. Purifying and potentizing the sperm and egg with rejuvenation therapies can help create children of extraordinary constitutional vitality. By uplifting her mind with beautiful surroundings and joyful meditation, a woman can influence the consciousness growing in her womb, and bring into the world a child of superior intelligence and creative capacity. By invoking blessings of the spiritual realms through prayer, chanting, and devotion, seeds of positive karma can be planted in the mind-stream of a child, to sprout later in its life as wholesome inclinations and good fortune. Many herbs provide high-quality nourishment to the placenta and developing fetus. Certain treatments, such as acupuncture with gold needles at the end of each trimester, can reduce transmission of constitutional imbalances from the parents to the child. This, rather than merely determining the sex of a baby, was the original and greater purpose of punshavan karma.

"The mind has no beginning, and no form," my old teacher continued. He was introducing the fourth factor needed for conception, the consciousness seeking rebirth. "All beings have the same kind of mind. It is called Wind Mind, because it has the nature of Air. All beings experience the Bardo, or intermediate state between death and rebirth, where the mind resides after leaving the old body and before entering a new body. Before conception the mind is not attached to a form: it cannot be seen except by highly realized beings, but it can perceive the forms of others. It can travel spontaneously with each thought. This is due to the presence of the Air element within the mind."

In Tibetan Buddhist medical teachings, reincarnation is considered a fundamental truth. This view is based on teachings given by visionaries and mystics, who have compiled such scriptures as the Tibetan *Book of the Dead*. The knowledge of what occurs during the process of dying, in the after-death state, and how consciousness returns to the world of form, is preserved in the transmissions of those who have achieved insight into these realities, either from meditative trance or near-death experiences. Tibetan medicine incorporates this larger view of cyclical lifetimes into its understanding of current and future health conditions.

One example of reincarnation philosophy applied to medicine appears in the teachings on karmic diseases. Illness can be classified into three levels: superficial, middle, and deep. Superficial conditions are those which are transient and affect the surface of the body, such as colds and flus; these are mostly related to fluctuations in daily routines and weather, and have relatively little mental or emotional significance. Middle-level illnesses are those that accumulate over a longer period of time and affect deeper organ systems; these are caused by lifestyle, such as liver diseases from alcoholism, and have a greater degree of emotional involvement. The deepest levels of illness are karmic diseases, spiritual and mental negativities that are carried in the stream of consciousness from lifetime to lifetime. They are brought from the last life into the current one, and become integrated into the embryo at the time of conception. These diseases are therefore intimately linked with the health and karma of the parents, in the sense that they provide the circumstances for the karma to ripen.

Dr. Chopel gave several examples illustrating the nature of karmic diseases. These include conditions caused by birth traumas, such as cerebral palsy; birth defects; and chronic constitutional disorders that are resistant to treatment or respond with paradoxical reactions. Cancer is a classic karmic disease, involving both individual negative karma and the fruition of society's harmful impact on the environment. Hereditary diseases unfold over generations and also involve collective karma. Karmic diseases can be described as a ripening of negative karma within the body, a sickness of the spirit, or both. Spiritual sickness is evident in diseases such as cancer, involving long-term repression of strongly negative emotions.

The philosophy of reincarnation is used not only to explain the origins of complex diseases, but to resolve them as well. In order to cure karmic diseases, the body must be treated, but more important, the causative negative karma must be removed from the mind. This is accomplished through the purification of consciousness by spiritual practices. In some cases the combination of physical and spiritual healing can cure the disease. In other cases the disease is incurable, because the illness is too powerful and the body too weak to recover. If the disease is in an incurable stage, then spiritual purification of the mind is said to help remove the karmic cause by the root, so that its seeds are not carried into the next lifetime to sprout again.

Dr. Chopel continued his comments. "For conception to take place, the red and white essences of the parents and the mind of the child must merge. Without the presence of the future child's mind, the body will not form.

"The mind of a being is propelled by its karma and emotions. A mind in the Bardo will be attracted to its future parents in sexual intercourse. The forces of karma draw the mind to the parents, and through the powers of emotions it perceives them. The mind must incarnate because of its karma, and because of its emotional tendencies it experiences attraction to the parents. If there is no former karmic relationship between the parents and child, there will be no conception."

This profound revelation about what occurs within the consciousness of a being before its conception required further elaboration. I interrupted my teacher's commentary.

"If there is no attraction within the mind residing in the Bardo, is there no rebirth?" I asked.

In reply, the doctor clarified the role of emotions in the process of incarnation. "The baby's form is due to its karma and its emotions. Emotions are the root of karma; if we give up our emotionality, then we do not have to suffer karmically. Emotionality is the force that turns the wheel of karma. Without emotions, karma has nothing to do. Even the Buddha had karma, but he was free of emotionality. Ordinary beings such as ourselves have karma as well, which continues to be activated by our emotional tendencies. For bodhisattvas the seed of karma remains inactive, but for ordinary beings it is planted in the field of the emotions.

"In the Bardo the mind is governed by emotions. Reincarnation for highly developed meditators is not like the reincarnation of ordinary people. These great beings are able to choose their future parents and incarnate under their own power for the purpose of benefitting others. Ordinary beings in the Bardo are driven by marigpa. The karma from their previous lives governs their experience, causing them to desire the future parents."

Almost a hundred years ago, in a Tibet that no longer exists, a woman was gathering roots, flowers, and fruits of medicinal plants from the forest. She glowed with joy and good health as she waited for the child inside her to arrive. Ever since the night he was conceived, her sleep had been filled with dreams of auspicious meaning.

The child moved, and the woman knew it was time to return to Precipice Hermitage, the hilltop retreat where she lived. Her son was born upright, feet first, amidst wonderful events that were seen by everyone in the vicinity. Above and all around the house, brilliant rainbows formed and snow fell gently like a rain of flowers. As soon as the baby entered the world, he looked around and smiled radiantly, then spoke. He prophesied the spreading of the Buddhist teachings of spiritual truth, and recited the six-syllable mantra of universal compassion, Om mani padme hum. Such was the birth of Kalu Rinpoche, Karma Rangjung Kunchab, Self-Arisen and All-Pervading.

Tibetan embryology describes four different levels of beings who incarnate. Ordinary beings enter the womb ignorant of their past and future lives, and remain so while in the new body. One who has entered the stream to enlightenment enters the womb with awareness of past and future lives, but forgets while in the womb. A novice bodhisattva will enter a new body with knowledge of the past and future, but will lose it after birth. Advanced bodhisattvas will retain the knowledge of their past and future lives. These highly evolved beings have gained the freedom to choose the conditions of their rebirth as a result of their past spiritual practices and strong motivation to spread the Dharma. In order to incarnate, it is said that they enter the father's mouth on his inhalation, descend through his body, and reach the womb through his semen. Wondrous signs occur at the time of conception, the mother has auspicious dreams during the pregnancy, and the newborn child displays remarkable behavior.

When the Chinese Zen master Hsu Yun, Empty Cloud, was conceived, his parents both dreamed that a tiger jumped onto their bed. They woke to find the air perfumed with an intoxicating fragrance. His birth was entirely different from Kalu Rinpoche's, but equally unusual. He was born in a membranous bag, which was left with the body of his mother, who died during delivery. The next day a wandering herbalist appeared, opened the bag, and removed the baby.

One of the primary goals of Tibetan Tantric meditation is to gain control of the subconscious currents of the mind and life force that lead to rebirth, in order to bring about incarnation in favorable conditions for developing one's spiritual practice, or close the door to rebirth entirely. These energy meditations mimic the movements of pranas and winds in the subtle nerves, and therefore allow access to states of consciousness that lie buried in the deeper recesses of the nervous system. By gaining mastery over these currents, advanced meditators conquer the forces that carry ordinary beings from life to life.

This type of meditation is used during initiations into the practices of Tantric deities. Students are instructed to imagine entering the mouth of the guru, who is in the form of a male deity, descending through the central channel of the guru's body, and being emitted through his reproductive organ into the "secret sky" of the deity's female consort. Within the secret sky of the womb—the internal dimension of infinite space where consciousness becomes clothed in flesh—they are made into a new form, that of a baby deity. This visualization follows the route of incarnation described for bodhisattvas. Through such mental experiences, the student gains insight into the processes of nature that lead to rebirth; by perfecting these practices, an adept can repeat the process during and after death.

Pregnancy and childbirth are difficult, sometimes dangerous, and accompanied with suffering for both mother and child. Birth, proclaimed the Buddha, is the first great suffering of this life, to be followed by sickness, old age, and then death. The recognition of this cycle, repeated endlessly through infinite realms permeated with various miseries and devoid of lasting comfort or happiness, is the root of renunciation. It has brought untold numbers of seekers to teachings and practices which lead to an ultimate state of emancipation: nirvana, the cessation of craving for becoming, which releases us from samsara, the whirlpool of existence.

"If there is no desire within the mind, there is no rebirth?" I asked Amchi-la again.

"Yes," he answered.

"Is the goal of meditation practice to overcome desire?"

"The goal of practice is to overcome desire," the old doctor replied patiently.

Classical embryology's description of the microstructure of sperm and ovum reveals an early understanding of genetics. Semen is known to consist of bijas, seeds, which are the sperm cells. Each bija is composed of bijabhagas, individual units responsible for creating specific organs and viscera; the bijabhagas in turn are made of subparticles, which can produce structural and functional disturbances if they are defective. This concept roughly parallels the description given by modern microbiology: sperm cells carry chromosomes made of DNA strands consisting of individual genes.

Tibetan medicine states that the sex of a child is determined primarily by three factors. The first is the relative strength of the red and white essences of the parents. "If the sperm of the father is more abundant," Dr. Chopel stated, "then a boy will be conceived, and if the blood of the mother is more abundant, then a girl will be conceived."

The second factor is the timing of conception. Dr. Chopel presented the view shared by both Tibetan and Ayurvedic gynecology: if conception occurs on the first, third, fifth, seventh, or ninth day of a woman's cycle, it will be a boy; if it is on the second, fourth, sixth, or eighth day, it will be a girl. Modern doctors would find it difficult to accept this numerological explanation of the chromosomal processes responsible for determining a baby's sex.

The third factor is attraction and aversion toward the mother and father existing within the mind seeking incarnation. If the consciousness feels attraction toward the mother and aversion toward the father, it will become male; if the attraction is toward the father, it will become female. While this concept is impossible to prove or disprove scientifically, it plays a role in the Tantric meditations relating to conscious reincarnation. Tibetan Buddhism, with its patriarchal and patrilinear views, generally maintains that enlightenment is possible only in a male body. It is for this reason that the Tantric meditator visualizes entering the mouth of the father, so as to relate to the female from the masculine side of attraction.

Dr. Chopel's lecture continued. "The human form is created by the three humors, which are formed from the five universal elements and the karmic links of the parents and child. Each of the five elements is needed if the fetus is to take form and develop: the air element sustains life by oxygenating fetal circulation; space provides room to grow; fire stimulates metabolism; earth gives flesh form; and water nourishes development.

"The earth element produces the sense of smell, the flesh, and the bones. The water element produces the blood, the sense of taste, and the body's moisture and fluids. The fire element produces the complexion, the heat of the body, and the power to see. The air element produces the breath, hardness and softness of the skin, and sense of touch.

The space element produces the holes and channels of the head and body, and the sense of hearing. With all of these conditions, the shape and form of the baby is created."

Ayurveda describes the embryo as garbha, the union of sperm, ovum, and atma (soul), nourished by rasa, the refined nutritive juices of the mother. Of all the factors influencing the vitality of the embryo, atma is most important. Atma is composed of mind and intellect, which transmigrate from the past life in an astral body composed of etheric forms of the five universal elements.

We are brought into existence through the merging of the maha-bhutas, the five psycho-physical aggregates and primordial elemental qualities. These are simultaneously matter, energy, and intelligence. Flowing unceasingly through the labyrinthine networks and passageways of the body, Creation's five atomic qualities form, in miniature, a mandala of the universe. Our bones are the clay and dust of the earth, minerals in continuous circulation shaping and unshaping our dense skeletal core. Water travels endlessly through rains and rivers, sweat and blood, ocean and dew, the unctuous liquids of life softly enveloping the hardness of our bony structure. Our breath moves invisibly, its clarity and lightness expanding and contracting through space. The sharp and subtle rays of the sun shine back in the light of our eyes and bodily warmth; the fire of digestion gives luster to our complexion. Our human body is a web of warmth, liquid, light, and breath, an ephemeral matrix of mutable forms.

Tibetan and Ayurvedic physicians, since the early days of medicine, have described the week-by-week evolution of the fetus. This knowledge is one of the many brilliant accomplishments of early naturalistic scientists working without sophisticated technology. Their observations, gathered from both accumulated physical evidence and contemplative insight, are remarkably consistent with what is known to Western science. Dr. Chopel explained this ancient knowledge.

"In the first week the blood and sperm will mix, and will have the consistency of milk and blood mixed together," the doctor said. "In the second week it thickens."

Twelve days after conception, the womb closes like a "lotus at sunset."

"In the third week the fetus becomes like yogurt, white in the middle with blood surrounding it. There is no form to the body at this stage. During this week the sex of the baby may be influenced by such practices as mantra, yoga, and various medicines. After the fourth week this is not possible. During the fourth week the form of the fetus is like that of a radish."

According to the medical theories of Tantric yoga, the first part of the body to be formed is the navel, through which the blood of the mother begins to circulate inside the embryo. This nutritious warmth and breath stimulates the formation of the embryo's primitive channels.

"During the fifth week the navel begins to form in the middle of the radish shape. In the sixth week the spinal cord begins to grow from the navel. The baby develops with the help of the umbilicus. The navel of the baby is connected to the main channels of the womb. Nutrients from the food the mother eats are passed to the baby through these channels. Without this nourishment the baby cannot grow, just as rice cannot grow without water."

When fully developed, the umbilicus contains a plexus of five hundred subtle nerves. Their function is to help the process of refining the marrow into red and white kua. These nerves also play an important role in Tantric meditations which activate the circulation of prana through the chakras, the energy centers of the etheric body.

Lacking tools of internal visualization such as ultrasonography, the ancient physicians relied on astute observation and deductive reasoning to develop their concepts of embryology. These doctors, like their modern counterparts, gathered together from distant lands to share knowledge. During one of these conferences, they debated theories of how the body is formed. Some postulated that the head developed first, because it is the seat of the senses. Others said it was the heart, since it is the seat of animation, intellect, and mind. The umbilicus was believed by some to be the original organ, because it is the inlet of nourishment. Others said the hands and feet, the primary instruments responsible for all sorts of movement, were first to appear. The large intestine was postulated because it is the seat of vata, which governs all activities in the body; others said the sense organs, because they are the faculties of perception. Still others claimed the trunk of the body formed first, because all other parts are connected to it. Dhanvantari, the physician-saint of Ayurveda, concluded the debate by stating that all organs develop simultaneously in different phases. He gave examples of things growing in nature, such as a mango fruit, to illustrate how various parts of organisms develop in stages, even as they are forming simultaneously.

"From the father the bones, teeth, and spinal cord are produced," Dr. Chopel said, continuing his explanation of the elemental stages. "From the mother the flesh, blood, and vital organs are produced. The consciousness of the baby produces the sense organs." The father contributes those elements that are hard and stable, and the mother contributes the soft organs and tissues.

Ayurveda says that an incarnating being inherits its constituents from the influences of the sperm, ovum, rasa, and atma. From the rasa come proper growth, invigoration, plumpness, strength, and other such aspects of nutritive power. The atma determines what realm of creature-hood incarnation will occur in, the life span, self-awareness, sense organs and sense consciousness, pleasure and pain, desires and aversion, understanding, memory, and so forth. The atma brings with it the influences of mind, such as character and emotional tendencies. The atma is also endowed with varying degrees of wholesomeness, which contribute to the health of the body, clarity of senses, virility, and other such traits.

"During the eighth week the eyes continue to form, and the shape of the head emerges. In the ninth week space appears inside the fetus, which becomes the stomach. Up to this time the embryo is referred to as a fish, because it lacks limbs."

We start as a seed planted in the soil of the womb, naked awareness being clothed in the flesh and blood of our mother. Drawn by craving for existence and the ripening of past actions, we emerge from the formless Bardo and traverse the evolutionary stages of life. In embryonic development, every human has passed through the vegetable, lower animal, and higher animal realms.

"In the tenth week the arms and legs begin to form. During the eleventh week the eyes, ears, nose, and mouth develop, and the sex organ and anus are more completely formed. During the twelfth week the five vital organs begin to form, and during the sixteenth the hollow organs appear. The arms and legs are further developed in the fourteenth week, and in the fifteenth the muscles of the arms and legs increase. In the sixteenth week the fingers and toes appear, and in the seventeenth the major nerves develop that connect inner and outer parts of the body. At this stage the human form is completed. During this time the fetus is referred to as a turtle, because it has limbs and a head."

During the last trimester, the growing fetus places the heaviest burden on the mother's organs of elimination, thereby adversely affecting the quality of blood and nutrients circulating in the womb. For this reason, the period between the eighteenth and thirty-fifth week, when the fetus is most exposed to these impurities, is referred to as the stage of the pig. Tibetan, Ayurvedic, and Chinese medicine regard some childhood illnesses, such as chicken pox, to be a natural and healthy process of purifying the prenatal toxins accumulated during those weeks.

Classical embryology describes not only the physical development of the fetus but various conditions the incarnating consciousness experiences as well. As might be expected, ancient medical authorities disagreed on when consciousness first manifests in a fetus: in the third, fourth, or fifth month. One reason for the differing viewpoints was that distinctions were made as to when the fetus begins to feel body sensations, when it begins to have emotions, and when it becomes mentally aware. There was a general agreement that consciousness is associated with the heart, and a consensus that as the heart begins to beat, the mind begins to function. Tibetan and Ayurvedic medicines both state that as the mind awakens, the embryo begins to experience emotional states, past-life memories, and longings. These thoughts and feelings are transmitted from the heart of the fetus through the bloodstream to the heart of the mother, who subsequently begins to develop cravings and aversions for different foods, smells, and so forth.

"During the fourth week, when the form of the embryo is like that of a radish," Dr. Chopel explained, "consciousness begins to enter into its form. In the seventh week the eyes begin to develop, which are the first of the sense consciousnesses. At week twenty-four the baby is fully formed. From that time on it experiences various kinds of suffering. If the mother takes hot liquids, then the baby feels burning sensations, or if cold foods, then freezing sensations. If the mother moves suddenly, the baby feels as if it's falling, and if she lifts something heavy, the baby feels as if it is being crushed. During the twenty-fifth week the currents of the Air humor begin moving, and in the twenty-sixth week the baby begins to remember its past life. During this time it will experience different types of emotions. During the thirty-seventh week the baby suffers from sadness and discomfort, and experiences itself surrounded by blood and body fluids. At this time the baby will begin to have negative thoughts as a result of its previous karma. Because of its ignorance it begins to experience desire and aversion."

The human being is now completely formed. Its consciousness is residing within its new home, waiting in its cramped quarters to be expelled into another lifetime.

"If the baby lies to the right side of the abdomen," Dr. Chopel said, "milk or tenderness are more apparent in the right breast, the mother dreams of men, and her body feels light, then the baby will be a boy. If the baby lies to the left side, milk comes first to the left breast, and the mother dreams of singing, ornaments and jewelry, and so forth, then the baby will be a girl." This description of polarities is based on the Tantric view of the nervous system, which describes the right nostril as the opening to the solar, masculine current of prana, and the left to the lunar, feminine current. Many traditional doctors and midwives are experts at using this system of observation to correctly predict the sex of the child.

Human beings emerge from a warm curdlike mass, undifferentiated, primordial, at one with the Mother. Shifting through animal shapes, we traverse the evolutionary stages of embryonic life. Floating, translucent, in this lightless liquid world, we feel every sensation, every thought, every emotion of the one who is giving us life. Finally, we are pushed through the birth canal, squeezed through the convoluted conch shell. With our first inhalation, the wheel of time is set in motion, with no knowledge of how many times it will turn before the last exhalation.

Our sense of self develops, with its dualities of inside and outside, heart and mind, self and other. Soon, we lose our ability to perceive the feelings of those around us, and gradually drift away from our inborn spontaneity and expressiveness. Our sense of separation increases until we find ourselves alone in the world. "Conceptualizing separateness is the source of all suffering," my wise old teacher said, concluding his comments on embryology.

Inside us there remains a translucent embryo, its dark eyes staring into the infinitude of space. In the recesses of our nervous systems, coursing through the channels of life force below the threshold of perception, the sensations of the world around us can be felt. Somewhere inside the deepest layers of our bodies and minds, we are still aware of our connectedness with totality, which has never ceased.

If we could peel away the illusory "self" we imagine within the dancing, streaming, vibrating mass of wind, water, fire, and earth we call our own, we would begin to feel again the life around us and within us. We would feel the pain and happiness of others as our own. We would naturally want others to be happy and free of suffering. The sleeping Buddha would awaken.

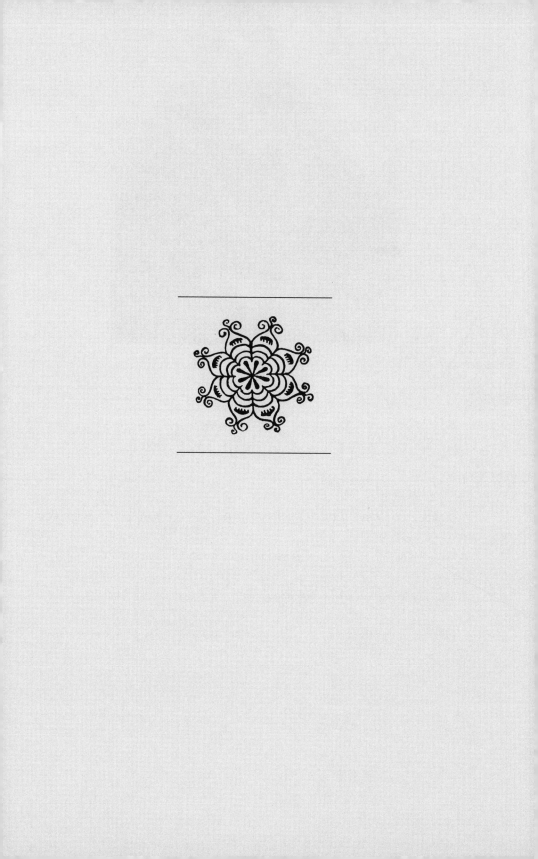

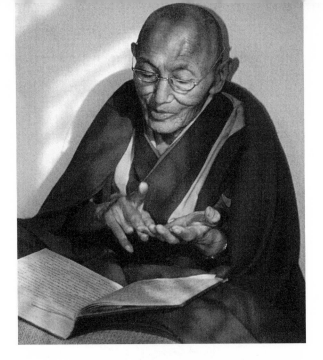

IX.

SATTVIC MEDICINE

Medicine is spiritual if the person who practices it, having recognized others as his or her parents in past lives, is motivated to liberate all beings from their suffering. The competent physician acting out of love follows the teaching of the Dharma. If the physician practices giving love and security, medicine can be made more efficient.

KALU RINPOCHE

The results of a doctor's treatments are a reflection

of his level of purity and virtue.

DR. NGAWANG CHOPEL

According to the Sankhya system of enumeration, from which the Ayurvedic principles of physiology are derived, Creation flows from the interaction of Purusha (primordial emptiness) and Prakruti (primeval nature's dynamic manifestation). Issuing forth from Prakruti's fertile matrix, all subsequent levels of the Great Mother's expressions, from the most subtle forms of mind to the gross external elements perceived by the sense organs, emerge as a triad of qualities, or gunas, which weave together the underlying reality of the cosmos. In their purest form, the three gunas can be seen in every moment and every dimension of Creation, which begins as a conceptual impulse within consciousness, comes into being through the movement of energy, and finally takes form in material substance. These stages, respectively, are sattva, rajas, and tamas. By gaining some understanding of the nature of the gunas and how they guide and influence the infinite unfolding of life, one opens the doors of perception to many secrets of the world, the body and mind, disease, and healing.

Nature's myriad activities can be qualified according to the functions of the three gunas, yet are inherently neither good nor bad; the violent rajasic powers of volcanoes creating new earth, or the tamasic decomposition of a rotting body, are all necessary processes of life. In the context of Ayurvedic philosophy, however, where the gunas are used to describe mental, emotional, and psychological characteristics and their impact on health and disease, it is necessary to differentiate between those attributes which are beneficial for human wellness and those that are not. Thus, sattva is generally recognized as ultimately positive, while rajas and tamas are regarded as inherently negative, although having useful aspects.

One way to illustrate the many attributes of the term *sattva*, especially in relation to healing, is by visualizing the Medicine Buddha. His lotus seat is the blossoming of sattva's upward-rising inner clarity; he sits in the most sattvic posture of perfect yogic self-control, padmasana (full lotus), upon a moon-disc of cooling sattvic love. Bhaisajyaguru's left hand rests in the gesture of sattvic equipoise, holding a bowl of immortality-bestowing nectar, the drink conferring sattvic liberation. With sattvic motivation to cure all sickness, his right hand offers a fruiting myrobalan branch, the supremely sattvic drug that causes no harm to anyone. Sange Menla's blue body of space permeates every cosmos with boundless sattvic presence, as his sattvic rays dissolve the poisons within the minds of beings. His golden robes emit the glowing warmth of sattvic virtues; around his body rainbows of sattvic purity form whirling fields of auric light. Such are a few examples of the rich meaning of sattva.

Based on the gunas, Ayurveda describes three realms of medicine. "There are tamasic, rajasic, and sattvic treatments," Gopal commented one afternoon, as we sat with Dr. Aryal in his laboratory. "Tamasic treatments come from the demonic realms; they are harsh methods that cause pain, fear, and bad effects, like surgery and toxic drugs. Rajasic treatments come from the middle realm of humans and the earth; they consist of the bitter, salty, sour, and astringent tastes, which aren't pleasant but have good effects. The sattvic treatment is rasayana, alchemical rejuvenation. This is brought from heaven, and has no bad tastes or negative effects. It is not just here: it is very popular in other galaxies, with the gods in heaven, the rishis, and divine beings."

Dr. Aryal concurred, adding that "medicines from the highest realm are alchemical elixirs, created by the union of pure spiritual practice and the outer transmutation of medicinal substances. The physician who creates these nectar medicines is renowned throughout the three worlds."

A striking example of the differences between sattvic, rajasic, and tamasic medicines can be found by comparing the roots of modern medicine and classical Ayurveda. The three original branches of allopathy, those of trauma medicine, surgery, and synthetic drugs, first sprouted during the era of toxic mercury compounds and indiscriminate bloodletting, grew in the battlefields of the world wars, then spread through the marketing of pharmaceutical discoveries. Consequently, the most valuable role for allopathy is symptomatically addressing the effects of society's rajasic and tamasic behavior, by utilizing heroic treatments for violent injuries and accidents, sophisticated technology for acute and life-threatening conditions, and biochemical management of symptoms.

Ayurvedic and Tibetan medical history, on the other hand, can be traced back to the mystic contemplations of ancient seers, who elucidated the universal principles of spirit and nature as perceived by meditation. Health, according to the ancient doctor-sages, goes far beyond the treatment of symptoms; it is defined as a state of equilibrium among the doshas, dhatus, and malas (humors, tissues, and wastes), along with happiness of mind, senses, and soul. Ultimately, the aim of Ayurvedic and Tibetan healing arts is enlightenment and salvation. As a result, these healing systems are primarily concerned with attaining wellbeing and longevity through harmony, balance, rejuvenation, and transcendent wisdom, and are therefore predominantly sattvic in quality.

Ayurveda, first and foremost, is the art of preventing illness with a healthy lifestyle. According to Dr. Tiwari, "Medicines and treatments are not the priority of Ayurveda. It first teaches how to achieve and maintain health with conduct, diet, and daily routines; only after that do we prescribe the drugs. The treatment of disease is the secondary objective. In modern medicine, we are not up to that level yet." This philosophy, and the roles for doctors and patients it implies, is an important distinguishing characteristic of sattvic medical systems. In doctor-patient interactions ruled by rajas and tamas, patients become unquestioning, passive recipients of treatments and medications; in a sattvic relationship, the physician is primarily an educator who supports positive transformation by teaching self-care and responsibility for one's health. Sattvic doctors are spiritual friends on a shared journey toward well-being, who elevate and empower their patients by assisting them in self-improvement.

For Dr. Singh, like most Ayurvedic practitioners, the Science of Life is not simply a system of medicine. "Ayurveda tells us how to use our senses and intellect in the proper way," he remarked during one of our philosophical discussions. "It is a very practical approach that doesn't try to get into the high levels, just daily life: don't do too much, don't do too little, just do the optimal level, and that is different for each person. All the Vaidye should do is help people choose what is best for them."

"The word *Dharma* in Ayurvedic philosophy means the conduct which is beneficial and necessary for you," Dr. Tiwari once explained. "Some define it as a way of life. Dharma teaches us what is beneficial and what is not beneficial. Things that are beneficial for you are your Dharma, your religion. If the doctor knows what is harmful and what is beneficial, he is able to advise you to do this and don't do that; you then learn your Dharma."

Ayurvedic health consultations place great importance on restoring equilibrium to an individual's constitution by cultivating a sattvic lifestyle. Almost every ailment has a cause, or at least several aggravating factors, originating from people's daily activities, which must be identified and eliminated before starting treatment. Without removing the sources of illness, all medicines become palliative at best; at worst, medications that suppress symptoms allow unhealthy behavior to continue and the roots of disease to proliferate. Unless a foundation of wholesome routines is established to support a cure, symptomatic medicine becomes futile and frustrating for both patients and physicians. The regimens prescribed by Ayurvedic and Tibetan physicians promote physiological balance, using sattvic approaches such as right livelihood, right conduct, right thinking, proper sleep cycles, appropriate diet, and nurturing relationships. Once these changes are implemented, many conditions disappear without medicines, and those that persist can be corrected with less time and effort. In the words of Ayurveda: "Those who have a good diet don't need herbs or treatment; those who have a bad diet don't need herbs or treatment."

Sattvic medicine is considered the highest realm of healing, which produces the best results with the least discomfort and fewest side effects. In order to be truly effective, however, sattvic methods must be supported with positive and sometimes radical changes, which many people find difficult to implement in their daily lives. "Sattvic means 'that which is good for everybody,'" Dr. Shrestha explained during one of our conversations about the spiritual aspects of Ayurveda. "But we can't apply sattvic treatments with everybody, because they are not that easy. A sattvic diet will certainly have effects, but people have to change their behavior also.

"One of the causes of diseases is pragyaparad, those things we know we should not do, but do. These things are done out of negligence and habit. People have samskaras [habitual tendencies] from birth, society, and education; to transform ourselves from one mental tendency to another takes a long time. In controlling those habits, we need strong determination, and strong determination is a function of the mind. Once our thinking process and activities are sattvic, then the impact of our behavior will gradually create sattvic surroundings. Sattvic transformation is completely possible, but it is not easy. It is a very high level of treatment." The scriptures of the seer-physicians encourage doctors to live sattvic lives, in order to provide exemplary guidance toward health.

Ayurvedic and Tibetan medical philosophy claims that the physician's degree of sattvic development affects the outcome of treatments and prescriptions. One of the most obvious examples is the influence of empathic attention in the patient-doctor relationship. Rajasic conditions of high stress, heavy workloads, impersonal interactions, and bureaucratic complexities all cause emotional and physical exhaustion for doctors and nurses, which in turn leads to dissatisfying interactions with patients and to mistakes and injuries. Doctors who take time to create and nurture sattvic relationships, based on genuine concern and undistracted attention, derive more enjoyment and fulfillment from their clinical work. They have more satisfied patients and a significantly lower incidence of malpractice.

In traditional Asian medicine, and even until recently in allopathy, a physician's sattvic clarity has been not only an important spiritual characteristic, but also a necessary requirement for successful diagnosis. A doctor's skill and success are based on the ability to perceive subtle external signs revealing the inner workings of the body. The colors of the complexion, profoundly complex tactile sensations of the pulses, thermographic patterns of the skin, intangible brightness of the spirit, palpable topography of the abdomen and acupuncture points, expressions of the body's movements, the patient's odors, the geography of the tongue, and numerous other diagnostic indicators reveal their secrets to the highly trained eyes, ears, nose, and hands of classical physicians. The procedures of diagnosis are a sattvic art of undivided attention, gentle touch, and receptive listening.

Modern technological sophistication has eliminated much of the human element in medical diagnosis. Lacking traditional diagnostic skills, doctors have become almost entirely dependent on laboratory testing, and no longer rely on their own powers of perception. In the process, many important lifestyle issues, such as the influences of stress and improper diet and their commonsense solutions, are overlooked in the quest for financially lucrative biochemical data. "The first duty of a physician is to use his own brain for diagnosis," Dr. Tiwari once commented. "At present, we are mostly using instruments, but I think it should be just the opposite: first diagnose, then use the pathological investigations to support your diagnosis. This is one of the basic differences between modern medicine and Ayurved."

Dr. Singh believes that reliance on technology is one of the reasons Westerners are becoming increasingly interested in Eastern methods and ways of thinking. "You go to the Mayo Clinic," he once said in a typically animated discourse, "and when you come out, you have all your health data from the computers, but you have never met a single doctor! Does that solve the health problem? Westerners feel alienated, and are just crying for some human touch." In many ways, physicians of old were better equipped to satisfy human needs using simpler methods.

Traditional Asian medical philosophy is based on seeing macrocosmic forces at work within the microcosm of the body. Perceiving this unity of body, mind, and environment is a sattvic quality, which gives physicians an understanding of the wide range of factors influencing an individual, and insights into the deeper causative layers of illness. Ayurveda encourages the study of diverse subjects as the means of increasing holistic knowledge, and warns that the more specialized doctors become, the less they understand. During my studies with Dr. Tiwari, he frequently emphasized how Ayurvedic thinking is holistic in nature, rather than specialized. "By becoming overly specialized," the herbalist once said, "we stop thinking of the whole body. Ayurveda regards all the circumstances of life, while modern medicine is only thinking of the sickness and symptoms."

Dr. Tiwari felt that if modern medicine used the diagnostic patterns and pathogenesis theories of Ayurvedic and Tibetan medicine, it would become more beneficial, and the treatment of disease would be easier. "Culture, daily routine, diet, surroundings, family condition, social status, and mental factors all influence our health," he explained. "If the cause of disease is nutritional, Ayurvedic and Tibetan doctors work as nutritionists, using their knowledge of specific foods for healing. Sometimes they work as hygienists and advise daily routines, sometimes as physiotherapists and prescribe certain exercises. All these disciplines should be incorporated in one person; modern medicine utilizes these approaches, but in separate branches."

One of the first diagnostic concepts taught in Chinese medicine is that of *shen*, spiritual presence. Its written character depicts a field of earth intersected by a vertical brush stroke; this ideogram conveys the concept of immaterial breath becoming infused within matter. Shen is described as that which gives cohesion to consciousness; in Ayurvedic terminology it is the luminosity of ojas and vibrant positive prana emanating from the heart and brain. Shen gives clarity to the eyes and confidence to the voice. When the spirit is bright, the patient is willing to listen to the messages from the body, accept responsibility for creating health by making lifestyle changes, and learn from the experience of illness. These sattvic manifestations of bright shen activate the immune system and hasten healing; with a shining spirit, even serious diseases can be overcome. When the shen is dull, the patient is said to have a "wooden" complexion and pessimistic attitude; with a weakened spirit, even a simple illness becomes difficult to treat.

Perhaps the greatest tragedy of modern medicine is the damage inflicted upon people's shen whenever doctors reinforce negative beliefs about recovery and healing. Patients feel helpless and hopeless after being told they have to live with their ailments, frustrated by the prospect of taking drugs for the rest of their lives, discredited as psychological cases because of doctors' diagnostic inability, pressured and manipulated into unwanted and unnecessary procedures, ridiculed for their interest in alternative treatments, and terrorized by dire predictions. The Hippocratic vow to "do no harm" can only be fulfilled when doctors avoid creating such negative feelings, and strive instead to elevate the patient's shen; once a person's spirit has been touched by sattva, the stage is set for the successful outcome of treatments and medicines.

"We develop healing power by giving hope to patients and invoking their willpower," Dr. Tiwari said. "Hearing encouraging words, the vitality of the body is increased, the effects of the drugs are strengthened, and the healing process is quickened. A doctor should have good willpower, confidence, and a commitment to treat the patient; he should have no confusion, no question of faith in himself. The patient should also think: This disease is curable. Faith between the doctor and patient is necessary; if the patient doesn't trust the physician, he won't be cured."

Healers who radiate a sattvic aura, whether they are doctors or not, are able to inspire religious faith in others. Recoveries attributed to divine influences are commonplace in a land where prayer, mantra, and blessings of holy people are part of everyday life. To a sattvic mind, curing by faith is a natural function of spiritual laws and the body's energetic sheaths, while to skeptics it is nothing more than the placebo effect; either way, patients feel better.

The use of mystical powers for healing was a favorite topic of late night discussions at Gopal's mountainside retreat. R. D. Mahatyagi, a physician trained in both Ayurveda and biochemistry, was one of the teachers who regularly visited to give teachings. "Many places in Nepal and India have no doctors," he said during one of his evening discourses. "There are only sorcerers who blow on water before you drink it. Sometimes a healer can just say, 'You must get rid of the sickness,' and the patient will get rid of the sickness without anything. There is a scientific theory behind this: if you are trusting, the secretion of hormones will heal your sickness. Sometimes the doctor is not capable of curing the patient, but a simple person can." These words echoed the commonly heard tales of yogis curing with only the pranically charged ashes from their fireplaces.

Although he had a skeptical attitude toward miraculous phenomena, Dr. Singh had witnessed demonstrations of such yogic powers and acknowledged the presence of forces beyond the rational mind; he once saw an old man materialize bowls of sweets in front of hundreds of scientists and professors at Benares Hindu University. "There is a saddhu baba who lives beside the Ganges," he said one afternoon in his Sinamangal office. "Every Tuesday and Saturday there is a huge crowd there, and you have to stand in a line to get to him. All of them have some problem, like 'I want to have a male child, sir,' 'My son is like this,' 'My company is not working.' All he has is two powders, a white powder and a black powder, two big jars. He says, 'Okay, you are going to have it, no reason.' Nobody knows which powder they are going to get. I know exactly what he is giving: the white powder is calcium carbonate, and the black powder is purified nux vomica. These are very common drugs. The old man has hundreds and hundreds of photographs of children he brought on this earth, so to say, and he has made so many people happy.

"How can you explain this? You cannot. I think there is something more than what your eyes see or what the drugs can do. When we are dealing in terms of physical chemistry only, we are bound by physical and chemical reactions; that's what modern medicine is. The moment we go to the spiritual level, the question of what is possible and not possible does not arise. If I wish, he will be cured. Both things are there, the physical and chemical laws, and certain situations where no laws apply."

Sensitive healers through the ages have observed that thoughts and feelings are composed of subtle atmospheric energies, infused with etheric gunas. By elevating the patient's shen with compassion, lovingkindness, and happiness, a sattvic doctor can increase the therapeutic effects of medicines and treatments. Doctors manifesting rajasic symptoms of stress and unhappiness negatively affect patients, who are already sensitized by pain and suffering. Ayurveda recognizes this phenomenon and encourages physicians to cultivate sattvic mental states in order to benefit their patients. For this purpose, nothing surpasses prayer and meditation. This is one of the great keys that unlock the potential of medicine as a spiritual path, for it is said that those who are able to communicate with the patient's inner being are the most effective healers. "Only those physicians who pray and meditate have the power to heal diseases of the mind and emotions," Dr. Jha had asserted in the early days of my studies.

"It is necessary for doctors to be spiritually devoted and trusting in God," Dr. Mahatyagi elaborated. "Ayurveda teaches that when doctors prescribe medicine, they must have a pure mind and a good spirit, with an attitude of giving blessings. By praying, good results are produced. When I give medication, I chant different types of mantras according to the sickness. I am performing my duty, but also praying to God, so it is more successful. Most of the traditional Vaidyes in India and Nepal believe in God, and chanting mantra is part of their lifestyle. To the degree they live like that, that much success they have."

Physicians become truly gifted when surrounded by the aura of their accumulated prayers and meditation. "If the doctor has some spiritual power or spiritual thinking, the treatment of the patient is more successful," Dr. Tiwari concurred. "In Hindu thinking, we consider ourselves only the tools, not the healer. The healer is almighty God. The doctor should think: 'God, help me to treat this patient.' That way the doctor has a divine force supporting him. If you have the blessing of God, you are very successful."

Sattvic healing philosophy believes that the more deeply we are connected to our inner divinity, the healthier we become; the role of medical treatment is therefore regarded in Ayurveda as secondary to the more important work of supporting a patient's spiritual evolution. "The basis of Ayurveda is spirituality," Dr. Shrestha explained. "This is because the Vedas are concerned with divine power. Divine power, spirituality, and mind are the deepest seat of our being." Traditional Ayurvedic and Tibetan physicians encourage their patients to engage in religious devotion and prayer, yogic techniques, and mental disciplines such as meditation and visualization.

The ancient doctor-sages taught that the practice of medicine is an excellent path for cultivating sattvic virtues, which can lead the physician to moksha, spiritual emancipation. This idea is clearly elucidated in the teachings of the *Tsa Gyu*, which state that by embodying the sattvic qualities of Sange Menla, a physician may reach enlightenment. When physicians integrate meditation and prayer into the everyday work of medical practice, healing becomes a spiritual path; thoughts, actions, and speech are purified with sattvic mindfulness, and the clinic is transformed into a sacred temple. Every interaction with the patient can become an expression of the six paramitas, the boundless disciplines of morality, generosity, concentration, diligence, wisdom, and patience, which lead to transcendent fulfillment. Upon the altar of uncontrived morality the physician places offerings of selfless generosity. With one-pointed concentration he performs the ritual of healing with tireless diligence. Guided by the wisdom of mental equipoise, he patiently nurtures the transmutation of sickness into health. Thus, the healing arts become a supreme vehicle for realizing meaningful inner refinement, and a profound sadhana that opens the secret lotus of the heart.

When patients return with worsening conditions caused by escalating numbers of medications, doctors' consciences are troubled. In order to harm no one, the physician must prescribe treatments and medicines that are wholesome and safe. The practice of Ayurvedic and Tibetan medicine is based on the doctrine of ahimsa, nonviolence. This aspect of sattvic medicine is beautifully illustrated by Bhaisajyaguru, whose right hand extends in the mudra of supreme generosity, offering us nature's curative power in the form of a divine myrobalan fruit. By this gesture, the deity reminds us that ultimately, the physician is not the healer: it is the plant kingdom that provides the different elements, qualities, and tastes which balance the body. By approaching the art of healing as a servant of Creation's compassionate intentions, generously sharing sattvic medicines given freely by the earth to benefit our bodies and minds, physicians can find personal satisfaction and professional fulfillment, and avoid suffering for themselves and others.

Herbal medicine, when practiced with conscientious skill and compassionate motivation, transmutes the primitive feeling-consciousness of the plant kingdom, which is ruled predominantly by the tamas guna, into a sattvic art and science. Most herbs used in clinical practice are sources of food-grade phytonutrients with minimal toxicity and are therefore unlikely to produce side effects; those that are highly toxic will create problems only if not properly purified and administered. The side effects of most common herbs tend to be mild and transient, and long-term use does not create the insidiously complex levels of iatrogenic complications seen with synthetic pharmaceuticals. The majority of herbs used as medicines possess the sattvic virtues of being nutritive and immune-supporting, regulatory and balancing to physiological functions, and cleansing and detoxifying, thereby addressing the root causes of disease. In contrast, synthetic pharmaceuticals are inherently hepatotoxic, immune-suppressing, and prone to causing physiological disequilibrium, rendering them incapable of curing chronic and degenerative illnesses.

Ayurvedic, Tibetan, and Chinese medicines recognize a distinct class of herbs with highly sattvic properties. Herbs that are capable only of curing diseases are considered inferior to those with powers to both cure and prevent illness, while those which not only cure and prevent illness, but also facilitate spiritual evolution, are regarded as supreme medicines. The "divine drugs" such as Soma, and purified mercury used for rasayana in Tantric alchemy, are considered the highest level of medicinal substances from this earth, capable of healing every disease and bestowing jiva mukti. For those resigned to mortality for lack of such mythical elixirs, a large number of supremely sattvic herbs are easily available for enhancing health, promoting longevity, and increasing wisdom. The most renowned examples from Chinese medicine are ginseng and shou wu (*Polygonum multiflora*), while myrobalan, amla, and brahmi are some of the most well known from Ayurveda.

Sattvic healing systems recognize that many common complaints can be treated with simple and nontoxic methods. Therapeutic massage, which requires no drugs or equipment, is an excellent example of a sattvic healing art. A good therapist must have meditative concentration, relaxing touch, and sensitivity to the patient's body and emotional state; these skills produce the sattvic results of bestowing numerous therapeutic benefits while doing no harm. Ayurveda considers massage the most effective treatment for many types of headaches, sleep disorders, and the multitude of complaints arising from tension and stress. Among the benefits are rejuvenation, increased nutritional intake by the tissues, removal of toxins, enhancement of self-awareness, balancing of emotions, giving luster and strength to the skin, increased immunity, longevity, and improved eyesight. The Ayurvedic form of massage, which utilizes oleation as preparation for pancha karma purification, is called snehan; one of the meanings of this term is "to give love and contentment."

Traditionally, Chinese and Ayurvedic doctors received training in massage techniques; this education not only enhanced their diagnostic skill by developing hands-on sensitivity to the human body, it also improved their bedside manner. As Ayurveda's astute simplicity observes, giving a massage is the best way to create rapport with a patient.

Acupuncture is another form of sattvic treatment, highly effective for activating the healing responses of the body yet free of harmful side effects. It is also a good example illustrating how the practitioner's mental status influences the outcome of treatments. To engage the chi, says the *Nei Ching* (*Yellow Emperor's Classic*), the shen of the doctor must become one with the needle. If the attention is not fully focused, the field of life force, which is itself composed of mind-matter, cannot be aroused or directed through the meridians into the diseased organ system. This same principle is found in the practices of qigong and pranic healing, which forgo the use of needles and emphasize direct transference of chi through the hands of the healer. The term *gong*, as in qigong, means "body and mind together," referring to how the life force begins to flow in tangible waves and currents when attention is fully engaged. Without deep and steady concentration, the bioelectric field cannot be focused and channeled for healing or any other purpose. Acupuncture produces wonderful therapeutic results through the relaxing effects of endocrine and parasympathetic stimulation; its benefits become more profound when practitioners follow the advice of the Yellow Emperor, and unify their shen with the chi field of the patient.

The ancient philosophies and sattvic treatment methods of classical Asian medicine are now receiving widespread recognition and acceptance in the Western world. I was greatly surprised to learn that many Ayurvedic doctors in Nepal had little interest in their own tradition and were more concerned with emulating their allopathic counterparts. Unfortunately, modern medicine in Nepal is dominated by indiscriminate prescribing of antibiotics and redundant lab tests.

One winter morning I took Dr. Shrestha to Mt. Shivapuri to escape the oppressive conditions at Naradevi Hospital. Himalayan kites soared on brown and black wings as we followed a trail through the rhododendron forest, dry and dusty like the streets far below. The conversation eventually returned to our ongoing dialogue about the status of Ayurveda in Nepal.

"Throughout Nepal there are many doctors practicing modern medicine in the name of Ayurved, who feel proud using synthetic pharmaceuticals," Dr. Shrestha said. "You will find very few Vaidyes who have faith and confidence in themselves; they don't want to say they are Ayurvedic doctors. You Western people are so interested in Ayurveda, but the people in our country are much more interested in modern medicine.

"Once I asked some of our students, 'Why are you so against practicing Ayurved?' They said, 'What do you and Dr. Singh get from

Ayurved? Other doctors have cars; Dr. Singh doesn't possess a single car.' Who will tell them that materialistic things are not everything?"

This was an important cultural lesson revealing how rajasic and tamasic concerns with prestige and social status affect sattvic forms of medicine.

"I will never forget one thing that happened in Par Ping that shows how orthodox we people are," Dr. Shrestha continued. "The lower-class people there are shoemakers. Because they are poor, they have more skin problems. The doctors and health workers were Brahmins, and wouldn't touch the patients. One day I saw a patient with a skin infection that had pus formation. The doctor was so afraid he would get something, he made the patient wait outside on the ground, and poured the medicine from high above. I asked, 'Why are you doing that?' The doctor replied, 'He is a lower-caste person. I can't touch him, and no one is here to clean him.' I lifted up the patient's leg, cleaned his wound, and did his dressing. That fellow cried because he had never seen such type of service, and would not have seen it otherwise. This is our Nepal."

One of the historical reasons Buddhism became the major vehicle for disseminating medical knowledge across Asia was its nonjudgmental attitude toward bodily wastes, while cleanliness was an obsession among Hinduism's higher castes. Even today, Tibetan doctors are taught to regard all aspects of the body without revulsion, and to view the concept of impurity as a fabrication of perceptual ignorance. During my most recent visit to Nepal, Lobsang Dhonyo described an experience he had while studying with Dr. Chopel. "Amchi-la instructed us to not be afraid of the patient's impurities," Lobsang said. "One day he asked me to check a patient's urine; as I examined the sample, I was feeling it was dirty. Amchi-la caught me and said, 'Don't think it is dirty. Always think about the suffering of the patient.'" This spiritual exercise helps overcome aversion caused by marigpa's discrimination; ultimately, it results in attaining a highly sattvic view that confers fearless immunity. While being no substitute for good hygiene and sterile technique, any practice which develops equanimity deepens the transformation of clinical work into a spiritual path.

Ultimately, the expression of sattva in medical practice is not dependent on the form of medicine being used. Although Ayurvedic and Tibetan medicine is generally sattvic in its gentle spiritual approaches, not all practitioners of these systems are sattvically inclined. Conversely, even though allopathic medicine carries a heavy karmic debt of iatrogenic suffering, and is by nature more suited to the treatment of rajasic conditions, there are countless physicians practicing modern medicine with sincerely altruistic and compassionate motivation. "If a doctor practices the Dharma," Kalu Rinpoche instructed me, "his medicine becomes Dharma medicine. It is not important whether it is Tibetan or Western."

During my studies with Dr. Chopel and other teachers, I often heard of the health benefits produced by meditation and spiritual practices. Meditation, prayer, and recitation of mantras increase the vital power, enhancing resistance to illness, Amchi-la told me. Sadhanas invoking the Medicine Buddha or other deities attract their healing blessings, sometimes curing people miraculously. Periods of fasting and abstinence from worldly activity can remove many diseases. Leading a simple life of contentment is a specific remedy for diseases of aggravated Air humor brought on by excessive desires. When one's life force is coming to an end, it can be renewed and extended by saving the lives of animals, practicing generosity toward the poor, making pilgrimages to sacred places, and performing ceremonies to drive away harmful spirits. I learned that all suffering comes from the darkness of marigpa, that disease-causing habits are created by the mind poisons of craving and aversion, and that sattvic religious activities can prevent and cure these sicknesses.

Spiritual disciplines have always played a major role in the healing of illness. Yet, paradoxically, every high lama I met or heard about in

Boudhanath was troubled by sickness; even Kalu Rinpoche, despite extraordinary yogic attainments, endured illness in the later part of his life. If meditation and Dharma practices were so effective, I wondered, why do so many accomplished practitioners suffer from entirely preventable diseases? Why are spiritual teachers, who have reached high levels of realization, often apathetic about their health? Knowing that the precious human form is the abode of deities, why do they eat foods that make them sick, neglect basic health regimens, or even abuse their bodies?

"Why do so many meditation masters, who have eliminated marigpa, have disease in their bodies?" I asked Amchi-la. We sat quietly, sipping our tea as the doctor reflected on the question.

"Spiritual teachers manifest illness as a way of enlightening their students," he replied. "By becoming ill and passing away, they demonstrate the truth of suffering and impermanence for the purpose of motivating disciples to practice Dharma.

"There are other reasons as well. An enlightened teacher has the power to take negative karma from the minds of disciples who have devotion. This is a mysterious thing that happens when a disciple has great faith and his mind becomes one with the guru. When there is this kind of relationship, the guru can purify the student's obscurations by creating illness in his own body. This form of taking the suffering of others is a unique and profound blessing."

"What is the nature of disease that makes it possible for a person to take it from another?" I asked.

"There are basically two components of diseases," Amchi-la answered. "The root cause is karma, or the part caused by actions in our past or in previous lives; the secondary cause is the activation of the three humors by the karma. That is, the karma is present, but it needs the three bodily humors to become actualized. Diseases taken on by lamas are usually those created by karmic causes, although they can take on any kind.

"Spiritual teachers are human beings. Even though they may have eradicated the root of karma from their mind-stream, thus closing the door to future suffering, the body is still subject to decay and death. They manifest illness and death to purify the last of their karma. We can reach the stage of development where we no longer cause suffering for ourselves or others, in this or future lives, but due to the power of past actions, negative karma continues to ripen. If we have committed any sin, we must suffer for it. Even high lamas have to suffer their own karma."

"If each person has to suffer his own karma, how can a lama take it away?" I inquired.

The doctor smiled patiently at my insistence.

"It is difficult to answer in a concrete way, and requires the Tibetan religious view to understand. This healing is based on the relationship between the disciple and the teacher. Usually lamas take diseases by giving blessings to people, which causes a kind of karmic connection between them. When a disciple seeks refuge in a lama, he tries to mix his mind with the mind of his teacher, making the exchange of blessings and karma possible. If the disciple has deep faith, his sins can be cleansed by prayer to the lama.

"In order to understand the nature of the mind and how these things are possible, we must practice meditation. During meditation the mind can be separated from the body. This is done by meditating on the body as composed of the five universal elements, and the red and white reproductive essences from the parents. Once the composite nature of the body is perceived, we then meditate on the mind having no beginning or end. It is also possible to blend one's mind into the mind of a deity, such as the Medicine Buddha, and the mind of one's guru, and then meditate until these three minds become one."

Amchi-la leaned back against his cushion and straightened the sleeves of his robe, looking at me intently over the rims of his dark glasses. "There are many stories of great practitioners who have taken on the suffering of others," he said. "This is the practice of Tonglen, 'to send and to receive.' It is the very essence of Buddhist practice. Tong means 'to send,' and len means 'to take.' One visualizes sending all happiness, prosperity, and blessings while exhaling, and taking all forms of suffering while inhaling. If one practices this method, its results can be realized."

"Sending and taking" is a form of meditation that develops metta, compassionate loving-kindness. One begins by contemplating how every sentient being, during the endless cycle of reincarnation, was once our mother. Now, throughout the infinite realms of existence, our past mothers are experiencing immeasurable kinds of suffering. Remembering the love and kindness they have given us, we inhale the black smoke of their sadness, breathing it directly into the center of our hearts. There, on a blossoming lotus, resides a radiant deity, or drop of luminosity, representing the essence of our Buddha-nature. Absorbing the darkness of universal pain, the heart-deity becomes filled with metta, which we exhale as purifying white and rainbow-colored light. Expanding the exhalation throughout space, we imagine that all beings are touched by these uplifting rays, and are spontaneously liberated into joy and happiness. Between meditation sessions Tonglen is further developed by putting the welfare of others before our own. Cultivating the desire for others' happiness alchemically transforms ego-clinging and self-cherishing into unconditional love.

The Sanskrit name for the heart is hridayam, which means "that which receives, gives, and circulates." This name accurately describes the organ's anatomical function, which is to receive deoxygenated blood from the veins, give back oxygenated blood to the arteries, and pump the blood through the circulatory system. This receiving of dark blood and giving back of bright prana-infused blood is the physical counterpart to Tonglen, a kind of unconscious "sending and receiving" occurring in the body with every breath and heartbeat. During Tonglen meditation, the heart also gives and receives, absorbing the suffering of beings, then emitting the light of compassionate consciousness.

Metta is the essence of our being, and the heart is the center of metta within the body. Tibetan embryology teaches that at the moment of conception, the blue spacelike light of consciousness seeking incarnation becomes infused into the merging red essence of the ovum and white essence of the sperm. Coalescing into an infinitesimally tiny drop, this mind-seed is gradually enclosed within three sheaths, likened to jewel boxes inside each other, dwelling invisibly inside the heart. This formless, indestructible, omniscient, and omnipresent awareness is the gem of potential Buddhahood within each mind. The entire alchemical journey from samsaric suffering to enlightenment is the rediscovery and liberation of this atomic particle of universal love that encompasses all beings. It is this innermost consciousness, mentally given form as a deity residing in the lotus of the heart, that is the source of infinite metta, the joy which transcends comprehension.

"Tonglen has special relevance to those who practice healing," Amchila continued. "Patients feel and respond to the influences emanating from the doctor."

Although largely unaware of the subtle exchanges occurring around us, we are in a continuous process of "taking and sending" on many levels. Body language, eye contact, the subliminal fragrances of pheromones that carry our emotions, and the electromagnetic field of life force that surrounds each person are all mediums of subtle communication. Consciously or unconsciously, every thought and feeling occurring within the mind and heart of the physician is transmitted to the patient, who is sensitized by illness, vulnerable to the damaging aura of stress and negativity, and frequently in need of human nurturing more than the miracles of technological medicine.

Tonglen offers a way to establish a mindful, positive relationship with the pain of the world, the daily challenge faced by those in the medical field. Cultivating metta gives birth to a warm and caring heart, which is an elixir of healing for those in pain and fear; as Kalu Rinpoche observed, love improves the outcome of medical treatments. This is the reason sattvic practices play such an important role in classical medicine, and why the doctor who prays and meditates achieves superior results. "When the conjunction arises between the physician whose heart and mind are filled with altruistic compassion, and the patient who has faith in his medicine," Dr. Chopel said, "there is no condition that is incurable."

"In the past, many people were adepts at Tonglen," Amchi-la went on. "Once there was an abbot of a monastery who became very proficient at this practice. One day, while giving an empowerment, he suddenly yelled in pain. When the lamas asked what was wrong, he told them that a dog was being beaten outside. Going out, they found an angry man with a stick chasing away a dog. The abbot called for the man to come in, then pulled down his robes to reveal his back. On the same place where the dog was hit were fresh cuts and bruises." My teacher waited quietly while I wrote my notes and pondered the meaning of his story, which seemed to imply that egolessness could be demonstrated on a physical level, that there is no separation between self and other.

The doctor continued. "There are many stories of epidemics ending after a high lama contracted the disease and died. Taking suffering upon oneself in this way is different from dying of ignorance and disease, and is often accompanied by miraculous displays.

"Many people in Tibet demonstrated their enlightenment in unusual ways. There was once a monk who lived at Shelkar Ling. He was quite ordinary, and spent his life going about his monastic duties. One year a terrible epidemic of smallpox broke out in the village, killing many people in the area; the monk also contracted the disease and died. It was the middle of winter, the ground was frozen and wood was scarce, so his body was taken to a lake and put under the ice. Shortly after this, the epidemic stopped. In the springtime, as the ice was melting, people noticed a rainbow over the place where the monk had been put. They went back and found his body floating there, perfectly preserved. He was brought back to the monastery and given a special cremation ceremony. As his body disappeared into the flames, rainbows came out of the pyre into the sky, and relics were discovered in the ashes. Everyone then recognized that this monk had been an extraordinary practitioner, and credited him with purifying the karma that had caused the epidemic by taking it into his body."

In the world of Tibetan Buddhism, sickness can be a manifestation of spiritual accomplishment, and a sacrifice made on behalf of others. This is something any mother can understand, who gives her own vitality to nourish her children. But is this really why so many sattvic adepts have poor health?

Over the years I have treated monks, nuns, Rinpoches, and saddhus; their illnesses are often avoidable, if they are willing to adopt healthier, more sattvic ways of caring for their bodies. Yet many—especially the most sattvic elders—are apathetic about their health. Is this disinterest a sign of spiritual evolution, a manifestation of detachment from the flesh, or simply stubbornness? Ironically, even when troubled by sickness, the elders of the Himalayan cultures are frequently stronger than many "health-conscious" younger Westerners, who are often unable to tolerate the crushing poverty, pollution, and malnutrition prevalent in India and Nepal. Under such difficult circumstances, sattvic ideals of health are often unattainable. When treating some of these wise men and women, usually at the request of their students or loved ones, I found myself wondering who was actually the doctor and who was the patient.

Dr. Chopel's comments revealed that spiritual maturity and physical health, although closely related, are not necessarily synonymous. Sickness is the greatest obstacle to a yogi's practice, and health the greatest comfort and boon; yet sickness is also the broom that sweeps away bad karma, say the wise, who embrace the hardships and suffering of the spiritual path as purification. Just as mystic realization does not always translate into health awareness, those preoccupied with physical well-being do not necessarily gain spiritual maturity. As Kalu Rinpoche observed, "If health itself were the cause of enlightenment, many Americans would be enlightened by now."

At the root of medical philosophy lies the assumption that illness and suffering are synonymous, and that health and happiness can be equated. When it comes to practices such as Tonglen, however, or other types of meditation which purify negative karma by manifesting sickness, the solidity of such paradigms dissolves. In ordinary life, clear and simple answers about why people are sick, why they get better, and what they gain from their experiences are frequently shrouded in bewildering uncertainty; in the context of spiritual development, illness and healing assume an entirely different, and generally more meaningful, purpose. In addressing my original question of why sattvic persons suffer from illness, my wise teacher responded with profound insight without providing a simple answer; instead, his words pointed toward greater mysteries and deeper unknowing. Only when the mind is opened by life's incomprehensibility do we begin to understand the truth.

Of all my medical teachers, Dr. Chopel practiced the most rigorous sattvic lifestyle. He was perpetually engaged in religious activities, slept very little, and ate a simple diet. As abbot of the Shelkar Monastery, he had administrative responsibilities, but was fundamentally disinterested in politics and worldly affairs; he preferred caring for people by giving medicines and Buddhist teachings.

Dr. Chopel was the holder of a unique and ancient sadhana, which had been conferred upon him by his primary guru, Chupsang Rinpoche. The beneficial effects of this ritual, my teacher explained, extended to every realm, from the lowest insects to the highest gods. The doctor's life revolved around the prayers and meditation handed down by this lineage; he performed these six times daily, three during the day and three at night. Amchi-la had maintained an unbroken discipline for many decades, even while incarcerated in concentration camps. Once, before the Chinese invasion of Tibet, he stopped his practice, because the monks of the old Shelkar Monastery thought his devotions were distracting him from his administrative duties; as a result of neglecting the sacred initiation oath to perform the prayers, he became ill. When Chupsang Rinpoche learned what had happened, he admonished Amchi-la to never miss a single session, even if he had to perform the ritual in his imagination only.

Dr. Chopel went to sleep at seven in the evening, then rose three hours later for his first Dharma session. The second session was at one in the morning, and the third at four. After completing the morning puja, he climbed to the monastery roof, gave the leftover ritual offerings to the birds, then descended to the prayer hall to perform liturgical chanting with the monks. He then walked to the Stupa and prayed while circumambulating the shrine. He returned to the monastery for a light meal of soup, and resumed recitation of scriptures. Around nine he went to the clinic and began his morning of diagnosing patients and prescribing medications; between patients, he chanted from various religious texts. After lunch the doctor saw more patients, taught medicine to his students, meditated, and then went to the Stupa again.

Amchi-la's monastic schedule was interrupted periodically when he and the monks participated in various Buddhist festivals. Sometimes these took place nearby at the Stupa; at other times the monks made pilgrimages to Bodhgaya or Dharamsala in India. The monks sometimes performed longer pujas involving days of fasting, which were attended by the old physician as well. Not surprisingly, my teacher viewed idleness and preoccupation with mundane distractions as a misuse of our precious human existence.

In spite of his monastic, spiritual, and medical responsibilities, Amchi-la made himself easily accessible as both a teacher and physician.

Generous with his time and attention, stern yet patient, humble but possessing remarkable presence, he set a striking example of goodness. He had gentle words of advice for his students, emphasizing the importance of cultivating a sattvic attitude toward everyone. "Think about others, and be compassionate to everybody," Dr. Chopel would say. "Whenever we see poor people, beggars, and animals, we should try to develop compassion. Even if you can't help someone, don't harm them."

Amchi-la would remind us to maintain an open mind, so as to be worthy recipients of the teachings. "Being a doctor is a great and noble job, but try not to be proud. If you are proud, there is no way to get knowledge from others; if you are humble, you will become a very educated and learned person. We should never think we are too great, because we never know what kind of rebirth we may have in the future."

Amchi-la stressed that practicing medicine was Dharmic activity. He encouraged me to provide selfless service, explaining that this was the essence of Buddhism. "Our life is short," he once said as I was preparing to return to the West. "Don't cling to worldly things. For endless lifetimes, our actions have been based on love of ourselves and hatred of others, but we should give this up. In this human incarnation we have the best opportunity to benefit others, as Lord Buddha has done. By benefitting others, you will accomplish your wishes and attain enlightenment." The doctor's words revealed an important truth: sattvic medicine is the path of spiritual self-improvement, even if the physician does not accrue wealth.

"When giving treatments, you must receive some money to pay for your medicines," Dr. Chopel continued. "Even if you lose money giving treatments to poor people, you should think only of how you can help them. When Westerners come, they give me extra money because the medicines are cheap by their standards. When Nepali and Tibetan people come, they often can't pay. But this is the way of the doctor. Please strive to do more for others than for yourself. With this attitude you will accumulate more spiritual merit, greater peace, and a happy life. I give treatments for this reason only. My only wish is to always benefit others." This sattvic philosophy was the fruition of Dr. Chopel's dedication to intensive Dharma practice, and the result of continual prayers, meditation, and service to the sick and poor.

As I listened to Amchi-la's words and watched how he went about his daily life, I often wondered about his past, and the influences that had shaped and nourished his compassionate intelligence. I knew very little about my teacher, but what I knew inspired my respect: he was an elder from an endangered spiritual culture, one of the last to live in a flourishing monastic age before the Kali Yuga cast its long shadows across Tibet. What training had Dr. Chopel received? I wondered. What doctrines had he studied, what words had his teachers spoken, what experiences had he gone through that now, in old age, gave him the gentle wisdom he shared freely?

It took a long time before I felt comfortable asking Amchi-la to tell me his life story. I knew that Tibetan people had endured genocide, torture, and famine, and I learned from Sonam, my translator, that my teacher had been a political prisoner for a number of years in concentration camps after the Chinese invasion. I was very curious about what Amchi-la had lived through, but his serious presence did not invite inquiries into his traumatic past. Unlike some of my teachers, who loved to talk about themselves, Dr. Chopel was reticent about sharing personal information; an accomplished scholar and meditator, he was not inclined to small talk. I could only imagine what he had experienced during those years.

Occasionally, Sonam and the old doctor would leave me out of the conversation; when I asked Sonam to translate, he would only say, "He's talking about what happened to him in Tibet." From what I understood of the language and felt in the room, I knew that the subject was painful and private—that the two men were troubled about their homeland and what was happening to friends and relatives. Amchi-la would gaze at us intently from behind his tinted glasses, or look silently out the window, and I wouldn't pursue the matter.

I asked Sonam for advice on how to approach the subject. "If you want to get specific information, ask him specific questions," he replied. "If you ask him to tell you about his life, he'll say something like 'There's not much to say.' A lot of older Tibetans are like that; they don't like to talk about themselves."

After a year of study, I asked my teacher to tell me the story of his life. Amchi-la looked bored, then replied, "There's not much to say, really. I was born about seventy-one years ago, but we Tibetans don't keep accurate dates of our birth." He smiled and went back to reading the text on his table.

"Tell me about your family, and the village you came from," I persisted, trying to be more specific. The doctor ignored my question for a while, then put down his glasses and sat back, bringing his memories into focus. In the ensuing hours of discussion, I would learn again how fortunate I was to have a teacher of such spiritual stature and sattvic demeanor.

"I was born around 1918 in the village of Patruk, in southwest Tibet, near Mt. Everest," Amchi-la began. "Patruk means 'Six Fathers.' It is a large district along the side of a river that flows from the mountain, which was the home of six families, each headed by an elder father. Among these, one was Kuyu Nangpa, who had nine sons. One of those sons was Khenpo Ngawang, who was my father. Among the people of Patruk, our family was the largest. I had five brothers and one sister.

"My father, Khenpo Ngawang, always spoke of religious things, like karma and life after death. Because he was a religious man, he wanted five of his six sons to enter monastic life, and one to keep the family alive. Two of my brothers entered Tsa Rimpu, which was a six-hour walk from Patruk; the other two entered Shelkar Ling, which was a day's journey by horse from the village. It was a rule of that monastery that all the families in that part of the country send one son there.

"Being the second son, I was expected to enter the monastic order. I became a monk of Shelkar Ling at age six, with the blessings of Lama Lingka Kanjupa. The monastery was the largest in that part of the country, with over three hundred monks and scholars, and a thousand-year tradition. The monastery was built on a precipitous peak of rock, and named because of its resemblance to a crystal cup. Its name also referred to a sacred object that had been at the monastery since its beginning, which was some kind of large volcanic crystal. It was believed that the power of the monastery was protected by this object."

From age six to thirteen, Dr. Chopel studied the required introductory courses. Monks could then choose to major in dialectics and debate or in Tantra. Amchi-la majored in the first field, which he studied from the age of thirteen to age twenty-eight. I had heard stories from the elder Shelkar monks about Amchi-la's intelligence; he was considered one of the most outstanding scholars among the three hundred monks of the monastery.

Amchi-la continued. "At the age of nineteen, at the urging of my father and because of the general recognition of my intelligence, I began medical studies. At that time there were two major medical schools in Tibet, Chokpuri and Menzikong in Lhasa, both of which had over a hundred doctors teaching medicine. Monasteries in the remote parts of the country usually had only one doctor, who trained his students. I was the only monk at the Shelkar Monastery to enter into medical training at that time.

"My first teacher was an aged monk-physician who had been an administrator of the monastery. I considered it very good fortune to be able to study with this old doctor, not just because of his understanding and skill, but because he had already entered strict retreat for the last phase of his life. My training, like that of all students of Tibetan medicine, began with the study of the *Gyu Shi*, the four medical Tantras. For a period of three years I worked with this teacher, memorizing the Tantras, receiving oral instructions, and studying the illustrations of the medical thangkas."

Amchi-la's teacher was Chupsang Rinpoche, who taught him both medicine and Dharma. Dr. Chopel said this man was his most important mentor, and that he considered him his guru.

"After Chupsang Rinpoche became too old to teach, I began studying with a second doctor, who lived on Jomolong Mountain near the village of my birth. For three years I studied with him, learning anatomy and how to find the blood vessels and nerves used for bloodletting and cauterization. We also took numerous field trips, studying and gathering the herbs used in the making of medicines. Because of the extreme cold in this area during the winter, I lived with this teacher half the year, and returned to the Shelkar Monastery during the coldest months."

The Shelkar medical lineage traces its origins to two physicians of mythical stature, Yuthog the Elder and Yuthog the Younger, who lived in the seventh and ninth centuries, respectively. Amchi-la knew the names of the doctors in his lineage as far back as seven generations; one of them had been the personal physician to the Dalai Lama Gyalwa Tubten Gyatso.

"At the age of twenty-five, after six years of medical training, I became an administrator of the monastery and began practicing medicine. During the summer I would gather herbs in the mountains, either alone if nearby or with groups of friends on longer trips. We would frequently go to the area of Tsi Bri, where there was a large forest. After performing a fire puja and making prayers, we would gather the herbs. In this way I could procure about fifty of the most important medicines for my clinic. Traders and travelers would bring other herbs from different parts of Tibet, and medicines such as myrobalan and spices from India.

"For sixteen years I practiced medicine as physician of the Shelkar Monastery, treating both the resident monks and the people from the

surrounding villages. I administered herbal medicines, moxibustion, cauterization, bloodletting, and trauma medicine. In general there were no
serious diseases, because of the good air, good water, and clean environment. The most common complaint was gastric distress from eating old
or rancid foods. Because I was a monk and practiced conscientiously, I
made no major mistakes, and generally had good success with my patients."

The practice of medicine helped my teacher cultivate sattvic awareness and reach spiritual maturity. "During this period I developed strong
altruistic motivation," Amchi-la said simply, characteristically understat-
ing the importance of his words.

"When I was thirty-eight I was put in charge of the treasury," the
doctor continued. "I controlled the expenses of the monastery, what
types of foods to buy, what to collect from the farmers, how much to
spend for the year, and so forth. I did this type of work for three years.

"In May 1959 the Chinese arrived. I was forty-one at the time, and
had had no previous contact with them except for some occasional
traders. When they arrived they attacked the soldiers of the village and
confiscated their weapons. All the officials of the village, the military,
and the monastery were called to a meeting in a large building, then imprisoned. For eight months we were tortured: we were forced to sit
completely still in one place for long periods of time, endlessly interro-
gated and indoctrinated, and deprived of sleep, food, and any opportunity to relieve ourselves. At other times we had to perform hard labor.
Eventually the Chinese forced the villagers to destroy the monastery by
hand, then finished the work with bombs."

Over time, from both Amchi-la and the other elder monks of the
original Shelkar Ling, I would learn more about the events which transpired in those apocalyptic months, as genocidal armies swept through
their land and lives. The Chinese surrounded the monastery, locked the
monks in the prayer hall, then killed the religious leaders. The monastery
was ransacked for its treasures of art, gold, and relics. The high lamas

were bound in chains, hung upside down from the ceiling, beaten, and tortured in other ways. Eventually, they were shipped off to the large prisons.

"After eight months of imprisonment in the village of Shelkar, I was transferred to several different places," Amchi-la went on. "I was first taken to Shigatze for three months, then to Lhasa, then to Jomolong, back to Lhasa for three months, and finally to Ningri in Khombu, where I stayed for two years. At this place was a great forest, which the prisoners were forced to cut down and replace with factories. Every day five to ten people would die from hunger, accidents, and beatings.

"The first year in Ningri I worked to clear the forest and build the factories. During my second year I was appointed to a group of doctors who cared for the dying prisoners. The dying would be given special meals, which they usually could not eat. The doctors would take this food and secretly distribute it.

"After this I was moved to Jomolong again for a month, where I worked as a farmer, and then transferred to Shigatze again for three years. In Shigatze there were thousands of prisoners performing different tasks. The younger prisoners carried stones and water, and the older ones worked mostly in a wool factory. The conditions were brutal and there was little food. Among the prisoners were forty Chinese, who had either resisted the invasion or had been married to Tibetan women."

Most of the people in Shigatze prison were religious leaders, military persons, and district officials who had had some rank before the invasion. They survived on a small piece of tsampa and a cup of tea daily, while forced to study Chinese political policies and Maoist ideology. Those who studied, appeared to respect Maoism, and followed the orders of the Chinese, were given some rank in prison. Those who tried to chant mantras or practice meditation were killed or tortured. Anyone who uttered the name of the Dalai Lama was shot. After being tortured, Amchi-la realized that if he wanted to survive, he would need to follow the Chinese policies outwardly while inwardly continuing his Dharma practice. "When Amchi-la was in prison," Lobsang Dhonyo once commented, "he never ceased his practice of meditation and making torma offerings, even though the ritual objects were not there."

Dr. Chopel continued. "After Shigatze, I was taken to Emakong. This was a place of even greater hardship than before, due to the extreme environment and the labor that the prisoners were forced to do. The Chinese had plans to develop this barren landscape into more factories and livestock farms. Although there was less starvation, more died from the conditions under which they worked, and many committed suicide. During my first year there, I built irrigation canals and worked as a farmer."

It was during this time that the Chinese recognized Dr. Chopel's medical skills. They gathered together the traditional doctors in the prison and asked them to be veterinarians. Amchi-la's first job was artificially inseminating sheep. He was later trained in acupuncture, and then served as a surgical assistant.

"When I was first imprisoned, I was not allowed to practice medicine at all," my teacher said. "As the years went by, the Chinese eventually trained me in the 'acceptable' forms of Chinese medicine. This was not traditional Chinese medicine, but what was adopted by Mao during the Cultural Revolution. It was basic Western medicine, first-aid methods, and simple acupuncture. The spiritual basis of healing was rejected and suppressed; I was forbidden to use any Tibetan herbs or treatments. The Chinese used propaganda to convince people that herbs from Tibet were all 'worthless grasses.'

"I was freed in 1980, after twenty-one years in various prisons. Returning to the village of Shelkar, I found the monastery completely destroyed and the monks gone. I stayed with relatives for a month, went to Lhasa to visit other relatives for a year, then returned to Shelkar for another year."

After Dr. Chopel was released from prison, the Chinese government asked him to stay in Shigatze because of his proficiency in medical techniques; at the same time, the people of Shelkar village asked him to return, because they had no medical practitioners. After receiving permission from authorities, the doctor traveled to Shelkar. He met with family members, and gave medicines and teachings to the villagers. "Dr. Chopel has a very good reputation in that part of the country," Lobsang Dhonyo later affirmed. "The people regard him as someone who took care of the poor."

Amchi-la concluded his story. "In 1983, I left Tibet and entered Nepal, coming to Solokumbhu, where some of the Shelkar monks were. I flew from Lukla to Kathmandu at the end of the year. After a brief visit I traveled to Dharamsala to consult with the Dalai Lama about my future."

I was deeply grateful to Dr. Chopel for sharing his life story. Over the coming years, I would learn more about my teacher from several other Shelkar elders, who remembered incidents the doctor was not inclined to share. Their stories concerned Amchi-la's unusual intelligence and compassionate nature, such as the time in prison when he risked his life to cure a Chinese officer of a debilitating condition. What touched me even more profoundly were the spiritual insights Dr. Chopel had attained as a result of his Dharma practice in prison.

"How was it possible to have loving-kindness and compassion for the Chinese while in prison?" I asked my teacher during our conversations about Tonglen, the practice of "taking and sending."

"My experiences were the fruition of my bad karma," the doctor replied. "They were a good opportunity to develop my mind. If I viewed circumstances in this way, and remembered that the soldiers, too, were being forced by their orders and their karma to do what they did, I could endure the suffering. I have no anger or hatred toward the Chinese."

These were remarkable statements, revealing a profound accomplishment. After his ordeal, Dr. Chopel had emerged as a dignified elder who embodied the spirit of Buddhistic metta.

"I was treated relatively well by the Chinese," Amchi-la continued. "Overall, I have learned much from my experiences. I feel that this is a pure view." I wondered what Dr. Chopel meant when he said he was treated "relatively well." Undoubtedly there were others who fared worse and didn't survive: "relatively well" probably meant just staying alive. As a monastery administrator who publicly spoke out against the invasion, he was subjected to more torture and longer incarceration than many.

"When I was freed, my relatives asked me how it was," the doctor continued. "I told them it certainly wasn't a good life, but I was all right. During those years we had to eat whatever food we could find, sometimes even eating grass in the fields like horses and cows. When I suffered, I practiced viewing it as the ripening of my karma; each of us must suffer the effects of our own deeds.

"The Chinese have done horrible things, of course," Amchi-la said. "Their bad actions are also the result of their ripening habitual tendencies. If we examine the situation, we find that Mao's actions were due to his emotional conflicts. Again, I feel this is a pure view, which is not necessarily shared by other Tibetans."

Dr. Chopel was not only an accomplished Tibetan physician; he was also a monk, whose faith in the Dharma had been put to the ultimate test. He had been confronted by death, torture, and despair and had emerged with utmost confidence in the truth of Buddha's teachings. He viewed his experiences as an opportunity to develop spiritual awareness, and made no claims of transcending suffering, saying only that compassion was the refuge that had helped him survive. I will never know the thoughts and emotions my teacher experienced during and after the atrocities he witnessed and endured, but his practice of mindfully loving, forgiving, and empathizing with his oppressors revealed to me a man who was accomplishing something remarkable for humanity. His words went beyond scholarly understanding, for he was living testament to the healing power of metta.

"It is not difficult to have compassion, once you have come to know the essence of the Dharma," I heard the elder monks say at different times. Now, after learning about Amchi-la's life story and the magnitude of Dharmic realization it revealed, my appreciation and respect for the soft-spoken physician increased further. In contrast to what my mentor had gone through with sattvic character, I could not help but see myself as selfishly preoccupied, rarely grateful for the good fortunes I took for granted, and frequently irritated by life's minor obstacles and insignificant troubles.

Because Amchi-la had survived prison with such dignity, his teachings were imbued with the authority gained by both profound practice and realizations achieved under unimaginable conditions. I was extremely fortunate to have a teacher who not only was gifted in medicine but also understood the spiritual causes of suffering and their resolution.

"From the smallest insect running around here and there to the highest god in a heavenly realm, nobody wants suffering," Dr. Chopel said during our discussions concerning karma. "If we observe how all beings are the same in this regard, we can develop our minds, and our understanding of the Dharma will increase.

"Everyone knows that after they are born they must die. When we die, the mind continues and seeks rebirth; this is based on our actions. If you do good in this life, its fruition will be peace and happiness. If our actions are negative, we will take rebirth in lower realms of existence and will have to suffer. Human beings are all looking for happiness, but so many are suffering, and they rarely find it; this is because of their karma. Everybody wants peace and happiness, but if we do not do good things, how can we find this happiness?

"I came from a rich family with many luxuries, and when I lived in the monastery I had a high position. When the Chinese came, I was put in prison without edible food, and lost all my previous forms of power. In the monastery I had beautiful blankets to sit on and nice robes to wear, but in prison I suffered from not having clothing or blankets. I understand something about the fruition of karma, because these things have ripened for me. You should believe in karma, and think about this."

The great festival of Shivaratri is held in Kathmandu at the temples of Pashupatinath, along the banks of the Bagmati. The faithful come from all over India and Nepal to celebrate this "Night of Shiva." At its peak, the twilight is filled with voices and music of worship, as naked ash-covered men with long braided hair pray and sing to the Lord, the King of Yogis, their devotion fueled by smoldering chillums. Phantasms from the worlds of myth dance among the shadowed sanctuaries of the deities.

I drifted through shifting shapes of people and stone, fluid sculptures carved in crimson firelight. Free of thoughts, my senses open to the textures of the ancient rituals, I descended to the footbridge. The water moved silently below, flowing past caves where meditators have sat through the millennia, past rooms carved in hillsides where the dying go to spend their final days, past the gilded pagodas, past the ghats with their burning corpses. The river's origin lay somewhere in the Himalayan snows, its destination somewhere in the steaming tropics.

A pyre was burning on one of the ghats. I made my way toward it until I could see a person lying in death's fiery embrace. The flames had consumed all but the rib cage, neck, and skull. The brightest burned inside the hollow chest, outlined by the blackness of the bones. I watched as this human like myself dissolved into heat, light, and smoke.

The bodies of two fortunate ones were brought out wrapped in saffron-colored cloth. They reached their journey's end, at this auspicious time, in this holy place, as they were laid on newly stacked pyres. White-robed attendants stepped forward and pulled back the cloth from each simultaneously, revealing the faces. Placing a handful of food, flowers, and oil inside the mouth of each corpse, they prayed for the deceased. The crowd began to grow. Suddenly, a torch was touched to each face, and plumes of fire rose into the air. Agni's soft tongues crept upward through the straw and wood, waking the souls asleep in their lifeless flesh, illuminating the mysterious journey ahead. The onlookers stood transfixed as the dead rose toward the afterlife.

I turned away, as if in a dream, and walked across the bridge toward the forest, up granite steps past the hazy silhouettes of the Shiva lingam shrines. Above me lay the abandoned ruins of old Pashupati, overgrown with moss and vines, home of monkey families.

From somewhere in the darkness came the voice of an invisible singer, accompanied by notes of a simple stringed instrument. The melody was from another lifetime, its rhythm from another age. Without knowing a word, I knew the song: the man was singing praises to the Creator. I followed the voice with unseeing eyes, my feet feeling their way across the stones, pausing to listen every few steps, the coolness of the evening breathing gently. Still the singer remained invisible, only a presence hidden in the shadows. Tiny rays of warm candlelight escaped through a wooden shutter above, leaving soft trails in my vision as I felt my way through the courtyard.

The mysterious song continued; I never found its source. Perhaps there was no singer, only a timeless hymn to God sung without a mouth. Perhaps it was the dead, rising from their pyres to make their way through the night. Maybe it was their guide, singing directions back to the source of life. Maybe it was just an old man, somewhere beyond the reach of my feeble senses, playing a simple instrument in the solitude of abandoned temples.

> "The doctor should not treat one who is in the mouth of Death.
> The sound of God's name is the medicine we should use. That kind
> of meditation will help the dying melt into God, and make the next
> life good. This is the last medicine."
>
> —Gopal, translating Nadi Parikcha (Pulse Diagnosis)

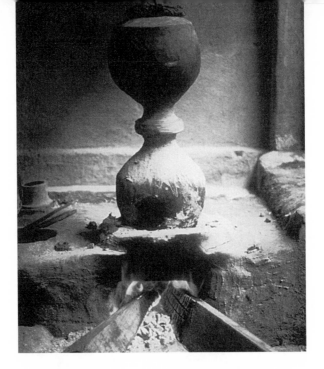

X.

THE SPERM OF SHIVA

A medicine prepared mainly from mercury and minerals is superior to that prepared from herbs; inasmuch as the former can be administered in much smaller doses than the latter, it does not give rise to aversion in the patient who takes it, it cures diseases more quickly than the latter, and it cures diseases which are considered incurable by medicines prepared from herbs. Medicines prepared from mercury, with or without the addition of other minerals or poisons, are the best of all the medicines known to the world. If used for a long time they can not only cure diseases, but also strengthen the body and cure and prevent senile

decay.

FROM RASA JALA NIDHI,
OR THE OCEAN OF INDIAN
CHEMISTRY, MEDICINE, AND ALCHEMY

Throughout my studies of Ayurvedic and Tibetan medicine, I encountered no subject more mysterious, complex, or controversial than mercury. The metal and its gases are a virulent poison, yet Vaidyes have claimed for millennia that when properly cleansed and sublimated, it becomes supreme among all medicines. Mercurial drugs have a long history of use in Asia, with over a thousand years of clinical experience, but virtually no modern research into their actions has been undertaken. Mercury toxicity is a dangerous global threat to human and environmental health, but generations of Ayurvedic physicians have confidently stated that without alchemically purified mercury, many serious and chronic diseases cannot be cured.

When I first encountered Rasa Shastra and Ayurvedic and Tibetan mercurial preparations, I was fascinated with their exotic history and intrigued with their uses, and I enthusiastically sought more knowledge and experience. The more I learned about the complexities and subtleties of alchemical preparations, however, the more I was confronted with formidable personal and professional dilemmas. Why would anyone want to explore and publicize the ingestion of medicinal mercury, knowing that the practice is fraught with medical controversy and legal ramifications, and filled with alchemical magic and religious superstition?

For years, these concerns prevented me from addressing a subject that is well-known in India and Nepal but almost unheard of in the West; I now believe it is important to discuss the following aspects of medicinal alchemy. The first is the major role mercurial drugs play in Ayurvedic and Tibetan medicines, which recognize their curative value for diseases unresponsive to other forms of treatment. The second is the extremely dangerous nature of mercury, its misuse in modern medicine, dentistry, and industry, and its poisoning of people and the environment. The third is the reverence alchemists and iatro-chemists have for mercury, a reverence which—if adopted by modern science and medicine—could halt their growing abuses of nature. Finally, and perhaps most crucial, is the question: What solutions do classical Tibetan and Ayurvedic methods of healing offer the countless patients who suffer chronic and acute disorders attributed to the ever-increasing presence of mercury in our lives?

Mercury and its gases are extremely toxic. These potent suppressors of the immune system are deadly to cellular functions, powerfully disruptive to the hormonal functions of the endocrine system, damaging to the cardiovascular system, and highly poisonous to the reproductive system. Mercury is now known to be used by pathogenic microbes to strengthen their resistance to antibotics.

Mercury is absorbed through the respiratory system, gastrointestinal tract, and skin. There is no place in the body this liquid metal and its gas cannot easily penetrate, yet our physiology is inefficient at eliminating it; it acts as a cumulative poison, since there are few pathways available to the body for its excretion. Mercury accumulates in the brain, liver, kidneys, heart, mucous membranes, and other tissues. As its levels increase, its potential to cause harm becomes greater. Mercury is known to damage the brain and nervous system; numerous studies have found that long-term chronic low doses of mercury cause neurological, memory, behavior, and mood problems.

Mercury has a special affinity for the glandular system. It gravitates to the pituitary gland, where it is stored in high concentrations. Even a minute amount can adversely affect the pituitary's hormonal manufacturing and regulating functions, which in turn influence all bodily processes. In addition to these endocrine-disrupting effects in the pituitary gland, mercury causes a reduction in thyroid hormone. Its adverse influence on thyroid cells can play a major role in the etiology of cancer in that gland.

Mercury is a potent reproductive toxin, suspected of playing a role in decreased sperm counts and defective sperm cells, and associated with infertility of animals living in areas contaminated with mercury. It is found in breast milk, and it accumulates in the fetus at much higher levels than in the mother's tissues. The highest concentrations are in the pituitary gland of the fetus, affecting development of the endocrine, immune, and reproductive systems. Mercury can cause birth defects and developmental problems in children, and is known to damage the brain and nervous system of unborn babies.

Mercurial drugs were first introduced to European medicine by Paracelsus in the 1500s; they later became, along with bloodletting and drastic purgatives, the basis of early American "heroic medicine." The practice of "touching the gums," or producing profuse salivation, was the treatment of choice for many diseases. Giving patients high doses of toxic mercury compounds produced an enormous flow of thick, ropy saliva, up to several pints a day. After this would come extensive ulceration or gangrenous inflammation of the cheeks and gums, which would begin sloughing and lead to loss of the teeth and rotting of the jaw. The treatment itself caused a new disease, hydrargism, or mercurial erethism, characterized by tremors, neuralgias, paralysis, convulsions, profound anemia, excessive purgation, and death.

By the late 1800s, countless patients had suffered and died from mercury toxicity. It was largely through the political efforts of the Eclectic physicians, the herbalists of the early twentieth century, that the Paracelsian compounds were abandoned. In the words of Dr. John King, one of the school's leading doctors, "There is no single remedy known to man which has produced a greater amount of mischief by its indiscriminate use than mercury; nor is there any other drug which has done one hundredth part as much to create a prejudice against scientific medicine, to destroy the confidence of the community in its practitioners, and to repel them from the physicians to the nostrum dealers." The Eclectic practitioners provided naturopathic remedies for those stricken with hydrargism, using astringent infusions like tincture of myrrh to control salivation and stop gangrenous ulceration of the mouth and throat, as well as botanical alternatives to mercurial drugs. For those suffering from the systemic effects of mercury toxicity, they prescribed herbal blood purifiers, tonics, and formulas to regulate the channels of elimination. The research and efforts of these American herbalists helped bring an end to a tragic chapter in the history of iatrogenic illnesses.

In spite of mercury's dark past, it continues to be employed in industry, manufacturing, and medicine. It is used in thermometers and other medical instruments, barometers, fluorescent lamps, advertising signs, electrical apparatuses, pesticides, chlorine production, paints, batteries, papermaking, metal refining, and numerous other products. One of its many uses in medicine is in thimerosal, a preservative added to vaccines, which has been linked to allergic reactions.

Mercury is the most common foreign material implanted in the human body: approximately 100,000 pounds are used by the American dental profession every year. It is now known that dental amalgams decompose in the mouth, in the process releasing methyl mercury, the element's most poisonous form. Dental amalgam mercury syndrome (DAMS) is becoming a medically recognized public health concern, and scientific evidence is mounting that so-called "silver" fillings are dangerous to patients, dentists, technicians, and the community.

The long history of Rasa Shastra is very different from the medical and industrial abuse of mercury in the West. Mercury was introduced into Ayurvedic medicine in the second century by Nagarjuna. Prior to this, many centuries of experimentation by alchemists yielded important discoveries about the metal's chemical properties. Seeking compassionate and painless alternatives to the surgical practices of the time, Dharma kings of the Indian Buddhist period promoted research into the use of mercury as a medicine. The result was Rasa Shastra, a medical system powerful and effective enough to replace surgery, yet conform to the Buddhist doctrine of ahimsa, nonviolence. By the 1200s, medicinal alchemy had spread into Tibet, where it was used to create the "jewel pills" of the Amchis.

Rasadis, mercurial medicines, have been made and administered for over a thousand years, with some family traditions continuing uninterrupted for centuries. Rasa Shastra has grown to become an academically established field of science taught in over 150 Ayurvedic colleges, and a branch of the government-standardized pharmaceutical industry. Mercurial medicines and tonics are prescribed by thousands of Ayurvedic physicians daily across the Indian subcontinent, and consumed by millions of patients both as prescriptions and over-the-counter remedies. Ayurvedic doctors claim that hydrargism, the gross mercury poisoning which once caused the rebellion against physicians in the West, is rarely, if ever, seen in clinics; properly prepared and administered rasadis, they assert, will instead cure the symptoms caused by hydrargism, such as kidney failure from nephrotoxicity.

For a millennium, Rasa Shastra has been regarded as the highest branch of Ayurveda's pharmacopoeia. Fifty generations of Indian and Tibetan saints, alchemists, physicians, yogis, kings and queens, and patients from all walks of life have relied on rasadis for curing serious diseases and maintaining good health. In contrast, the mercuric salts of the "quacks" (those who dispensed "quacksilver") in the West, quickly fell into disrepute and contempt because of severe poisoning in the population. The reason for these historical differences is that Vaidyes and Amchis use different mercurial compounds than those prescribed by early Western doctors, and in a different way.

There are three important differences between Rasa Shastra and the Paracelsian approach to iatro-chemistry. First, the compounds used by practitioners of heroic medicine were caustic salts, such as calomel, mercurous chloride. Ayurvedic mercury preparations, on the other hand, are inert forms of HgS, mercuric sulfides; these were not utilized by Western doctors because they seemed to lack any physiological effect whatsoever. The Vaidyes, however, observed that sulfides did indeed have therapeutic benefits. The Ayurvedic materia medica describes the primary physiological action of mercuric sulfides to be an alteration of the secretions from the mucous membranes of the intestines. These secretions create a detoxifying effect in the colon by controlling overgrowth of pathogenic microbes and supporting healthy flora. The most important secondary effect from this altered glandular function and rebalanced microbial ecology is the production of a pure golden yellow bile by the liver. The restoration of beneficial intestinal bacteria and stimulation of liver function are fundamental to curing disease and maintaining good health, and one of the reasons Vaidyes regard mercury so highly.

The second difference between the two traditions of mercury is in the preparation methods. Rasa Shastra utilizes unique and complex purification processes to render the metal a consumable ash. Many of these procedures cannot be duplicated outside of Himalayan countries, because they rely on indigenous plant materials.

The third difference is in the methods of administration. Western physicians routinely prescribed mercurial drugs in high doses, perhaps mistaking the symptoms of mercury poisoning for signs of healing. Vaidyes, on the other hand, prescribe their mercuric medicines in minute doses for short times. In addition, Ayurvedic physicians rarely use sulfides as a single drug; instead, HgS is compounded in formulas as a yoga vahi, a substance which potentizes other substances, such as herbs.

These chemical and clinical differences in mercuric use have allowed Ayurvedic and Tibetan physicians to utilize mercury extensively without, they claim, causing harm to their patients. According to Dr. Bhagwan Dash, one of the foremost scholars of Ayurveda, "It has been clinically observed that mercuric sulfide compounds, even if used for a considerably long time, do not produce any toxic effects." Ayurvedic physicians acknowledge, however, that if not prepared according to traditional methods, or if improperly prescribed, mercurial medicines can be extremely dangerous.

The first time I encountered mercurial medicines was at Dr. Chopel's clinic. I was sitting in the pharmacy one rainy monsoon afternoon, watching the old doctor read his patients' pulses and prescribe remedies. Sonam was late; maybe his motorcycle was stuck in the flooded streets. Outside the windows, Nepali families, knee deep in mud, were singing a rice planting song.

On the bench beside me were bowls of herb mixtures waiting to be ground to powder in mortars by the young monks. The largest bowl had a label, which I deciphered as "Dashel Chenmo." These were the ingredients for the Great Purified Moon Crystal Pill, one of the "jewel pills" of the Tibetan tradition. Many of the herbs were easily identified— green cardamom, cinnamon bark, pomegranate seeds, licorice root. Others were mysterious, such as a large ball of powdery white rock and spikes of purple flowers. The doctor listed their names in Tibetan as I pulled them out.

Sonam arrived as the last patient left. Dr. Chopel began explaining how he was preparing the ingredients of the Moon Crystal Pill. "I have just received some gems and precious metals from Tibet," he said. "They were alchemically prepared there. I can now make this medicine in its original, more potent form. Since living in exile, most Tibetan doctors are unable to prepare these medications with the proper proportions of ingredients, so their efficacy is lessened. The powder I received has a high percentage of purified gold, and a unique Tibetan gem called the tzi stone." These ingredients would be added to the herbs in the bowl, along with another crucial substance which the doctor had prepared: purified mercury.

Reaching over to his herb cabinet, Dr. Chopel removed a small jar with about a half cup of fine black powder in it, and offered it to me. I took it from his hand, noticing its heaviness. "Eat a little bit," he suggested, "it's completely nontoxic." I blackened the tip of my finger and tasted it; it lacked any distinct flavor. What I had just consumed was the most famous ingredient of countless Ayurvedic and Tibetan formulas, renowned for its ability to restore immunity and destroy disease. Would it be possible to see how this medicine is made? I wondered, intrigued and excited about watching Rasa Shastra in practice.

"We will have to wait until after the monsoon," the doctor replied, "because it must be done outside in the open air and under bright sun." I sat back and assimilated my first lesson in alchemy: patience.

Over the years, I would receive lessons concerning rasadis, ask questions of my teachers, read whatever material was available on the subject, and participate in mercurial preparations. Gradually, I acquired a rudimentary knowledge of the basic concepts and practices of Rasa Shastra.

What Dr. Chopel had given me is described by the early pharmacopoeias of Western medicine as "hydrargyri sulfidum nigrum," black sulfide of mercury. King's *American Dispensatory*, one of the important textbooks of the Eclectic physicians, describes this compound as a "heavy, somewhat grayish black, inodorous, tasteless, amorphous powder, insoluble in water. It acts very mildly, and may be continued for a considerable length of time in doses of several drachms without producing scarcely any sensible effect." This substance, known in Rasa Shastra as kajjali, is the basis for almost all mercurial medicines used in Ayurveda.

Kajjali is made by smelting alchemically purified mercury and sulfur together in a hot mortar. I witnessed this basic process of medicinal alchemy several times during my studies. "In mercurial preparations, sulfur and mercury must be mixed into a black paste," Dr. Tiwari explained one afternoon as we prepared to make kajjali. "We add different ratios of sulfur, one to one, one to two, one to three, and change the form of the medicine. It may be mercuric sulfide, mercuric disulfide, mercuric trisulfide."

This process, like all aspects of alchemy, is regarded as having spiritual and mythical dimensions, as well as a scientific basis. The Sanskrit names of mercury, such as parada, the "sperm of Shiva," allude to its great power. To make parada safe for consumption, it must be mixed with a substance of equal power: sulfur, the orgasmic vaginal secretions of Parvati. Mercury and sulfur have a natural attraction, say the alchemists; when melted in molecular union, their poisons are transmuted into healing nectar. Sulfur is also considered the elemental embodiment of menstrual blood, and the womb which gives birth to kajjali. Kajjali is the alchemical child of Shiva and Parvati, and the basis of other medicines.

Kajjali is insoluble and seemingly inert, yet is considered by the

Vaidyes and Amchis to be one of the greatest remedies for humanity's ills. "Kajjali is called a yoga vahi," Dr. Tiwari went on, explaining this apparent contradiction. "Mercuric sulfide influences the absorption and action of medicines, making them more available for specific tissues."

The probable physiological explanation of this phenomenon would be threefold: enhanced intestinal secretions help digest the herbs; improved colon function increases their assimilation; and stimulation of liver activity promotes metabolism, which strengthens the herbs' inherent affinity for specific tissues and organs.

Another doctor who had decades of experience preparing and prescribing mercury-based medicines was Uprenda Thakur. "Kajjali is never used by itself," he told me as we watched his technicians preparing formulas. "It is mixed with herbal medicines and other bhasma. Parada goes to every organ, but you have to add different herbs to direct it. Mercury controls everything, but we have to use a medium to carry it. You have to modify it according to the pulse and the nature of the disease."

"When we prescribe mercurial medicines, we suggest a specific type of diet," Dr. Tiwari explained, emphasizing the symbiotic role mercury has with other substances. "To balance mercury's actions, we generally advise a cool-natured diet. According to our view, paro is hot in nature; eating spices and hot foods increases the heat of the rasadi and leads to unwanted effects."

Dr. Tiwari was describing the activity of mercury's elemental fire, tejas, the solar and atomic light and heat, which gives mercury its alchemical affinity to gold. According to Ayurvedic philosophy, parada's fire strongly increases the digestive transformations of the body, mind, and senses, helping to eliminate accumulated toxins, providing nutrition to the cells, and generating energy. Rasadis also provide an immense amount of prana, the current of vital force, which in turn is the basis for rejuvenation of ojas. If used correctly, mercury can increase prana, tejas, and ojas, which then restore the equilibrium of the three doshas, thus producing harmonious functioning of the body's elements. Ultimately, if used for rasayana purposes to bring about jiva mukti, parad can induce the flow of Soma, the sweet nectar of spiritual consciousness. If used incorrectly, however, mercury's intense energy, like the uncontrolled awakening of kundalini's bioelectrical current, can wreak havoc in the body.

There are many ways rasadis can cause side effects, including being administered in the wrong dose or with an improper vehicle such as hot-natured herbs and foods. By far the most serious concern for physicians and patients is the correct purification of the metal's elemental toxins. Both modern scientific research and Ayurveda's long lineages have documented mercury's dangers and poisonous effects. The texts of Rasa Shastra describe the metal's deadly aspects and how to remove them by alchemical methods.

Mercurial drugs were a frequent topic of discussion with Dr. Shrestha. I once questioned her about what Ayurvedic colleges taught about hydrargium. "Mercury has different types of poisonous effects on various levels of the body," she answered. "It can cause delirium, burning, restlessness, hematuria, and other reactions. All of these symptoms were taught to us during our medical training. We also learned how to remove those toxins from mercury with asta samskar, the traditional steps of purification. If we strictly follow those purification methods, we will not have to face the problems of side effects or toxicity."

Rasa Shastra utilizes many methods for purifying mercury; these are classified into either eight stages, for standard level rasadis, or eighteen, for superior medicines. Many of the preliminary sequences involve removing the opportunistic impurities of other metals, like lead, tin, and zinc. These are cleansed from the mercury by repeatedly mixing it with various substances such as wool, brick dust, charcoal, turmeric, lemon, and datura seeds, for prolonged periods of time, distilling the metal after exposure to each substance. After the metallic poisons are removed, further procedures cleanse the mercury's remaining impurities. Finally, the mercury is mixed with the juice of ginger, garlic, and lemon, three times each, and distilled after each rubbing in the mortar. This makes the mercury ready for standard-level medicines. If a doctor wishes to make medicines of a higher quality and potency, more procedures follow; there are countless recipes in the alchemical manuscripts.

"Purification is most important," Dr. Shrestha continued. "If we are even a little careless in these procedures, we will do harm both to the patient and to the field of Ayurveda. But once it is properly purified, the classical books say parada is the 'king of all medicines.'"

"Working with paro is very dangerous," Dr. Thakur warned, both during our laboratory sessions and in his lectures concerning the prescription of rasadis. The successful use of mercurials, the physician taught, depends on a high degree of expertise, an impeccably prepared product, a precise diagnosis, and an exact dose. "It is crucial that rasadi medicines be prepared properly," he said. "Otherwise, they are toxic and harmful. There must be a correct evaluation of the disease according to the doshas, and proper dosages must be prescribed. If rasadis are used in this way, they are like nectar; if not, they become poison." The doctor's words were similar to those of Paracelsus: "All things are poison, and nothing is without poison; the dose alone makes a thing not poison."

"When I prescribe, I always think about potential side effects," Dr. Shrestha answered in response to my inquiries about the safety of rasadis. "I won't say that Ayurvedic medicines don't have side effects; the degree may vary, but every medicine has side effects, whether it is herbs or rasadis."

The more potent medicines become, the greater the power to heal, and to harm. All doctors, whether using allopathic or Ayurvedic medicines, carry a heavy responsibility for the consequences of their actions. "The shepherd picks up his lunch bag and goes to heaven," Dr. Chopel once remarked. "The doctor picks up his medicine bag and goes to hell."

All the doctors I studied with had success stories about the efficacy of rasadi medicines. Hearing these accounts, it was impossible to not consider the role mercurial medicines could play in treating conditions unresponsive to modern medicine.

Of all my teachers, Dr. Singh was by far the most cautious and skeptical when it came to using rasadis. Even so, he had seen dramatic cures. One afternoon the doctor shared a story about a famous preparation of black mercuric sulfide called parpati. "We had a regimen of parpati in our Institute [at Benares University]," he said, "where it was used for ulcerative colitis. You know the range of pathology that may occur in this disease, that it is precancerous and that you may have to do a colectomy and live with an ileostomy. We have treated this with parpati alone, given with milk, and nothing else.

"There was a boy of about nine years who came to us as a last resort, otherwise he would have had to live with an ileostomy his whole life, and this was a miserable proposition. I am a very cynical man, and I don't believe in things I have not seen for myself. With my own eyes I have seen that boy consuming eighteen liters of milk a day, having formed stools, and gaining weight. Now after twenty years he is married and well settled in life. I have seen the effect, but even there I must put a question mark. Was it the sulfide that did the trick, or was it all of us treating him, because the psychological component is there in all these diseases? I don't know, but I can assure you that he did not die of mercuric poisoning!"

The red and black sulfides are described in the Ayurvedic materia medica as "extremely efficacious in liver complaints," such as cirrhosis of the liver, and dysenteries where there is a deficiency of bile in the stools. They are direct chologogues (stimulating bile secretions), and are considered to have no equal in the treatment of chronic dysentery. Their action is said to detoxify the large intestine and stimulate the liver to secrete golden yellow bile.

Like Dr. Singh, Dr. Thakur had had remarkable successes. When I inquired about the potential for mercurial drugs to cause toxicity in the kidneys and liver, the doctor responded by describing some of his experiences with rasadis in the treatment of serious conditions of those organs. "Modern medicine has no treatment for cirrhosis of the liver, and considers it incurable," he said. "I have had many cirrhosis patients, and am currently treating five cases. I have given them mercuric medicines for over a year and a half. They are almost completely recovered; their general symptoms are gone, and liver function tests are within normal limits. I have never seen any nephrological problems or other pathological changes in the reports, so I am confident from my own experience that mercuric preparations do not harm the body. If rasadis are harmful, they would have harmed those who have been taking them for more than a year."

This was a powerful testament. I wished that others could see and hear the doctor's demeanor of absolute confidence as he spoke. His authority was not simply age, experience, and medical certainty accumulated from years as the government's Chief of Ayurvedic Medicine; it was a palpable conviction that emanated from the core of his robust constitution.

"I had a unique experience with one patient," he continued. "He was in the Bir Hospital hemodialysis department with kidney damage. At that time the intervals of dialysis were every three days. I examined him in the hospital and said, 'Whatever procedure you are undergoing, please continue. You should also take my medicine, one dose in the morning and one in the evening.' The patient agreed and started the medicines, which were rasadis and bhasmas. After one week the interval of dialysis went to seven days, then fifteen days, then one month. After one month his nephrologist discharged the patient, and he came to me. I gave him a full course of medication, with rasadis and herbal preparations. After three months he went back to Bir Hospital, and the doctors were surprised. All his renal functions had become normal. People say that mercuric preparations are very dangerous and will destroy the kidneys. How can I believe that, when I have cured a patient suffering from an extreme condition of renal failure?"

Dr. Thakur is a highly qualified physician, who claims without doubt that mercury can bring about such pronounced therapeutic changes in the body that allopathic doctors are amazed. I knew from my own clinical experience that, when confronted with unexplainable good results from natural medicines, some practitioners dismiss the outcome by unscientifically reasoning that "it would have happened anyway," while the more curious and open-minded are interested in what happened and how they might be able to repeat it.

"There was another case," Dr. Thakur went on, knowing he had my undivided attention. "The mother of a prestigious family was suffering from severe diabetes with dangerous complications. She was being treated by doctors from here to Delhi, at renowned places. The medicines were not working, and she was taking many injections of insulin. After that she came to me and started treatment. The main drugs for this in Ayurvedic treatment are the mercurials. The diabetes became normal, there was no sugar in the blood, and the patient is living without any medications."

Very impressive results, I thought. Not too many physicians claim they have cured diabetes. But could this be substantiated?

"The history of rasadis goes back to five hundred years before Buddha," Dr. Thakur said. "I am doing nice work, but there is a lack of scientific documentation. The motherland of Ayurveda is India and Nepal, but these countries don't have much money. They are struggling with food for the people and many other problems, so this type of research has not been properly established. This is unfortunate.

"In my opinion, research into these mercuric and metallic preparations is very essential. Modern doctors claim that Ayurvedic practitioners are harming patients by using metallic medicines. This is a serious and dangerous allegation. We should have documentation to be rid of this blame."

I agreed. If charges of toxicity are to be made, they should be proved. Without documented evidence, unsubstantiated accusations have no more credibility than unsubstantiated claims of cures.

Considering mercury's toxicity, it is not surprising that the rasadis of Ayurveda are controversial. Some modern allopaths in India and Nepal are critical of mercurial medicines, an opinion also shared by a minority of allopathically oriented Ayurvedic practitioners. The controversy revolves around rare cases of mercury poisoning which have occurred as a result of poorly prepared or administered medicines. Quality-control problems and misuse of drugs affect every pharmaceutical industry, including Ayurveda.

All my teachers praised the efficacy of rasadis and claimed to have never seen toxicity in their patients, but they also admitted that mercurial medicines can poison people when manufacturing processes are not followed carefully. For that reason, they either make the medicines themselves or rely on long-established, reputable companies. The doctors agree that clinical research into the safety and effectiveness of rasadis is needed to disprove the negative allegations of critics, and that quality control in the Ayurvedic pharmaceutical industry is crucial to protect its reputation.

Even though their use is discouraged by some practitioners, mercurial medicines continue to be an integral part of health maintenance and medical treatment throughout the Indian subcontinent. Each of the 150 Ayurvedic colleges in India teaches rasadis as a major part of its curriculum, with each school graduating between fifty and a hundred doctors every year. Between the combined prescriptions of these physicians and the large number of major reputable companies providing rasadis to the public over the counter, the quantities of mercurial drugs consumed per year must be huge. These compounds have been the most renowned medicines in this part of the world since at least the days of Nagarjuna, if not a thousand years earlier, as some claim, making the number of people who have used them through the centuries uncountable. Rasadis have been consumed for so many generations, and so many people have seen their parents and grandparents routinely using them, that there is widespread skepticism regarding modern doctors' claims of toxicity.

My teachers all used mercurial medicines extensively throughout their careers. Among them, these ten doctors had hundreds of years of combined clinical experience, and had given these drugs to possibly hundreds of thousands of patients. Dr. Thakur alone estimated he had given them to over 40,000 patients.

Dr. Shrestha's comments concerning the accusations of toxicity were typical of many other Ayurvedic physicians. When I asked whether she had encountered any cases of hydrargism caused by rasadis, she replied, "We have not seen mercury poisoning in patients taking these preparations. I am getting good clinical results: in some cases patients are relieved, and in some cases they are cured, so I am satisfied with my prescriptions of rasadi medicines. I have never seen any bad side effects."

"What about other physicians?" I asked.

"In India and Nepal, most of the traditional doctors are practicing with these medicines," Dr. Shrestha replied. "Every classical Vaidye uses mercury."

"Are those doctors seeing cases of mercury toxicity?"

"In Nepal this type of study has not been done. There are only rumors and controversy about the toxicity of these medicines, but nobody has observed it, because patients are not presenting this type of problem. We have so many problems in Nepal, but it is very rare that patients come with kidney toxicity or other symptoms which could be from mercury. I know so many people who are using mercury, and gold preparations also, and they are living without any problems. How can we say there is toxicity?

"Sulfur and mercury are said to be renal toxic," Dr. Shrestha continued. "But we give those medicines in renal diseases. Previously, we rarely did ultrasonography, but now we are doing it more. Patients come to us after going elsewhere, so they have a lot of records already. Using those records, we start their treatment, and afterward prescribe another ultrasound. In many cases of renal calculi, patients have passed the stones using rasadi medicines."

Dr. R. D. Mahatyagi's practice in Thamel is based mostly on the use of rasadis. He claims to have prescribed mercurial medications to thousands of patients.

"Have you ever seen any side effects of mercury toxicity?" I inquired during a class at Gopal's. His answer was typical of every doctor I studied with.

"Never. I use them myself."

At ninety-three, Dr. Siddhi Gopal is the eldest Vaidye in Kathmandu, and a veritable fountain of vitality. One day Dr. Shrestha and I sat with the old man in his tiny office in Patan and questioned him about the practice of Rasa Shastra.

"How many years have you been working with mercury?" I asked.

"I have been doing this job since childhood," he replied. "I am my family's twentieth generation of Ayurvedic practitioners. When I was in Benares for my studies, I used to prepare the paro, because I had already been practicing. Everybody used to ask me to do this work, because I could do it in a better way. One who has not practiced before may spoil it or get afraid."

"Have you ever seen anybody get sick from mercury toxicity?"

"I have never seen it in my life."

"And you have given it to a lot of people."

"Many, many people."

"Have you ever heard of cases of mercury poisoning?" I asked Dr. Tiwari as we prepared kajjali.

"Never," he replied. "With Ayurvedic processes you can change the molecular constituents of mercury so it has different types of actions; some forms of mercury are not toxic.

"The *Ayurvedic Pharmacopoeia* is an important government publication," the herbalist went on. "It deals with the methods of preparation, the ratios of each ingredient in a specific preparation, and which disease it is indicated for. The pharmacopoeia has the preparations of all the major mercury medicines. If rasadis were toxic, the government would ban them. Most of the Ayurvedic pharmaceuticals, both herbal and mineral, are government standardized, because there are so many companies manufacturing them. To control the quality, these standards must be met."

"Do you think companies are following those standards?" I asked, somewhat skeptical.

"Mostly, yes."

In the course of our discussions on medicinal alchemy, Dr. Mahatyagi also raised the possibility that new companies could be manufacturing low quality or dangerous rasadis. "Our texts warn that mercury which is not finely incinerated is very toxic," he said. "All the famous bigger companies know this and are trustworthy, but many new companies are being established. I only utilize companies that I know very well, that have been practicing a long time."

"Have you seen any problems from impure rasadis?" I once asked Dr. Thakur.

"People have come to my clinic with edema from using bad quality paro medicine," he replied. Just as he was not hesitant to claim dramatic cures from mercury, Dr. Thakur was also unafraid to admit that bad medicines have made people sick. Knowing that, I imagined that his care in prescribing mercurials would certainly be accentuated.

"To compete in the market, people are going commercial," he explained. "It is better to make rasadis yourself. With outside medicines, maybe it is high quality, maybe not. If you don't make it with your own hand, there is no guarantee."

Greed and incompetence lie at the root of iatrogenic illness, whether caused by synthetic or natural drugs. The safe preparation of mercury, like all pharmaceuticals, is based on wisdom and integrity, essential qualities that are easily neglected in commercial competition. Without the skill, knowledge, and spiritual maturity of the old alchemists, the safety of rasadi drugs and the validity of their use in Ayurveda become questionable.

Even if extensive research verifies the safety of properly prescribed mercurial medicines, and manufacturing standards can be fully guaranteed, it is unlikely that the sulfides of Rasa Shastra will ever be medically or legally accepted outside the Indian subcontinent. For patients suffering from illnesses unresponsive to other forms of treatment (such as cirrhosis of the liver, colitis, diabetes, and asthma) who could potentially be helped by rasadis, this is unfortunate. Advocating the use of mercurial medicines would be foolish, however, in the absence of modern scientific assessment, assurance of purity, and qualified physicians to prescribe them. What, then, is to be done with the precious alchemical wisdom and experience of the ages, which accept the efficacy of rasadis as medical truth in the land of Ayurveda?

Perhaps an even greater discovery than Rasa Shastra's methods of making medicines, and of more importance and relevance for the modern world, are the alchemical manuscripts containing recipes for curing mercuric poisoning. Even with recent efforts to restrict mercury in manufacturing and improve its collection from recycled materials, vast amounts continue to be released globally into the air, water, soil, and food. Ultimately, it becomes biomagnified in the human body.

Mercurial waste from medical, industrial, and consumer products finds its way into landfills, is discharged into rivers and lakes, applied to soil in sludge used as fertilizer, and emitted into the air by incineration. Studies estimate that the total amount of "accounted for" and "unaccounted for" mercury released into the environment over a recent fifteen-year period from dental sources in the United States alone is almost 2 million pounds; other research shows that 5,500 tons, primarily from manmade sources, is emitted globally every year. It is impossible to know completely what long-term effects this will have on the environment and on human health.

What is known is that a very small amount of mercury can do a great deal of damage. One pound of mercury, a few spoonfuls, will contaminate an eighteen-square-mile lake enough to warrant fish consumption advisories. When mercury enters lakes and rivers, it is chemically transformed by bacteria into methyl mercury. Methyl mercury biomagnifies as it moves up the food chain, so large predator fish can carry concentrations in their flesh up to a million times higher than those found in the water. Thirty-nine states have issued health advisories in recent years because of high levels of methylated mercury found in fish from numerous lakes and waterways; mercury is the principal cause of fish contamination in North America and Scandinavia. Mercury may be a contributing factor to the worldwide epidemic of mutations occurring in amphibians.

As the combined effects of toxic chemicals, radiation, and heavy metals rise through the animal kingdoms and begin affecting human populations, physicians will face increasingly complex mutagenic disorders, immunological deficiencies, and allergenic syndromes. Until now, detoxification methods for cleansing the metallic poisons from the body have been less than satisfactory. If there is anyone who would have knowledge of how to efficiently remove mercury from the organs and tissues, it would be the alchemists. Their methods could potentially have profound implications in the treatment of other toxicity problems as well.

My teachers were unanimous in their opinions about the treatment of mercury toxicity: the primary medicine is sulfur, which must be administered according to the individual's symptoms.

"What is the most important medicine for paro toxicity?" I asked Dr. Thakur during one of our discussions about mercury preparation and use.

"Gandak Rasayan [purified sulfur]," he replied, "supported with different herbs. Sulfur is used in any kind of blood purification treatment." Blood-cleansing therapy was also the choice of Eclectic physicians, who were well acquainted with mercury.

"What is the theory behind using sulfur?" I wondered.

"To digest mercury, sulfur is the only one. Mercury is the sperm of Mahadeva [Shiva], and sulfur is Parvati's raja."

When I posed the question to Dr. Mahatyagi, he replied, "In our texts there are different chapters on how to detoxify the poisonous effects of mercury. You must treat according to its specific manifestations. Sometimes there is vomiting tendency, sometimes headaches, sometimes pain, sometimes skin diseases. Gandak Rasayan is important; you can mix it with other things, so the medication will work in different ways. If there is heat, with boils and burning sensations of the skin, you can give sulfur with praval pisti [pearl rubbed with rose water under the full moon], and it will pacify it very nicely."

Using sulfur for treating mercury toxicity is a fascinating possibility, considering its role in cellular metabolism and its molecular relationship to mercury. Sulfur is essential for liver detoxification, enzymatic reactions, hormone functions, nerve tissue conduction, and red blood cell activity. As the alchemists have explained, using their mythical sexual terminology, mercury and sulfur are chemically attracted to each other. Mercury blocks sulfur's enzymatic activity, causing many of the metal's toxic reactions in the body. Could it be that supplementing the body's supply of sulfur leads to the "digesting" of mercury and the restoration of sulfur's metabolic activity? Some progressive physicians involved in mercury detoxification are now using sulfur compounds in their treatments.

Sulfur in its native state is toxic; in order to be used internally it must be purified. The process is relatively simple, requiring only sulfur, milk, and ghee. I witnessed this alchemical procedure several times, finding it performed almost identically by different doctors.

One day Gopal brought a saddhu to my house, explaining that the bearded baba had spent many years working in Ayurvedic pharmacies and was adept at the preparation of minerals for medicinal use. Following the guru's instructions, Gopal and I melted several kilos of fresh butter in an iron vat, skimmed off the froth until only the clear ghee remained, then poured in yellow sulfur crystals.

The crystals sank to the bottom of the vat and melted, becoming a deep-purple liquid. The undulating mass began releasing golden metallic globules, which rose slowly to the surface. Our teacher explained that these were the poisonous impurities of the mineral that had to be skimmed off.

After the sulfur had been cleansed by boiling in ghee, we poured it through a cloth. The bright oily mineral sizzled and spat as the brown sludge seeped away. We put the resulting sulfur cake in a pot of milk and brought it to a low boil. When finished, the milk was poured off and the cake washed with water. The entire process was then repeated two more times.

The purification of the sulfur was now complete. We ground it to a fine powder in a mortar. It had a whitish yellow-brown color with a light earthy smell, without any of the original sulfur aroma. Our guru explained that like most alchemical preparations, the more we repeated the cleansing, the more refined the sulfur would become. The sulfur we now had, he said, was safe for internal consumption as a medicine.

Ayurveda offers more than sulfur for the treatment of mercury toxicity. Pancha karma therapy also holds much promise as an approach to detoxification, especially purva karma, oil massage followed by herbal steam bath. The combination of tissue oleation, improved circulation, and perspiration produces excellent results for many of the symptoms associated with DAMS. Nasya, nasal insufflations of decoctions, juices, oils, and powders, is also an important part of treating mercuric symptoms originating from the teeth. Both of these "karmas" can be infinitely modified according to the patient's needs by using different combinations of ingredients.

Using a few basic principles of Ayurvedic medicine and the remedies from Rasa Shastra, it would be possible to create a highly effective mercury detoxification program using entirely natural substances and therapies. A program of this type could be located at a sulfurous hot spring, be based on pancha karma, and utilize foods and herbs known to have significant mercury-clearing powers. As long as mercury and other environmental contaminants continue to be abused, naturalistic physicians capable of removing them from the body will be in great demand. Like the early Eclectic doctors facing the ravages of "heroic medicine," modern herbalists have a major role to play in the future of medicine.

"Why don't we talk about mercury," I said to Dr. Singh. Dr. Shrestha and I were sitting with the professor in his home office in Sinamangal. I took a hard straight-backed chair in front of his desk, and Dr. Shrestha sat cross-legged on the treatment table against the south wall. The doctor leaned back in his reclining chair, dressed in his usual natty brown suit.

"Well, I don't think I'm competent enough to talk about paro. I've never had much of an interest in it," he replied, with the typical reticent attitude which preceded an erudite discourse.

"You prescribe mercurial medicines, don't you?" I insisted.

"Oh, rarely."

"Approximately how many patients in your career do you think you have given rasadi medicine to?"

"Oh, I don't know, it must be running in the thousands. I prescribe them once in a while. My first priority is no drugs; that is the best treatment. Second is a few drugs, and if that doesn't work, then gradually increasing medications.

"I admit that I use them, but I am totally against promoting them," the doctor said bluntly. "There is no question that we believe in their effectiveness, but I would not let everybody use them. They are very potent, and should not be used as common over-the-counter medicines. The minerals should only be prescribed by competent and trained Ayurvedic physicians in a hospital setting. You cannot give them to people to use indiscriminately. The Ayurvedic companies of India and Nepal are selling these compounds over the counter, but I don't believe this is the right way to do it. Mercury may provoke reactions in our body which we still don't know.

"I myself use these mercury medicines, but I have to be sure they are processed in the proper way. I am not talking about chemical processing; you may have chemically pure mercury, but that is not the kind of purity we want in Ayurveda. It has to be processed with many herbs before it can be used. For us, shodan, purification, means 'to be made fit for human use.' It is a long process; I think that is where the clue to understanding these drugs lies, why they are effective, and why they do good.

"I am not against the use of these mercurial preparations, and I am not concerned at all whether you can prove it scientifically or not. They have been in use for centuries and centuries, and I have seen the effects myself. But it should be done with the precision and methods described in our texts. I am not sure that with modern technology they do all these procedures. I have seen people suffering from kidney problems from using rasadi medicines, and I believe it was because they were not prepared in the proper way."

If rasadis were manufactured according to strict Ayurvedic protocols and administered by trained professionals, Dr. Singh could endorse them, but would not promote their use in the West.

"These rasadis may be totally nontoxic, they may be very effective, but for God's sake, I would like to be very careful," he insisted passionately. "Who's giving them, where have they come from, how have they been prepared?"

The doctor paused. "When I was a child, my father, my great uncle, and some of the others, only they were allowed to handle the mercury. Nobody would touch it. That care was taken, it was instinctive. It was not for the toxicity, but for the regard. It is a very valuable thing; it should be done with reverence. It was a sort of puja they used to do with it."

"Mercury is Mahadeva," Dr. Shrestha said.

"Mahadeva," the surgeon agreed. "It was reverence which they had toward this mercury."

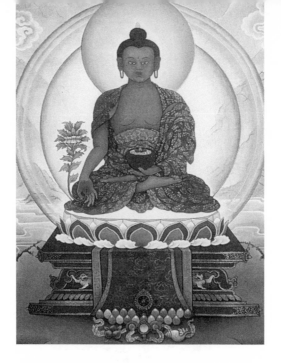

XI.

BEAUTIFUL TO BEHOLD

Then this thought will occur to these beings: "As a consequence of our evil deeds, we have suffered this heavy loss of our kith and kin. It would be well if we were to do good deeds. And now, what good deeds should we do? Let us refrain from taking life. It would be well to perform that good deed!" So thinking, they will abstain from killing; they will perform that good deed. In consequence of performing such good deeds, their life span will expand; their physical appearance will improve. When their life span thus expands and their physical appear-

ance improves, the children of those people whose life span is ten years will live for

twenty years.

BUDDHA,
CHAKRAVARTIN SUTRA

The land that gave birth to the Medicine Buddha was once a world of natural splendor. In the living pharmacies of primordial jungles, luscious hanging gardens of perfumed orchids dripped green nectars, tonics, and poisons. Vast forests of medicinal trees sweetened the pristine air with fragrances of camphor, sandalwood, cinnamon, cedar, and pine. The empty solitude of the arid mountains sheltered strange and unusual species, their flesh bitter with potent alkaloids suspended in the gel of morning dew. In turquoise lagoons, teeming aquatic life drifted through embryonic worlds of fluorescent coral reefs. Prairies undulated in waves of color, roots of all flavors burrowing into the fertile soil; the sky above was as vast as the plains below, where herds of wild animals grazed contentedly.

Places legendary for the diversity and strength of their herbs were the destination of physicians and their disciples on medicine-gathering pilgrimages. In alpine meadows, yogis prepared longevity elixirs from profusions of wildflowers watered by melting snow, singing praises of their wilderness hermitages and the beauty which inspired them to the highest levels of meditative joy. Merchants carried cargoes of herbs and spices along great trade routes stretching from the Mediterranean across the Himalayas to China. Weary travelers found relief in steaming mineral waters, where crystals of salts and sulfur grew. The ground was filled with veins of precious metals and gems. Temple-hospitals, some magnificent and others humble, provided the skilled services of the region's most accomplished physicians, and centers of medical learning prospered under the patronage of Dharma-kings. These are the scenes that unfold across the geometric dimensions of Bhaisajyaguru's mythical world, Sudarshan, Beautiful to Behold.

The mandala of the Medicine Buddha's kingdom is not only a transcendent pure land; it also portrays, in Tibet's unique artistic style, the ecological grandeur and wealth that flourished across the Indian subcontinent until recently. Now, the iconographic vision of the deity's healing realm is becoming a fading memory of vanishing creatures and botanical wonders, a dream of nature's beauty and power from time immemorial that is evaporating like a mirage from the soul of humanity.

We are living in an age of biological extinction. From the perspective of our infinitesimally short human lifespan, global changes appear to be unfolding slowly and imperceptibly; in the larger context of recent history, however, the extent and rapidity of these events are nothing less than a precipitous collapse of the biosphere. Over the course of only two generations, the woods our parents knew became the fields of our youth, and now those are covered with suburbs and pavement, and the songbirds are gone. The land covered by the freeways of Los Angeles was home to abundant botanical and animal diversity, as recently as our great-grandparents' generation. Their great-grandparents saw what we will never know: a continent whose ancient forests stretched unbroken from the Atlantic to the Mississippi, sheltering cultures whose original ancestors walked out of the mists at the dawn of Creation. If changes of this magnitude have transpired so recently, it is unimaginable what kind of world our great-grandchildren will be born into.

No one knows with certainty the full range of endangered and recently extinct forms of life, or how their functions are entwined, for we have only begun to glimpse the immense web of complex interrelationships among the microbial worlds, animal kingdoms, plants, and the behavior of the planet's elemental systems. Recent studies estimate that within twenty years, over 10 percent of the world's botanical species will be gone: tens of thousands of plants, representing millions of years of evolutionary development, which cannot be replaced. What is certain is that innumerable medicines will never be discovered among those extinct trees, grasses, shrubs, ferns, cacti, and orchids; we will never taste countless foods and valuable nutrients; and we will be deprived of new sources of energy, fibers, cloth, paper, woods, oils, resins, and other valuable necessities.

Nor does anyone know what impact the loss of this many plants will have on the microbes, insects, and animals they symbiotically sustain, and in turn, how humanity will be affected. Modern research is finally revealing what indigenous people have taught their children for millennia: our lives depend on the small and seemingly insignificant forms of life we ignore, take for granted, and mindlessly annihilate. With the disappearance of butterflies, birds, and other tiny treasures, plants will be unable to pollinate and reproduce, and the earth's crucial life-support systems may no longer function sufficiently to support humans. The breakdown of wastes will become slower, oxygen regeneration will diminish, soil fertility will weaken, and atmospheric balance will be disrupted.

Plants are the basis of all life, good health, and prosperity. If we destroy the foundation of botanical diversity that purifies the water and air, protects and regenerates the soil, supports animal populations, and provides food, medicine, clothing, and shelter, civilization is destined to decline into sickness, poverty, and violence. If the waters are fouled with turbid waste and tainted with carcinogens; if the atmosphere is burning with petrochemical vapors and ultraviolet fire; if the oceans are poisoned, the forests stripped, and the streets full of hungry people, the outcome is certain: deteriorating health standards, culminating in epidemics that make no distinction among nations, races, religions, or economic status. We all eat from the same soil and sea, breathe from the same sky, and drink the same rain.

In Nepal, these are not hypothetical problems in a distant future. Over a period of thirty years, the Kathmandu Valley has gone from a pastoral kingdom reminiscent of Sudarshan, to a place of asphyxiating pollution, miserable overcrowding, and cultural decay. Kathmandu's degradation is a reflection of afflicted cities everywhere, and the decimation of the country's forests, jungles, and farmlands is typical of the disappearance of natural resources around the world. Physicians in Kathmandu are facing rising tides of illness brought by undrinkable water, unbreathable air, and unlivable social conditions, from which they, too, suffer. Medicine is becoming palliative at best, and disease-producing at worst. If these trends continue to worsen, all medical systems, both modern and traditional, will ultimately be rendered futile, and health care meaningless.

The limitations of modern medical advances, the weaknesses of allopathy's symptomatic methods, and the dangers of utilizing powerful drugs without a strong scientific and moral foundation are starkly evident in Kathmandu. Like many physicians in undeveloped countries, Nepali doctors indiscriminately prescribe multiple antibiotics for almost every condition. The latest generations of antibacterials are sold over the counter and used haphazardly, thus contributing to the creation of superinfections and medically resistant diseases. Most benefits of modern clinical treatments are economically unavailable to those who need them most, a problem which will increase as the gulf widens between rich and poor. In the villages, obstacles to distribution, inadequate storage, and lack of trained personnel hinder effective delivery and utilization of drugs and treatments. Government health-care policies have been dictated by multinational pharmaceutical companies that have no inhibitions about engaging in unethical and dangerous practices, such as selling drugs banned in First World countries. Under these conditions, allopathic medicine is not only powerless to prevent or control the coming epidemics, but is actually complicit in their generation and spread.

Even under the best medical conditions, synthetic pharmaceuticals have an inherent flaw which renders them incapable of curing the diseases of the future: they can neither cleanse toxins from the body nor regenerate vitality. Ultimately, all sickness is related to these two physiological processes, which are now under increasing stress from environmental pollution and degradation of the food chain. Without agents to remove the rising accumulation of chemical, metallic, and radioactive poisons in our bodies, especially the liver, and without compounds to enhance and strengthen resistance and immunity, allopathic medicines will become increasingly ineffective and inappropriate. Doctors everywhere are already seeing the human face of the spreading ecological crisis, as more patients come with complex allergic and immunological disorders caused by the multitude of poisonous substances pervasive in our homes, workplaces, and diets. Many physicians are unaware of the origin and scope of these problems, lack the training and methods to treat them, and further complicate the underlying causes by prescribing drugs that add to the body's toxic burden.

Now, more than ever, we need the healing gifts given freely by the plant kingdom, to protect and strengthen, nourish and revitalize, cleanse and detoxify, both our bodies and the environment. Plants not only are the medicines which can cure the toxicity syndromes and nutritional deficiencies of the future; they also have the power to purify the earth's elements and remove the environmental causes of future epidemics. When the era of antibiotics has ended and synthetic medicines have failed, the wondrous creators of photosynthesis can heal us with the sunlight, blood-purifying chlorophyll, antibacterial essential oils and alkaloids, vitamins, and complex trace elements stored in their bodies. They also provide, on a global scale, what technology and science cannot: drinkable water, breathable air, and fertile soil.

As the earth sickens and increasing numbers of people are afflicted with illnesses unresponsive to modern drugs, the demand for botanical medicines will increase, and skilled practitioners of natural therapies will continue gaining respect and recognition. Herbal products are already a rapidly growing multibillion-dollar global industry and one of the fastest-developing fields of agriculture. But classical Asian medicines and their holistic philosophies are not merely medical and economic trends; more important, they are helping countless people find healthier, more satisfying lifestyles, and raising collective awareness of our dependency on the wellbeing of the environment. The growing need for herbal medicines and traditional healing knowledge could bring about a revolutionary change in social priorities and become a catalyst for the preservation of wilderness, development of nonpolluting plant-based economies, and establishment of sustainable ecosystems. "Of all the new frontiers of agriculture," says a World Bank report, "the cultivation of medicinal plants is among the most powerful for doing good in the world."

Plants are sustenance for all creatures and, when conjoined with human intelligence and compassion, are the basis of civilization. A global horticultural renaissance, motivated by deteriorating collective health, economically stimulated by lucrative botanical markets, and guided by the holistic philosophies elucidated by Ayurveda and other traditions, could transform destructive ignorance into life-sustaining wisdom, and bring about the blossoming of an earth-centered spiritual culture. This is the symbolic meaning of Bhaisajyaguru's kingdom of Sudarshan: enlightened consciousness governing a sacred society, which lives harmoniously within a flourishing and healthy natural environment.

Is it possible to create an ecological paradise that nurtures humanity's highest potentials? If this utopian dream cannot be achieved, can nations enjoy prosperity and good health by building their economies on the peaceful and meaningful use of nontoxic renewable resources? If this idealistic goal cannot be reached, can enough people find sustainable livelihoods that will at least ensure a livable world for coming generations? Each of these scenarios is founded on our relationship with the plant kingdom.

If we were to ask the Medicine Buddha, "What can you offer us to protect and restore the earth?" we need only look to the deity's hand and heart. The mandalic geometry of Sudarshan converges at Bhaisajyaguru's heart, proclaiming that for civilization to thrive, it must be governed by love and wisdom. The deity's hand reaches toward us in the mudra of supreme generosity, showing us the antidote to the greed that has impoverished the world and endangered our children's future. Graceful lapis fingers hold a fruiting myrobalan branch, symbol of the botanical realm's restorative fecundity—upon which rests the success of all human endeavors—reminding us that the earth provides freely, asking nothing to sustain her fertility but gentle care given in gratitude.

When Buddha taught the art and science of healing, the world became a medicinal realm, luxuriously endowed with an abundance of trees, shrubs, bushes, grasses, vines, tiny herbs, and creatures large and small. Sudarshan is not only a mythical kingdom where divine physicians carry on their noble sattvic labors, alchemically procuring elixirs to remove the suffering of beings. Beautiful to Behold is also the answer to the environmental crisis threatening the future of humanity; it is the forest-garden of a spiritual civilization, waiting to be replanted, cultivated, harvested, and shared by all. Here, in this green mandala, is a vision not only of past splendor, but of hope for a renewed world.

I am driving with Gopal along roads and alleys filled with dirt and sewage, smoking cars, and weary crowds. At one time, before Kathmandu became choked with staggering pollution and human despair, I found pleasure in the exotic flavors of this ancient land. But now, aching with fever and coughing with burning lungs, I seek only dispassion and equanimity. Our car crawls through gridlocked streets, windows shut against nightmarish fumes and noise.

My sense of self is dissolving, as I see my illness reflected in the gaunt faces and sunken eyes around me. I am suffering, yet how much more intensely others must feel the same misery, the same persistent burning in the throat, the same headache, the same twisting of the bowels. In this feverish delirium it is easy to understand the warnings of wise renunciates: from its glamorous heights to its terrifying depths, samsara is a sea of fire and a battlefield of razor-sharp weapons, in which we shall ultimately find nothing but sorrow.

I turn a corner, and our car is immobilized in a seething mass of yelling people.

"What's happening here?" I ask Gopal.

"They are fighting to fill two government seats," he replies.

During the last few years the Nepali government has changed from a corrupt monarchy to an even more corrupt Congress, and political unrest is growing. The country is sinking deeper into economic decline, and municipal services are breaking down. Crowds gather around blaring loudspeakers as rallies and marches occur all over town. On election days the voting districts are sealed off to prevent rioting. Maoist guerrillas are bombing police stations, and violence is spreading across national borders; in Bihar, the land where Buddha taught the doctrine of universal peace, the wealthy are decapitated in retaliation for their atrocities against the poor.

Our car inches through the storm of emotions and blaring horns, while Gopal muses about the ineffectual and corrupt politicians who are destroying the country. "Everybody is saying they are going to do something," he explains. "But the money just keeps on disappearing. All kinds of foreign aid comes here. They will put down a cornerstone for a new building, make a big deal out of it, then nothing gets finished. But it is also the ignorance of the people. They think that because there is democracy now, they can just do anything they want."

The crowds swirl away behind us as we enter the stream of traffic along Durbar Marg. I sweat in the humidity of my fever, too hot to keep the car windows closed, too fearful of the noxious air outside to open them. Behind us the Himalayan peaks are barely visible through the smog. High on their slopes, global warming is melting the glaciers, threatening to flood the alpine lakes and bring disaster to the villages below. At the same time, deforestation is causing drought. In the Kathmandu Valley, water is scarce; until recently the Bagmati ran throughout the year, but now it is a dry riverbed. People wait in long lines for a few precious liters, and household plumbing is useless.

We pass the stone spigots that used to provide water for washing and drinking. Legends about these fountains tell how Tantric sorcerers performed pujas, made sacrifices, and water came. It has flowed continuously for as long as people can remember, all over the valley. The fountains' sunken alcoves are still decorated with little shrines built in gratitude for the life-giving element, but their flow has stopped. The women no longer gather to wash their bright saris, then modestly bathe, fully clothed, at the busy intersections.

The stone taps are dry because people are drilling wells and pumping out the reserves of ground water. With water tables sinking, sewage systems failing, and contamination increasing, people are forced to drink water poisoned with foul-smelling chemicals, petroleum products, heavy metals, fecal material, pathogenic microbes, and parasites. Soon, waterborne epidemics will afflict every continent, and wars will be fought for water instead of oil.

I remember the words of Dr. Jha, eloquently paraphrasing the ancient teachings of Charaka. "The origin of epidemics is dishonest governments," the Vaidye once said. "When the leaders of governments become dishonest, people begin to think this is the virtuous way of living. When families are influenced by this dishonesty, and people adopt sinful lifestyles, their behavior releases heating influences into the world. These impurities mix with the atmosphere, disturbing the water and rain elements. This in turn causes droughts and poor crops, and the whole country begins to suffer from hunger and thirst. As hunger and thirst afflict the people, they begin eating bad food and become malnourished. From this come epidemics of various diseases."

"Ayurveda teaches that people should speak the truth," the doctor continued, describing how this desperate cycle can be broken. "We should make offerings to the hungry and thirsty, make sacrifices and pray, be involved with spiritual activities, and be kind."

It is prayer, especially giving fragrant sacrificial offerings during fire pujas, that induces the skies to bring timely rains. When societies live harmoniously, care for nature, and ceremonially feed the celestial gods and goddesses, the deities become delighted and shower abundant nourishment upon us. When we forget our primary relationship with the earth and sky, arrogantly imagining we can desecrate them as we wish, nature sends diseases to reawaken us from our ignorant slumber. "Beings exist from food," says the *Bhagavad Gita*. "Food is brought into being by the rain god; the rain god is cherished through sacrifice; sacrifice is brought into being by Dharmic action. He who does not cause to turn here on earth the wheel thus set in motion, lives in vain."

What Dharmic sacrifices will we make to bring the world back into balance? Will we give up our addictions to the fossil fuels and petrochemicals burning the atmosphere, the nuclear plants waiting to explode from old age and sabotage, the tons of carcinogenic pesticides sprayed on the soil, the toxin-spewing industries flooding the world with unnecessary consumer products? Will corporations abandon their ambitions to invent ever more dangerous technologies? Who will renounce the thirst for political power over others? What nation will lay down its weapons to feed its poor? I look with aching eyes at the scene around me, a strange and pitiful dream of hungry beggars and homeless children roaming the streets, living with their diseases among piles of rotting garbage. It seems we have chosen to sacrifice the earth and her inhabitants upon the altar of fear and greed.

The atmosphere in Kathmandu is apocalyptic, heavy with the scent of pestilence waiting to emerge from the bleak poverty of these rat-infested alleys. Pneumonic plague has erupted in India, and fear has spread its tentacles into Nepal. What will happen when waves of global epidemics begin to rise from cities drowning in their own waste? The local clinics are already understaffed, poorly supplied, and overwhelmed with the sick and dying. There is not even enough firewood to burn the dead on the ghats. This once-beautiful Himalayan kingdom has become a terrible vision of the world's future.

We drive past Bir Hospital, its dark windows and dank concrete walls speaking of the impending collapse in medical services. Like hospitals everywhere, it is a breeding ground of bacteria resistant to every known antibiotic, and the birthplace of hideous contagion. Uncountable cases of AIDS have been spread by places like this, through such practices as reusing hypodermic needles without sterilization. How do impoverished hospitals dispose of their medical waste and radioactive material, I wonder, when the entire country is a dumping ground for developed nations? A young man with deformed legs crawls along the sidewalk; is this the price coming generations will pay for living in the shadow of technology?

We drive around Swayambhu Hill, cross Ring Road, then head west away from town. The roadside is cluttered with broken-down vehicles, the air heavy with toxic campfires. Year by year, the beautiful rice paddies of the countryside have disappeared as neighborhoods spread across the valley. The lush green fields that once graced the Kathmandu

Valley have succumbed to leprous scabs of concrete. To meet the demands of construction, brick factories have sprung up everywhere, spewing raw black smoke into the mountain air.

We pass the military checkpoint at the edge of the valley, park the car, and slowly climb the mountainside behind Chagdol. Below us, the road to India is jammed with trucks, climbing and descending along hairpin curves. All we can see of the Himalayas is one peak, floating faintly in a haze of exhaust fumes. Even from our vantage point high above the highway, the greasy smell of diesel permeates everything. We sit quietly as the sun sinks through the orange and brown shades of evening, and a cool wind comes up. The jewel of the Himma Leh lies tarnished under the gathering darkness.

"What is the fate of Kathmandu?" I ask Gopal.

"In ten years Kathmandu will be a dead city," he replies.

How paradoxical that so many wonderful medicines can be found in this poisoned land. Nepal is a bittersweet mirage of the wonders and potential benefits Ayurveda holds for the world. There are brilliant and generous doctors, treasure troves of old manuscripts, a wealth of botanical resources, and alchemical laboratories; what more could those seeking healing and knowledge of classical medicine wish for? But Kathmandu has become a living tragedy. Many Nepali people would leave the country at the first opportunity.

Gopal is philosophical, as always. "The Kali Yuga is everywhere, Guruji," he says. "Every place is finished now."

What I see happening around us is the same in many ways as what is taking place in my own homeland. Towers of brown smoke rise from the once fertile San Joaquin Valley, the heart of California agriculture. The air is thick with pollution as the dry fields are burned off. Farmers dressed for chemical warfare sit in billowing clouds of poisonous vapors as their sprayers creep along rows of vegetables. Day after day I would listen to the stories of patients seeking help for their deteriorating health.

"I'm so exhausted by midmorning that I have to go back to bed."

"I got a cold last winter, and six months later I'm still fighting it."

In spring and summer, orchards of blossoming fruit trees are repeatedly sprayed with chemicals. Children play in toxic canals, or lie bedridden in the cancer wards of local hospitals, victims of agriculturally poisoned groundwater.

"When we were children, we used to run behind the sprayers because we loved the smell of DDT. Now I have hundreds of lymphatic tumors throughout my body."

"My daughter has had brain tumors since childhood. She suffers horrible migraines and doesn't get her period regularly."

"My fifteen-year-old son has a bone tumor growing on his femur."

"First they thought it was an ovarian cyst. Then they thought it was something wrong with my fallopian tube. Later they thought it was Crohn's disease. The pain continued to get worse. Now they've found a lymphoma."

Low-flying planes make aerial applications of pesticides, unconcerned about the lives of the people below.

"I would suffer from blinding headaches for days after the planes sprayed over our house. I finally had to move away."

"I never suspected that handling those chemicals would disfigure my hands."

"I've been deathly sick since cleaning that chemical tank, and no one can find anything wrong with me."

"All my elderly friends are either debilitated or dying horrible deaths."

The wind blows across expanses of barren land, whirling through abandoned farm equipment, rotting chemical tanks, and empty corrals, lifting the dead topsoil into the sky.

On Chagdol Hill, darkness arrives. Gopal and I stand, absorbed in our own thoughts before descending back to the road. What medicine can save us, now that the earth is poisoned?

Somewhere in the evolution of the modern mind, we lost our connection with the simple, sensitive intelligence of the heart and our affinity and empathy for the land, its plants, and its creatures. This dissociation from spirit and nature affects all areas of culture, including medicine. Altruistically seeking to alleviate illness, yet desensitized by reductionistic science in pursuit of financial profit, medical research has both battled diseases and inflicted new suffering. In its complex relationships with industry, agriculture, the military, and biological sciences, modern medicine has given birth to valuable creations, but has also spawned inventions and practices that should never have been released into the world. By ignoring the voice of higher intuition, the deeper guidance of conscience, and the feelings of other sentient beings, researchers have perpetrated dangerous, painful, and fatal experiments on people, animals, and the environment. Physicians have taken the Hippocratic vow of ahimsa, nonviolence, yet the institution of allopathic medicine is troubled with a legacy of iatrogenic sickness, political corruption, and toxic wastes, the dark shadows of marigpa that poison the sacred art of healing.

One of the deepest wounds inflicted upon the world by the loss of sattvic wisdom in medicine is the adverse mutation of microbial intelligence caused by modern antibiotics. Antibiotics from botanical sources, such as mushrooms, algae, lichens, and alkaloid-producing plants, have been used throughout history. Undoubtedly, people have perished experimenting with some of these substances, and others have suffered at the hands of incompetent herbalists and physicians. Unlike the mass-produced synthetic drugs of modern allopathy, however, classical Asian medicines have never been a source of widespread iatrogenic sicknesses, a threat to the health of large human and animal populations, or a danger to the food chain and environment. Instead, holistic medical systems such as Ayurveda, and the gentle paradigm of unity their philosophies teach, are emerging as important solutions to the declining effectiveness of antibacterial medications and rising microbial virulence. Traditional indigenous plant-based medicines and therapies, unlike the biologically aggressive compounds created by our nature-dominating society, are nourishing, strengthening, cleansing, and rejuvenating, and promote individual, social, and ecological equilibrium.

The "germ theory" of allopathy is an excellent example illustrating the differences between the contrasting paradigms of classical Asian and modern medicines, the worldviews they evolved from, and their consequences. Pathogenic bacteria, when they interfere with normal physiological functions, are responsible for many of the most serious diseases of humans, animals, and plants. With the advent of microbiology and the development of the germ theory of pathogenesis, a new world of pharmaceutical possibilities emerged, based on the creation of "miracle drugs" to kill bacterial invaders.

In the land of Ayurveda, where contagious febrile diseases born of poverty and pollution are an everyday part of life, physicians have also developed medicines which are highly successful for treating bacterial infections, using plants and minerals with antibiotic properties. Yet, surprisingly, Ayurvedic philosophy places relatively little emphasis on the microbial origins of sickness or eradication of bacteria; instead, it promotes immunological development through dietary measures, herbal supplementation, and hygienic daily conduct.

During an afternoon class with Dr. Singh and Dr. Shrestha, I inquired about the Ayurvedic views concerning microbial pathogenesis. "In nature there are bacteria, viruses, everything," Dr. Shrestha began. "Human beings are always exposed to them, but we don't always get sick. According to Ayurved, whatever pathogens we have inside our lungs or digestive system don't matter until our immunity is decreased.

"There is a TB patient in every neighborhood in Nepal. According to the germ theory, if you come in contact with them, you will have the same problem. But not everybody is a tubercular patient, because people have different immunity, resistance, and prakruti [constitution]. According to Ayurved, the causes of diseases are either external or internal factors; these create imbalances of the doshas that manifest themselves as symptoms. The bacteria are secondary; they are not the root cause or primary concern. When the doshas are in balance, your body will be able to fight against the secondary causes." Traditional medical philosophy asserts that germs will proliferate only when there is prior weakness and disequilibrium in the body, and are therefore not the ultimate cause of disease.

"Sushruta has specifically mentioned the infectious conditions," Dr. Singh elaborated. "He has given stanzas that describe several ways diseases are transmitted from one person to another, 'by body contact, by the breath, by exchanging used articles, by flies.' He has also given examples and descriptions of the diseases, like leprosy, conjunctivitis, and TB. So you see, Ayurveda has some concept of infectious diseases, as well as worms and bacteria.

"But it is like this: for a disease to flourish, several factors are important. The rishis have given the example of a seed growing in the field. Having just the seed is not enough; you need to have proper soil, water, air, and all these things, for it to grow. Diseases are not there because the bacteria are there. Meningococcus and pneumococcus are all over our body, but we don't all suffer from meningitis or pneumonia. It is our body's reaction which constitutes a disease."

We live on a planet that belongs to bacteria. They are the most abundant organisms on earth, whose collective weight is greater than all other forms of life combined. The human body is inhabited by highly intelligent microbial communities composed of hundreds of types of bacteria, viruses, yeasts, and other organisms, in unimaginable numbers. On one square inch of intestine there are more microbes than humans on the planet. A trillion bacteria live on our skin, 10 billion reside in our mouth, and 100 billion are flushed down the toilet after every bowel movement. Over 300 different types of bacteria swim in the digestive tract. Overall, about 100 trillion individual organisms consider each of our bodies as their home. Almost all of them live a harmonious synergistic existence with the others, and with us.

These organisms play an important role in sustaining our health. The microbes of the digestive tract help digest different classes of foods, manufacture vitamins needed by the body, and break down chemical toxins. By attaching themselves to the intestinal wall and competing for nutrients, they form a protective colony against invading organisms. They produce natural antibiotic substances, stimulate the production of antibodies to fight infection, and destroy pathogenic organisms. We owe our health, digestive capacity, and immunity to the complex intelligence of the microbial communities within us.

"Three basic causes of disease have been given in Ayurveda," Dr. Singh went on. "The first is the improper combination of our senses with the sense objects, that is, excessive, deficient, or perverted. The second cause is if you do something against your conscience, your innate knowledge. And the third cause is time factors, like the seasons. Now, in all these three, where do the bacteria come in? The bacteria will grow only if these conditions are conducive. So the emphasis is on the field, the proper soil, the proper climate, rather than on the seed. The old physicians described bacteria—there is no question about it—but their emphasis was on the building of the body."

Louis Pasteur was the father of microbiology and the originator of modern science's germ theory. His ideas about germs being the causative agents of disease were widely debated by scientists of his day. At the end of his life, Pasteur expressed his final views, which were the same as Ayurveda's. "The microbe is nothing," he declared, "the terrain everything."

Although the Ayurvedic pharmacopoeia contains numerous botanical drugs with highly effective antibiotic properties, developing the body's resistance by restoring equilibrium within the terrain of tissues and humors is the primary goal of treatment, while subduing microbial toxins is secondary; most formulations for infectious febrile conditions simultaneously "attack" pathogens and "support" vitality. The emerging pharmaceutical industry in the West, however, found the pursuit of a "magic bullet" that could simply eradicate germs far more lucrative than preventive measures such as lifestyle modifications and enhancement of immunity using natural methods. Four antibiotic generations later the long-term consequences of this "attacking" philosophy are now appearing in the microbial kingdom.

Survival of the fittest has always been nature's law. Fossil records show that bacteria have been on this earth at least 3.5 billion years. Bacteria are found in all types of environments, and can survive where no other life can: they are at home in the boiling water of hot springs and in the ocean's depths. Live bacteria, estimated to have been dormant for a million years, have been found in Antarctic ice. Bacteria have been adapting to environmental challenges and noxious substances from competitors since the first appearance of life on this planet, and are highly skilled at resisting man's chemical onslaughts.

Under the influence of antibiotics, the weakest strains of bacteria die off and the hardiest mutate to survive. These increasingly virulent strains pass on new genetic information to their offspring, and more powerful substances are required to control each succeeding generation. Common types of bacteria have mutated into a wide variety of new forms, appearing in outbreaks of "superinfections" and medically resistant forms of old diseases such as tuberculosis and gonorrhea. While strengthening unwanted organisms, antibiotics also weaken the beneficial ones by eradicating the healthy microbial communities of the body. The combined results are decreased immunity and vitality, susceptibility to overgrowth and reinfection by invasive microbes, and accumulation of disease-promoting toxic residues. Using Chinese medical terminology, these effects can be described as "treating the stem while weakening the root." This symptomatic approach does not address causative factors, such as poor diet, that allow pathogenic bacteria to flourish within the terrain of the tissues, does not remove preexisting underlying impurities or those created by the disease process, such as excess phlegm congestion, nor does it regenerate or revitalize the "root" of immunity and resistance to subsequent reinfection.

If scientists had deliberately set out to radically alter the global microbial environment, they could not have found a better way to do so. In the space of a few decades, we have planted the seeds of virulent disorder in the microbial soil; now those seeds are coming to fruition, bringing the end of the antibiotic era. The fundamental shortsightedness of the allopathic paradigm—overlooking and underestimating the far-reaching repercussions of biochemical interference with nature's complex intelligence—is more apparent now than ever. The painful lesson to be learned from medically created diseases is that therapies which compromise human ecology must at least be supported, if not replaced whenever possible, by treatments which strengthen resistance. As modern drugs lose their effectiveness, the spiritual wisdom of the physician-sages and their vitalistic methods of healing will once again play a central role in medical practice. A holistic paradigm emphasizing harmony and compatibility with other forms of life will deepen in the psyche of the world, accompanied by a renaissance of traditional plant-based healing systems such as Ayurveda.

"I'll tell you a story," Dr. Singh continued, "about how I became more convinced about Ayurveda. I have treated all kinds of UTI [urinary tract infections] at Benares University; originally, we diagnosed the condition, then gave Ayurvedic drugs that would get rid of the infection. Isn't that the objective? The whole framework of looking at the disease was from a completely modern scientific point of view: you have a urinary tract infection caused by some bacteria, and you are giving some antibacterial drug that will get rid of it. I tested several Ayurvedic drugs and we were able to get rid of the symptoms, but the bacteria would refuse to go. With the antibiotics, bacteria and symptoms both went away; the only difference was that a couple of weeks after the antibiotics, the infection often came back.

"There was one particular patient, who was an important person in Benares. He had a kidney stone the doctors could not remove, so they removed the kidney, as simple as that. He had only one kidney left, and that kidney was infected. They had treated him with all kinds of antibiotics, but the infection was resistant to everything. He came to me, and the Ayurvedic drugs relieved his symptoms, but the bacteria wouldn't go.

"After some time he came with an attack. I had to scratch my head; what am I going to do? I realized that we were doing something wrong. We were diagnosing and treating the disease according to the modern viewpoint; we were not considering the three humors, or any of the parameters of classical medicine. This was not Ayurveda. I thought, 'Let me treat him according to strictly classical Ayurvedic ways. Let me analyze him according to his vata, pitta, kapha. Let us go from that point of view for what should be done.'

"The prominent dosha for diseases of the urogenital tract is apana vata ['downward clearing' Air humor]. Apana vata controls the ureters, all the excretory functions, and the status of the pelvic organs. If that is malfunctioning, then all the excretory activities become deranged. I said, 'All right, I will treat his apana vata.' Now the whole conceptual framework changes. I am not treating urinary tract infection, I am treating the deranged apana vata.

"So what is the best treatment for apana vata? There are three treatments, one for each dosha. If it is kapha, it is emesis; if it is pitta, it is laxatives; for vata, the best treatment is basti, medicated enema. I thought, 'All right, I'm going to treat him with basti.' I went to the people in the internal medicine department, to find out which is the best basti we could give. I decided on two: dashmool is a classical herbal preparation from Sushruta himself, and another was narayan tel, a famous oil.

"I admitted the patient into the hospital, stopped all the antibiotics, and did this basti treatment. After fifteen days my student came with the urine culture report and said, 'Sir, it is negative.' I just looked at him and said, 'Do you think you have done a miracle in fifteen days? You must have juggled the results. Did you tell the pathologist to make it negative? I don't believe you. Send it to another fellow.' So it was repeated twice, and it was working.

"There was no direct treatment for the kidney, bladder, or bacteria. He had symptoms caused by apana vata, so I was treating apana vata. Very logical. I knew the symptoms would be relieved, but his bacteria went away, and that was a miracle for me. I really didn't believe it. So we got another patient, and another, until we had thirty or forty. All of them had positive culture, and they all became negative.

"Then my modern colleagues said, 'You are talking bullshit, doctor. You are putting that thing into the rectum, and telling us you are getting rid of the bacteria in the bladder. Utter nonsense.' So we made a pact. I said, 'You diagnose the cases of UTI with a positive culture, and let my student treat them. I guarantee that no antibiotics will be given. Then you watch it yourself.' They did that. Now it has become standard therapy, and everybody uses it."

Holistic treatment of humoral systems using nontoxic methods, such as the therapy for apana vata described by Dr. Singh, is the medicine of the future. Highly specific synthetic substances that target and overpower microbial and biochemical imbalances supplant and interfere with the body's healing mechanisms, thus setting the stage for iatrogenic complications by weakening immunity and damaging humoral integrity. Ayurvedic practices, on the other hand, are based on the principle of restoring equilibrium among the humors' interrelated physiological systems, thereby activating the body's inborn capacity for self-healing. In the face of rising global pollution levels, doctors will be called upon to make a transition from synthetic substances which compound the toxic burden on the body, to plant-based formulations which reduce it.

While working as a surgical assistant with Chinese doctors, Dr.

Chopel learned about the early generations of antibiotics, and was able to synthesize the Western and Tibetan understandings of infectious diseases, with important applications in the prevention and treatment of emerging immune disorders. In recent years consumption of antibiotics by children has reached unprecedented levels, resulting in a generation of allergic youth burdened with medically resistant bacteria. According to Tibetan medical philosophy, the use of antibiotics to suppress common childhood fevers is inhibiting the development of people's immune systems.

"Many doctors think fevers are easy to cure," Amchi-la explained to me. "By prescribing cold-natured medicines, such as antibiotics, they cause the fever to spread. This leads to more serious diseases later." The premature use of antibiotics in the treatment of "unripened" fevers, the doctor elaborated, causes toxins to migrate through the body, where they become the source of recurring illnesses and, eventually, more serious diseases. Dr. Chopel claimed that one of the causes of chronic degenerative conditions and cancer was mismanagement of earlier febrile conditions. His assertions are consistent with the principles of other holistic medical systems such as homeopathy, as well as modern research findings that validate the importance of fever in the development of the immune system.

According to Amchi-la, when an "unripe" fever is prematurely suppressed, it is transformed into a "hiding fever." "When colds and flus are mistreated with strong medicines, they can become unresolved conditions that hide in the interior of the body. The illness may appear outwardly cured, but due to its hidden nature it is actually difficult to heal." The analogy used to describe hiding fevers is a fire that has died down, leaving a tiny ember glowing under cold ashes. This ember contains the dormant toxins of the unresolved fever, which gradually consume the body's vitality and leave it susceptible to reinfection. Secondary factors, such as poor diet or insufficient sleep, function like wind blowing on the ember, which can reignite into a recurrence of the previous illness.

With this simple concept, my teacher provided the key to understanding one of the most common conditions encountered in clinical practice: unresolved childhood illnesses with fever that have been treated intermittently for decades with repeated courses of antibiotics. The range of pathologies and secondary syndromes caused directly or indirectly by this chronic consumption of drugs would fill a volume, from asthma to autism. As scientific investigation validates the importance of fevers in developing the body's resistance, I appreciate more fully how this old physician from a remote Tibetan monastery understood the principles of healing in a way many modern doctors fail to grasp.

The proper management of the early stages of febrile diseases, according to the wisdom of traditional physicians, is to first "ripen" the fever; this brings the fever to a state of maturity by allowing the body to activate its thermogenic defenses. Following this stage, a fever is then "consolidated," meaning the toxins are brought together so they become centered in one location in the body. When this has been accomplished, the final stage is referred to as "killing" the fever, when medications to subdue and neutralize the toxins are administered. The successful treatment of fevers in this system is based on careful observation of subtle changes within the pulse, tongue, urine, and symptoms, and continual modification of medications. It is a way of practicing medicine that is more personal and time-consuming than is possible in modern clinics.

"One who follows the above three stages can be considered a good physician," Amchi-la told me. By following this protocol, the immune system is strengthened and developed, the pathogens destroyed, and the phlegmatic "soil" in which they are thriving restored to health. The result is that children's fevers are completed in childhood, and not perpetuated into adulthood as unresolved allergic syndromes, immune deficiencies, and conditions of chronic fatigue.

The future will require strong immunity, for even in the healthiest environments the world places heavy demands on the body. As this Kali Yuga unfolds, these challenges will only increase.

At the conclusion of his discourse about germs, Dr. Singh asked, "Have you read the book *A Doctor at Large* by George Bernard Shaw? In one place he said that the day will come when we will have a drug that treats every disease, and we will all be free from sickness. But that has not happened. All the antibiotics are there, the bacteria have outgrown them, and we still have the diseases. We have got to take care of this field after all. It is in this context that we can see the strength of Ayurveda. We cannot get rid of bacteria from the body, whatever amount of antibacterials are used. They are there with you, and you had better learn to live with them. I say: let's lead a symbiotic life, rather than an antibiotic life."

Every one of my sojourns in Kathmandu has been an ordeal; journeys through illness back to health were the price paid for time spent with my wise and wonderful teachers. When I lay burning with fever, woke gasping from pleurisy and painful lung infections, or endured another bout of acidic diarrhea, it seemed supremely ironic to be studying Ayurveda while afflicted with miserable sicknesses.

But I was not sick because of any weakness of Ayurveda, nor did I recover because of the strengths of modern medicine. I was sick for the same reasons everyone in this mountain valley suffers: the water is contaminated with viral, bacterial, and parasitic pathogens, and the air is permeated with poisonous dust from streets filled with open sewage and noxious smoke spewing from vehicles, garbage fires, and unregulated industries. My immunity was weakened from the devitalized condition of Nepalese food, while my humors, imbalanced by the multitude of pollutants, nutritional deficiencies, and climatic influences, became fertile ground for opportunistic infections.

The myriad diseases affecting humanity arise from a small number of underlying causes: malnutrition, weakened immunity, biotoxicity, and microbial pathogenesis. These fundamental roots of sickness are primarily the results of ecological and social degradation, which is created by human behaviors originating within the mind. In Nepal, as in most places across Asia and the Indian subcontinent, individual and collective health is threatened by the spread of two crises: obsolete patriarchal reproductive customs creating overpopulation, and deforestation with its destruction of ecosystems and biodiversity. From these disturbances come soil erosion, desertification, drought, flooding, and mass migrations to overcrowded cities. These conditions, in turn, lead to poverty, pollution, crime, corruption, and broken families, and culminate in epidemics and struggle for survival. The ultimate cause of these miseries, according to Ayurvedic and Tibetan medical philosophy, is ignorance: the confused bewilderment and shortsighted self-interest of marigpa, which prevents us from effectively utilizing our innate intelligence to liberate ourselves from suffering.

The prevention of sickness is the primary objective of medicine, I heard repeatedly from my teachers. Physicians who teach their patients how to avoid illness by following the health-promoting regimens of right living, thereby transforming society one person at a time, would be praised by the sages of old as supreme healers. A person who waits until he is sick to think about his health, says Chinese medicine, is like a person who waits until his house is on fire to dig a well. Ideally, we should strive to enhance the natural resistance provided by humoral integrity and balance. But when the body is weakened by malnutrition, when every breath and each meal is potentially the source of fecal and chemical contamination, no one can escape disease indefinitely. The success of preventive medicine depends on collective wisdom skillfully addressing the environmental roots of illness, for our lives are symbiotically related to the wellbeing of the entire biosphere.

"In the outside world we can see the earth, water, sunlight, wind, and sky," Dr. Jha once said, pointing out our physical interdependency with the environment. "These external elements are also present in our bodies. The body temperature, such as the fire in the stomach, the warmth of the blood, the liver metabolism, and the light of the eyes, are all forms of sunlight. The body openings, internal cavities, organ spaces, and the different channels are all aspects of the sky, the space element. Our speaking and respiration, movements, and the sounds of our intestines are all the activity of the air element. Our weight, bones, and other forms of solidity are the earth element. Phlegm, blood, lymph, and other bodily fluids are the water element. We first study the outer world, and by doing so we can understand the inner body."

Such contemplations develop appreciation for the immediacy, magnitude, and relevance of humanity's relationship to the planet's living systems. By meditating on the pancha mahabhutas as they circulate through the body and the world around us, we can learn to perceive these universal elements that compose the fabric of our internal physiology, and gain insight into the inseparability of the inner and outer environments. Mindfulness of the composite nature and therefore impermanent basis of existence decreases our false sense of selfhood and inspires the "wisdom of not possessing" by helping us feel how we are part of everything, yet utterly devoid of any substantiality. This biological spirituality, and the sattvic view of life it awakens, is the antidote to marigpa's greed and violence, and the damage they have done to the earth.

Ancient medical traditions contain a vast array of methods for treating diseases, practical knowledge of how to eradicate their causes, and sophisticated philosophies to guide efforts to restore a healthy environment. Perhaps the most valuable contribution Ayurveda has to offer the world is its definition of health: equilibrium among the humors, tissues, transformations, and wastes; and happiness of mind, senses, and soul. True health is the result of living harmoniously with the forces of nature, and the fruit of a culture's flowering spiritual maturity. Long-term ecological equilibrium, the global foundation of individual health, can be brought about only through sattvic consciousness guiding a society that loves, respects, and nurtures human, plant, and animal life. This is

Bhaisajyaguru's kingdom of Sudarshan, a vision of the flourishing natural wealth bestowed upon civilizations that practice compassionate Dharma for the benefit of all living beings.

Like a mirror of our Buddha-nature, Sudarshan reflects humanity's capacity to create thriving, enlightened cultures. Integrating universal truth, ecology, and medicine, the iconographic symbolism of the Medicine Buddha's mandala contains layers of teachings to assist us in becoming skilled and gentle guardians of the earth's healing treasures. Gazing upon Sudarshan's radiantly jeweled geometry, we can see the botanical opulence of past civilizations, the beginnings of a new era of ecological restoration, and the means to bring that restoration to completion. Sudarshan is the beauty, health, and happiness which await us, when the human mind has assumed its proper place in the pattern of Creation, and our lives once again follow the ancient rhythms of peaceful coexistence with nature.

Now, too many people are awakening to an unnecessarily desperate existence, eking out diminishing crops from dying fields, destroying the last of the local forests for sustenance and fuel, struggling to survive in overcrowded cities. We are losing the ancient botanical world our ancestors knew for so long, but the forest-gardens live on inside our cells and psyche, waiting to be brought back to life. Although much of humanity greets the dawn sick, hungry, and in rags, the quintessence of human consciousness is eternally divine; Bhaisajyaguru lives within every mind, and the mandala of a sacred world filled with healing foods, waters, and medicines converges at every heart.

In compassionate response to our suffering, the Medicine Buddha reaches down from his celestial abode, offering a branch of the heavenly myrobalan; he holds within his lapis fingers a silent commandment for realizing ecological salvation: trees. If we heed the deity's instructions, we will someday find ourselves at home in Sudarshan's magnificent medicinal forests.

Beautiful to Behold is luxuriously endowed with trees of all kinds.

Sandalwood and camphor infuse the air with sensuous energizing fragrance, aquillaria gives precious oil of oud, willowlike branches of pepper trees offer their spicy berries, cinnamon exudes its sweet pungence, and towering neem provide bitter antibiotics from their leaves and bark. All types of myrobalans grow plentifully, as well as sour amla, the master rejuvenator. Pomegranates and other fruits burst with ripe juices, essential oils, and medicinal seeds. The caroblike pods of cassia trees dangle in the breeze; pines, cedars, and junipers release their aromatic breath; rhododendrons paint impressionistic scenes with pastel flowers.

The wondrous trees that once graced the earth made a way for human life to emerge, and they continue, even as we destroy them, to silently sustain us. Trees feed us, cure us, protect us, and bless us with an abundance of resources. They bring rains, yet keep them from becoming destructive, hold the soil, regenerate its fertility, purify the toxins we spread across the land, give us oxygen, and cleanse the sky. Because of trees, all beings can drink pure water, and breathe. As we destroy the trees, springs stop flowing, wells run dry, vegetation withers, animals disappear, storms intensify, and desert sands begin to arrive. If there is to be a home for coming generations, nations must replant their trees and care for their arboreal heritage. Replanting forests, both around and in our cities, will enrich and sustain civilization and fulfill the Medicine Buddha's compassionate commandment.

Again, the deity extends his translucent lapis lazuli hand, the fruiting myrobalan speaking on behalf of every botanical species that contributes to environmental restoration.

All plants use their toxin-transforming physiology to purify the earth's elements. Many kinds of trees, shrubs, grasses, and herbaceous plants are being effectively utilized to cleanse the poisons we have thoughtlessly dumped in every part of the globe. Certain species, such as alpine pennycress and datura, hyperaccumulate toxic metals and chemicals, either converting them into less dangerous forms or concentrating the substances for further reprocessing. Poplars are being used to decontaminate soils ruined by dry-cleaning chemicals and petroleum products. Sunflowers bred to absorb strontium and cesium are being tested as a way of neutralizing the radiation around Chernobyl, and water hyacinths are used in sewage treatment. As the chemical, metallic, and radioactive wastes of modern culture multiply and their pathogenic effects increase in the population, phytoremediation will become one of humankind's most important livelihoods. Crops with specialized curative powers are appearing on military bases, around nuclear plants, and over chemical spills, bringing us one step closer to the pure land of Sudarshan.

By taking care of plants, we will in turn be cared for. As sickness, hunger, and chaos come in rising waves, the reintegration of civilization and the botanical kingdom will become an increasingly urgent necessity, and the fertile ground from which Sudarshan could emerge. A collective awakening to our dependency on the plant kingdom for nourishment, medicine, clothing, and shelter may catalyze societies to abandon obsolete, dangerous, and wasteful habits, and begin a new era of botanical stewardship. In urban gardens, agroforests, and eco-villages, families once isolated and estranged from nature's rhythms could again participate in the plants' eternal cycles of germination and fruition, and gradually reenter the stream of harmonious existence. When that age arrives, we will know another level of meaning in the mudra of the Master of Remedies: those who plant with a sattvic heart reap sattvic foods and medicines. As community forests and garden cities flourish on every continent, nations may begin resembling those in the pure lands of Beautiful to Behold, where devic caretakers labor peacefully around the jeweled palace of enlightenment. If we skillfully sow seeds of ecological compassion, we will harvest abundant blessings, and our life spans will increase.

Like emanations of the Medicine Buddha, we hold in our hands the medicinal branches which banish illness: an Australian distiller prepares fragrant eucalyptus for steam extraction, supplying a sweet camphorous essential oil with respiratory-strengthening powers to the growing world market. An Indian farmer collects neem for its insecticidal, antibiotic, and spermicidal substances. Caretakers of precious sandalwood groves select the finest grades of heartwood, fulfilling the demanding tastes of the most discerning perfumers. Nepali villagers harvest sour amla, with the highest concentration of natural vitamin C of any fruit, generating income for their community by sharing the rejuvenative medicine of the jungle. Innumerable gifts like these from the forests and gardens of Sudarshan are the foundation for healthy societies.

The healing of humanity's ancient wounds and the rebirth of Dharmic culture rests upon ecological renewal. Environmental restoration is a unifying purpose that brings together families of diverse racial, ethnic, economic, and religious backgrounds in a common struggle against the threat of biospheric collapse. By following the Medicine Buddha's wordless commandment to plant trees, cleanse the skies and seas, and harvest the fruits of sattvic planetary caretaking, the divisive conflicts carried through the ages can be forgotten. As communities and nations join hands in mutual concern for plants, animals, and coming generations, the long history of inflicting pain on others may cease, and true spirituality reawaken. If we are able to create a garden world, the all-curing golden myrobalan from heaven will become ours. From the desolate soils, urban squalor, and bleak poverty of this harsh Kali Yuga, the seeds of Sudarshan are sprouting, and tender leaves of hope are reaching toward the rising sun of a new day.

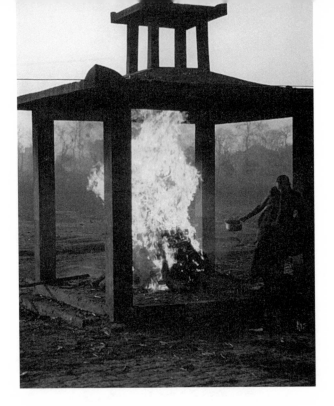

EPILOGUE

The esoteric medical and yogic teachings state that the black and white Life Nerves continue to circulate their energies for a period of time after the outer breathing has stopped at the time of death. From the brain, the activity of the white Life Nerve gradually diminishes downward toward the heart, while the activity of the black Life Nerve diminishes upward from the abdomen. When the activity of both diminish within the heart, consciousness leaves the body.

DR. CHOPEL'S TEACHINGS ON THE SUBTLE
NERVOUS SYSTEM, FROM THE *LATER TANTRA*

Amchi-la was dying. "Your teacher is lying on his deathbed with stomach cancer," came the news from an acquaintance in Boudhanath. Gopal
called from Kathmandu. "You must come quickly, he is very sick," he
said. He was going to the monastery every few days to check on the old
doctor. "He cannot eat, and is not speaking much. He said only that he
will try to wait for you."

I arrived a few days later. In the monastery courtyard a few young
monks were doing their chores. Ngawang Soepa, one of Amchi-la's students, greeted me. "He is upstairs," Ngawang said. "And how is he?" I
asked as we started up the stairs. "He's gone," the monk replied quietly.
"He died this morning."

I stood on the steps, letting the news sink in, waiting to feel some response. Emptiness, filled with the sounds of the monastery courtyard; uncertainty as we looked at each other, trying to know what to do next; sadness, but no surprise; loss, but completely expected. The sound of chanting lamas drifted through an upstairs window.

"Go talk to his brother; he can help you," Ngawang said. We walked quietly to Lobsang Samten's room. The old monk grabbed my hand and pressed his forehead to mine, then burst into tears. We wept together, surrounded by a roomful of old Tibetan relatives.

"About fifteen days ago he stopped eating food, and we had to feed him with an I.V.," Lobsang said. "Then about three o'clock this morning his circulation began to slow, and within an hour he died. Before his death, his face was very dull, but now it has a luminosity and brightness. The lower part of his body has become cold, but the upper body around his heart is still warm. We feel that these are signs that he is in his final meditation." Lobsang's eyes met mine, filled with grief and love for his brother. "He spoke of you in his last days, and told Gopal to tell you to come quickly." He put his head down and sobbed again.

Amchi-la sat on his couch, wrapped in blankets and covered with silk scarves. A pointed yellow Gelugpa hat had been placed on his head. He looked very small. His face wore an expression of stern sincerity, as if he had gone into death with every intention of mastering the illusion of phenomena and waking to final liberation. I remembered what Lobsang had said of his continuing meditation in the afterlife. The old physician's presence was palpable. It was awe-inspiring and bewildering to see someone so dead, yet feel him so alive. I bowed down in front of my teacher's body, my forehead to the floor, my hands in prayer above my head.

I stayed at his bedside, kneeling with humility and respect in front of this remarkable teacher. Here was a man whose life was truly meaningful, whose efforts and attainments, labors and realizations, sufferings and inspirations were towering mountains of accomplishment. I thought of how his spiritual discipline and purity of moral commitments had helped him endure inhumane suffering with compassionate nobility, how he had cured so many people, how the Shelkar Monastery had risen from the ashes of cultural destruction because of his strength and dedication to the Dharma. I felt small and transparent, contaminated by worldly impurities, pretentious and self-cherishing.

There was no escape from the presence of death, the omniscient mind residing in the heart of the corpse, the lamas chanting all around, or from myself. The only path was surrender. I thanked Amchi-la for all he had given me, for all he had given so many others, and for the Dharma work he had carried out for countless people around him. Standing slowly, I walked to a seat in the corner, then sat quietly. The Gelungs (senior monks) continued praying in deep voices, my body stopped shaking, and a deep peace and warmth came over me.

I returned the next day to pay my respects again and find out from Lobsang what the cremation plans were. Resonant chanting drifted through the hallways of the monastery. Inside Amchi-la's room the old Gelungs were continuing their prayers for his attainment of enlightenment in the afterlife. I entered quietly and sat down close to the deceased doctor. A trickle of blood was seeping from his right nostril, a sign that his consciousness was beginning to leave the body.

I sat absorbed in the comforting sound of sonorous voices, my heart listening attentively to Amchi-la's presence. He was far away now, sinking deeper into the unknown, returning to the source. Even in death, his teachings continued.

I spent the night before Amchi-la's cremation at his monastery. He lay resting in the room next to me, his mind freed from day and night, floating on waves of ritual bells and rhythmic prayer. The lamas chanted continuously, invoking Buddha's compassion. Throughout the monastery his spiritual family worked around the clock on his behalf, making the preparations necessary for the old doctor's final ceremony. Here was the fruit of his life's labor: community from near and far, young and old, coming to honor his worldly and spiritual accomplishments. I lay under heavy Tibetan blankets, listening to the prayers as I drifted into sleep. We would be leaving at five, departing before dawn for the cremation ground where his body would go into the fire.

I woke suddenly and looked out the window. The sun was already rising and the clock said seven. How could this be? Had I overslept and missed Amchi-la's departure? Had the monks forgotten and simply left me sleeping? As I sat in bed in disbelief, the dream I had been in began to fade. I opened my eyes again. The phosphorescence of the clock said four thirty; it was pitch-black outside. A moment later the wakeup gongs went off, the Gelungs resumed their praying, the monks ran up and down the stairs, and a young nun brought tea and breakfast.

At five the doctor was carried from his room, where he had spent the last five years dispensing medicines, giving teachings, practicing the Dharma. His body was wrapped in orange robes, his face covered with yellow silk, and a crown of Buddhas placed on his head. The monks set him upright in a silk-wrapped box and covered him with a brocaded canopy. A final procession began, accompanied by conch-shell trumpets, crashing cymbals, beating drums, and waving incense. We proceeded down the stairs and into the cold darkness of the courtyard, where Amchi-la was hoisted into the back of a pickup. Everyone piled into vans and trucks and drove through the deserted streets of Kathmandu's winter dawn.

"This place is called Ramadan," Lobsang Dhonyo explained when we arrived at our destination. "It is considered a holy place by Tibetans, because it is where the Vishnumati and Bagmati rivers meet. Nepali people prefer to go to Pashupati, but this place is sometimes used for funerals by lower-class people." We stood nearby while the monks assembled the pyre, unrolled carpets for the ceremony, and lifted Amchi-la out of the truck. By the time the preparations were completed, dawn was brightening the eastern sky, where the last crescent moon of the old year glimmered. Finally, it was time to put the doctor on the pyre. His body was unwrapped, lifted semi-naked to the top of the log pyramid, then lowered inside and covered again with his robes and crown. The lamas sat down across the courtyard facing the river, and began their prayers.

Dr. Ngawang Chopel was cremated on February seventh at sunrise. A young monk brought a torch from the Gelungs and ignited the pyre. A column of smoke rose into the turquoise sky, lifting the old teacher's spirit into the space of final rest. As the flames reached upward an eagle appeared, floating slowly across the ghat, circling low, then coming back to perch on a nearby wire. Ravens called, flocks of white birds swirled and landed, herds of water buffalo sat idle, visitors to the local temple came and went.

I watched as Amchi-la's body underwent its final transformation. He was melting, changing into billowing waves of brilliant heat. His life was rising before us, like a mirage reflecting the memories of his experiences. Echoes of his words and teachings floated through the air, then sounds from a Tibet which no longer existed, ceremonial music, chanting. Incandescent sparks spiraled from the ghat as his consciousness returned to the formless realm.

Periodically the monks poured offerings of ghee, frankincense, and cedar into the blaze, and stirred the coals. When the embers died out, they found tiny pieces of the doctor's skull in the ash, holy relics. Then it was over. The sun burned bronze in the Kathmandu sky. The monks rolled up their carpets, packed their ceremonial instruments, ate the food donations given by the monastery, and climbed into the truck. As everyone was leaving, the eagle flew from its perch, circled the morning sky, and disappeared.

I fly away again, through the haze over Kathmandu, circling the neighborhoods and terraces, through silver fleece and dark peaks, over the muddy rivers draining into the deltas of the Terai, fading into the brown horizon toward Bengal.

Where is Dr. Shrestha? I wonder, her heart absorbed in the suffering and pain of her patients, who come seeking her calm presence and reassuring touch as their last recourse. Somewhere in the tangle of horrible medieval streets, she may be thinking of me, of our discussions about a better life for her, personally and professionally, of coming to America with her wealth of wisdom and kindness and her bags of herbal nectars for women's ailments, of establishing her garden, her hospital.

And Dr. Singh? Probably at his computer with his academic hopes and frustrations, wondering how to overcome the stupidity, corruption, and apathy that pervade the world of Nepalese medicine. I can imagine Dr. Thakur sipping chai as he shares his knowledge and experiences, Dr. Tiwari going through some index on endangered Himalayan species, Dr. Jha reading a patient's pulses, Dr. Aryal melodically chanting a beautiful Sanskrit verse. Gopal is sitting in the bamboo grove at the Om land, no doubt, thinking of his Ayurvedic aspirations and how they will come to pass with alchemy's powers, God's blessings, and the hard work of his languid employees.

Below, rivers weave like petroglyphic snakes across the plains, dazzling mercuric colors in the afternoon light. I am free to go, but so many can only imagine what it is like to leave Kathmandu behind. Soon my lungs will be cleansed and healed of the soot, the noxious vapors, the powdered sewage inhaled with every breath. My cough will subside, the pain in my ribs disappear, my digestion return to some regularity. The dogs will howl all night, the crows will greet every sunrise, and I will be gone, alone in other mountains with my thoughts and memories. I will be free: free of having to be skillful with starving beggars and homeless children who pull at my heart, of negotiations with dear friends desperate to come to America at any price to work for minimum wage to amass a pitiful fortune to take home. Free of shopkeepers demanding my attention, of tuktuks filled with exhausted eyes going to work in some unimaginable environment. Free of squatting on stinking toilets, of garbage fires burning below my window.

The plains have vanished under layers of mist and pillars of thunderclouds. My mind is strangely discontent. I remember the feel of silk scarves draped around my neck by the gentle monks of Shelkar Ling, the tobacco-animated business meetings about saving the herbs of Nepal, the warm greetings and farewells. I see Dr. Shrestha's sad eyes as she tells me that a difficult time lies ahead of her, and hear the kind words of her family's hospitality. I imagine Raman sitting in the sun as he rubs the cinnabar in a black stone mortar. I remember the water falling in the forest of Mt. Shivapuri. The Indian Ocean appears through an opening in the clouds, its current running copper in the tropical heat; then everything is gray, suspended, motionless. My attention turns to how quickly I can return.

Fire is one of the necessities of life. The one in my fireplace comes from cliffrose wood, which is similar to manzanita in shape and hardness, with an intense heat that is excellent for cooking. I carried the branches up to this cave—in my arms, over my shoulders, and strapped to my pack—through meandering patterns in the shrubbery of the Mojave Desert. One gains a new respect for the preciousness of fire when the fuel has to be carried up steep hillsides. I thought of the Nepali villagers as I sweated along the trail, and of how their everyday supplies come only in backbreaking loads.

Now the day is done, the calls of the turtledoves have ended, and coyotes are making their evening rounds. I sit in royal ease in my humble dwelling, surrounded by massive granite boulders forming graceful contours of cheerful firelight, flowing breezes, and pale blue moonlight. The stone surfaces are peeling ever so slowly; perhaps every century another small slab falls to the ground. Their designs and textures vaguely resemble aboriginal art. The smoke drifts gently into the main chamber and out the southern entrance, instead of being pushed by the fierce cold downward current out the north door. It is so quiet I can hear the stars sprinkling dew on the sleeping wildflowers.

Moving aside the flat stones used to hold my cooking pots, I prepare the fire for prayer. The poles are placed in a ceremonial pattern, four pieces in a *V*, with two on each side. This is the symbol of love between man and woman, male and female. From their union come glowing off-spring of bright embers. Periodically, I gently roll the coals outward to form a half-moon, releasing their radiance into the evening chill. The embers grow old, turn ashen gray, and give the last of their heat to the soil, water, and sky.

The Ancient Power, as Dr. Aryal referred to God, expresses itself with fire. Millions of empty interplanetary miles from the solar inferno, it streams through the moist envelope of the sky to caress the leaves of vegetation everywhere on earth. In response, they transform the feast of rays into sugars, proteins, fibers, oils, alkaloids, foods, and medicines. This smoothly burning blessing cradled in the stone altar has traveled a long way. When and where did fire originate? It has seen an infinity of time and space, yet has never existed before.

Taking care of fire is a Way of learning. Fire is an Elder that has its own ways, its own relationship with the wood it dwells in, its own con-versation with the wind, its own consciousness. It is connected to our mind, body, and awareness in ways we have never considered. The smoke from offerings of pungent sweet plants carries away our prayers, opening the doors between realms so they can be heard, seen, and felt by those forces that take care of us. Our thoughts travel on fragrant trails, whispering in subtle conversations between minds.

The flames burn bronze yellow, with dancing wisps of occult blue where they escape the wood. These hard, dry, and gracefully twisted branches give embers that flow across the spectrum from soft gold, through bright orange, to deep ruby, then back as they breathe in and out. "The fire is the guru," Gopal once said. "It is the mouth of Shiva, and its flames His tongues." It communicates to us through the natural intuitive and visionary function of our minds. I spread the coals, focus my attention on the solar current glowing in the altar, and wait for it to speak.

I remember my teachers, who so generously shared their knowledge and wisdom. What can I do to repay their kindness? If I had the wish-granting powers of Mahakala, or the siddhis granted by mercury to those of spiritual merit, I would use them to provide sattvic medicines to the world. I would bestow gifts of freedom upon my mentors, so they could manifest their dreams.

Dr. Singh would be given the government's blessings to promote and develop Ayurveda as an officially sanctioned health care system. Herb gardens, a small hospital of natural medicine, generous sponsors of village health camps, and welcoming audiences of many countries would appear for Dr. Shrestha, and a long vacation. Gopal would wake to find an alchemical laboratory, the purest mercury, and gurus waiting to reveal the secrets of compounding the philosopher's stone. Lobsang Dhonyo would be endlessly supplied with the finest Tibetan medicines, to continue Dr. Chopel's dedication to serving the poor. Boundless resources would be showered on Dr. Tiwari, to finance the programs needed to save the plants he loves. Dr. Jha would be blessed with many grateful patients, successful Ayurvedic sons, and good digestion. Dr. Thakur would be granted many opportunities to advance his nation's great medical heritage. Dr. Aryal would be given good health, and many more years to share his precious medicines. For Kamala and Jagadis, a new life of opportunity would unfold in the West. For Amchi-la, now gone beyond the concerns of this world, I can only wish that he know my deepest appreciation.

But I have no such magical abilities, nor the wealth to accomplish any of these things. How do I follow the way of the Dharma, I ask the fire, and be unconcerned about the world, yet moved by its suffering? What is to be done with this desire to benefit others that frustrates my heart?

I have nothing to give but a bag of fragrant cedar from the mountains, and gratitude. I will offer them to Shiva's tongues dancing in the fireplace, in memory of those who have enriched me with precious drops from the ocean of knowledge. I hold the cedar leaf powder in my palm, empty my mind, and ask the light of the world to shower blessings on my teachers, wherever they are, in this world or the next. Tiny flecks of resin dust fall from my fingers across the molten landscape, transformed by my imagination into billowing clouds of offerings. As the smoke dissolves I see in the fire the connectedness between the hearts of beings, the life-giving power of the sun, and the dynamic creation of the galaxies.

I spread the embers and watch the breezes play across them. I think of the wild foods and herbal medicines that I have studied, tasted, and harvested, and how they have nourished and healed countless generations in every culture throughout human time. I hold the holy evergreen cedar in my hand, my heart communing with the living warmth before me.

The fire speaks to my inner vision, showing me how the sun's rays awakened the plants from their winter slumber, called forth their stored life force, stirred their innate desire to stretch, sprout, root, grow, expand, drink, breathe, multiply, and exhaust themselves in the procreative act of forming nourishing seeds. It shows me how, when winter returns, all the plants and animals will go inward toward the earth, protecting and storing their precious fluids and body heat, dreaming subterranean dreams of springtime. Now I know that putting an offering in the fire is giving directly to the power that awakens life. The cedar glows a soft lime turquoise for an instant as it falls like snow onto the embers. Its smoky fingers wafting into the atmosphere reveal how thoughts go everywhere through fire's transforming power.

The flames die down, the cavern is cast in blackness, and the stillness penetrates the depths of my mind. The embers glow, their warmth soft yet piercing. I throw a last offering into the magenta coals, and re-alize that prayer transcends concepts, words, and comprehension.

I sleep cradled in the earth's womb, warmed by fragrant drops of sunlight in the hearth. The wind carries me in its belly through the night. Under Venus rising, I am delivered safely into the outstretched arms of dawn.

List of Illustrations

INDEX

channels of the body, 99, 125, 146, 174

Charaka, 70, 196, 336

chi, 5, 272, 273

Chinese invasion, 283, 285, 289–93

Chinese medicine, traditional, 4–5, 39, 40, 53, 55, 125, 272, 351

Chintamani, Siddha, 176, 177, 180

Chopel, Ngawang (Amchi-la), 3, 7, 22–25, 30, 31, 35–38, 41, 43–45, 47–54, 56–58, 71, 72, 86, 102, 161–68, 185, 202–8, 238–42, 244, 245, 248–50, 252, 254–55, 259, 274–76, 281–85, 306, 307, 347–49, 358; death, 358–63; life story, 286–94

Chupsang Rinpoche, 282–83, 288

civilization: and spontaneity, 225, 227

compassion, 10, 22, 278, 280, 353, 354 (see also Mahakala)

concentration camps, 283, 285, 289–93

conception, 239–43, 245–49 (see also embryology; incarnation; reproduction); healthy, 240–43

consciousness, 163, 166, 237; obscured by limitations of body, 162–63

contemplation, 7, 30, 46

contentment, 188, 189

contraception and family planning, 198–201, 203–4, 210, 211, 213

contraceptive herbs, 203–5

coral powder/pisti, 115

Creation, 45, 151, 232, 250, 259, 271, 329, 353; stages of, 259–60 (see also rajas; sattva; tamas)

Creator, 105, 156, 169, 197, 232 (see also God)

Dalai Lama, 50, 288, 290 (see also Avalokiteshvara)

death, 98, 183, 185, 186, 243, 248, 277, 280–81

delusion. See poisons, mind

dental amalgam mercury syndrome (DAMS), 303, 321

desire(s)/craving, 161, 172 (see also poisons, mind); freedom from, 161, 167, 191, 248

detoxification, 26, 99, 172, 308, 349 (see also mercury toxicity and poisoning, treatment)

Dharma, 4, 7, 23, 105, 181, 207, 246, 262, 283, 292, 336, 353, 361

Dhonyo, Lobsang, 205–6, 274, 362, 367

diagnosis, 53–55, 57, 67–68, 264–66, 271 (see also humors; tree of knowledge)

dibir rasayan, 111

diet, 140–41, 263, 308, 309

digestion, 170–71, 240

doctors. See physicians

dong quai, 40

drug use, recreational, 77–78, 230

drugs, pharmaceutical, 271, 322–23 (see also allopathy; antibiotics)

duality(ies), 25, 255

dutsi, 25

egocentric thinking, 162, 228

egolessness, 280

embryology, 236–37, 239, 246, 248–55, 279

emptiness, 29, 232, 237, 259

enlightenment, 98, 111, 246, 261, 270, 279, 280, 355; attaining, 22, 34, 168, 177, 181, 249, 284

environmental crisis, 328–30, 333–39

environmental restoration, 354–56

equilibrium, 261–63

essential oils, 65, 75, 76, 174

faith, 29, 267, 277

fevers, 172

fire, 169, 172, 308, 365–69 (see also Agni)

flow, 28–29

Flower Ornament Scripture, 191

Four Tantras, 22, 24

fragrance, 174–76

frigidity, 89, 90

Gandak Rasayan. See sulfur

Gautama. See Buddha

generosity, 178

germ theory, 341–43

ginseng, 40, 272

God, 121, 227, 228, 269, 366 (see also Creator); communication with, 120

goddesses, 149, 222, 223, 231, 237 (see also Shakti)

gods, 231 (see also visualizations, of deities); Vedic, 219, 220

gold: purified, 37, 87, 88; true alchemical, 173

gold transmutation, 69, 97, 114–17 (see also alchemy)

Gopal, Siddhi, 316

Gopal Upreti. See Upreti, Gopal

Great Purified Moon Crystal Pill, 37–38

greed, 12, 162, 178–79

gunas, 259, 260, 268

Gyamtso, Sangye, 50

gynecological problems, 214–15

gynecology, 72, 196–99, 203, 209, 249

Gyu Shi (Four Tantras), 21, 24–26, 48–50, 55, 241, 288

hatred/anger, 172 (see also poisons, mind)

healing, 34, 244–45 (see also specific topics)

health, 170, 171, 178; defined, 70, 261

health-care delivery problems, 209, 215

heart, 278–79

herbal medicine, 180, 271 (see also specific topics)

herbs, 8–9, 45, 123–24, 140–45 (see also specific herbs); color and flavor, 150; essential attributes, 41, 47; mythical qualities, 146–48; preparation, 37, 47, 75–76, 106; types, 271–72; used in offerings, 148

Hindu culture, 61, 160; women's role and status, 196–200

ABOUT THE AUTHOR

David Crow, L.Ac., is an acupuncturist, herbalist, and practitioner of naturalistic healing systems. He is the founder of the Center for Sattvic Medicine, which provides holistic therapies derived from his studies with Chinese, Ayurvedic, and Tibetan doctors. He is dedicated to promoting the Dharmic principles and earth-based wisdom of traditional healing arts as a path to ecological restoration and revival of spiritual cultures. He divides his time between his two clinics, which are located at the Growing Edge, a residential retreat center in Big Sur, and in Venice, California. David Crow can be contacted at www.medicinecrow.com.